HAVING FAITH

HAVING FAITH

An Ecologist's
Journey to Motherhood

SANDRA STEINGRABER

A Merloyd Lawrence Book
PERSEUS PUBLISHING
Cambridge, Massachusetts

Permission of W. W. Norton to reprint four lines of "Diving into the Wreck," by Adrienne Rich (on page 39), is gratefully acknowledged.

Many of the designations used by manufacturers and sellers to distinguish their products are claimed as trademarks. Where those designations appear in this book and Perseus Publishing was aware of a trademark claim, the designations have been printed in initial capital letters.

ISBN: 0-7382-0467-6

Library of Congress catalogue card number is available.

Text design by Trish Wilkinson
Set in 11-point Janson Text by Perseus Publishing Services

1 2 3 4 5 6 7 8 9 10—03 02 01
First printing, September 2001

Perseus Publishing is a member of the Perseus Books Group.
Find us on the World Wide Web at http://www.perseuspublishing.com
Perseus Publishing books are available at special discounts for bulk purchases in the U.S. by corporations, institutions, and other organizations. For more information, please contact the Special Markets Department at the Perseus Books Group, 11 Cambridge Center, Cambridge, MA 02142, or call (617) 252-5298.

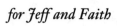

for Jeff and Faith

Contents

Preface

*E*very woman who becomes pregnant brings to the experience her various identities. I am an ecologist, which means I spend a lot of time thinking about how living things interact with the environments they inhabit. When I became pregnant at age thirty-eight, I realized, with amazement, that I myself had become a habitat. My womb was an inland ocean with a population of one.

So I turned my scientist's eye inward and began to study in earnest the biological drama of new life being knit from the molecules of air, food, and water flowing into a woman's body from the outside environment. I looked also at the environmental threats to the bodies of pregnant and breastfeeding mothers. How do toxic chemicals cross the tough sponge of the placenta? How do they find their way into amniotic fluid? How do they enter the milk-making globes in the back of the breast? What are the effects for the child of these earliest encounters with synthetic chemicals? The answers to these questions seemed essential to my new responsibilities as an expectant mother. And they all pointed to a simple truth: protecting the ecosystem inside my body required protecting the one outside.

This book is the result of that most personal of ecological investigations. Part I describes the unfolding events of fetal development, month by joyful month, the nine chapters named for the traditional names of each month's full moon in the agricultural cycle. Along the way, I explore various mysteries: the puzzling malaise of morning sickness; the historical failure to recognize fetal toxicants; the experience of holding in my hands a tube of my own amniotic fluid; the origins of birth defects; and the ways in which certain chemical contaminants can sabotage fetal brain development. As birth nears, I turn my attention to the ecology of the birth process itself. As I try to plan for a natural childbirth within a large research hospital, another one of my identities—cancer survivor—plays a key role in my decision-making.

Next, *Having Faith* takes a close look at the symbiosis of breast-feeding. Part II thus begins with the reestablishment of the biological bond between mother and child as the breast takes over from the placenta the task of nurturing the infant. In Part II, I also take a close look at the evolutionary origins of human breast milk, with its disease-fighting properties and unsurpassed ability to guide the brain development of nursing infants. Finally, I examine how the goodness of breast milk—and indeed a mother's very ability to produce it—is now being compromised by the presence of toxic chemicals in the human food chain.

The source notes at the end of the book direct readers to the many hundreds of scientific papers, monographs, reports, and texts that informed my analysis. Those interested in more detailed biological descriptions can seek them here. All this research, however, can really be summed up in a few simple sentences. In the words of Katsi Cook, a Native American midwife, a woman's body is the first environment. If the world's environment is contaminated, so too is the ecosystem of a mother's body. If a mother's body is contaminated, so too is the child who inhabits it. These truths should inspire us all—mothers, fathers, grandparents, doctors, midwives, and everyone concerned about future generations—to action.

January 31, 2001
Ithaca, New York

PART ONE

September 26, 1998, late morning

In the hospital solarium, sunlight pours through the glass like a warm shower. I have brought you here, little one, to show you the sky, blue as cornflowers, and the stone buildings of Boston, city of your birth. But you are sleeping and show no sign of changing your mind about sleeping.

You spent last night nestled in the crook of my arm. I curled around you so that the curves and bumps of your body, familiar to me as my own, pressed against my belly, pressed against me now from the outside instead of from the inside. (I recognize especially the curve of your heel. For many weeks I felt it through my own skin, just under my left rib.) At 3 A.M. you awoke. Your father said he looked over from his cot and saw you staring at a square of light on the wall. While I slept he held you in his arms and made shadow puppets for you. He said that you watched intently—he emphasized "intently"—and that, after he had run through his entire repertoire, you turned your attention to his face, holding him in a calm gaze. He said he knew in that moment what kind of person you would become. He said you have an observant, inquisitive spirit.

Your left hand wriggles out now from the top of your swaddling blanket, but still you do not wake. The pattern your veins make on the back of your hand is identical to my own. I cannot stop staring at you. No wonder mothers claim they cannot remember their labors clearly. You fill all my brain cells. Just the sound of your breathing—which is a miracle—requires my complete attention. The sea smell of your hair. The pulse behind

3

your ear. The butter of your skin. I am so busy memorizing you that I cannot recall anything about my life before today.

In the world outside this glass room, songbirds are feeding and resting in the trees. Some will take off tonight and not land until they reach Venezuela. Sandpipers, plovers, and broad-winged hawks have already left for Patagonia and Panama. Bats are heading for caves in Kentucky and Tennessee. Out in the Atlantic, humpback whales pass by on their way to the Caribbean. Even now, Canada geese are honking toward us from Quebec. It is a good day for the beginnings of journeys.

Every time I look at you, I think, Now I cannot die.

I decide your name is Faith.

1

Old Moon

JANUARY

*I*n a faculty bathroom on the campus of Illinois Wesleyan University, I am trying to pee on a stick. Outside, the first snowfall of winter is coming down thick and fast, which is a good thing because I have a seminar to teach downstairs in five minutes, and the snow—with all the required stomping of boots and shaking of scarves—should keep the class preoccupied for a while.

When I was a student here myself, twenty years ago, I always wondered what went on in private, professorial chambers like this one. Now that I have returned for a semester as a visiting writer-in-residence, accompanied by my visiting artist-in-residence husband, I've been walking through lots of familiar old buildings and opening doors to rooms I never knew existed. The provost's inner office, for instance. The faculty dining hall. And now this dark-paneled, wide-windowed lavatory with its crooked floor and oversized porcelain fixtures.

I focus on the chortling sounds of the radiator. Urine splashes over my fingers, and I feel the stick bend down like a divining rod.

In my office, a few minutes earlier, I finished an interview with the alumni magazine editor, during which time I was completely absorbed with the question of whether or not I was pregnant. My period is not due for another two days, and yet I have a hunch. So as soon as he left, I walked across the street to the pharmacy where, as a college student, I had bought contraceptive devices. I used to stand in the checkout lane and worry that one of my professors would walk in and see me with a handful of condoms and spermicides. Today, with the same air of fake casualness, I sidled up to that identical counter holding a home pregnancy test kit, hoping that none of my students would walk in before the clerk could slip that too-pink box safely into a bag.

I lay the wet stick on the cool, curved lip of the sink basin. White on white, it seems to vanish.

I hadn't really planned to do this right now. But I was amazed, after reading the directions on the back of the box, how simple and quick the test is. Pee on a stick, and three minutes later you have your question answered. It was too irresistible. In 1986, as a science writer for the *Detroit Free Press*, I had researched a story about diagnostic home test kits and raised eyebrows in the features department by keeping a stack of pregnancy tests piled on my desk. The idea of women diagnosing their own pregnancies was still disconcerting back then. The kits themselves contained entire miniature laboratories. They required first morning urine, a willingness to follow complicated instructions, and a half hour of waiting. "Am I going to have a baby?" a woman asked the little chemistry set. The appearance of a ghostly brown ring in a mirror mounted under the test tube meant "Yes." It was like reading tea leaves.

Before the advent of home tests, women handed their urine over to medical technicians to foretell their futures. The Aschheim-Zondek method was developed at a charity hospital in Berlin in 1927. It involved injecting a virgin mouse (later a rabbit or a toad) with the urine of a possibly pregnant woman and then dissecting the animal to see whether it had ovulated. If so, the test was positive. This took weeks. Before Aschheim-Zondek, women relied on their own bodies to tell them they were pregnant. For some, this could take months. Now, a positive pregnancy test means that two colored lines appear on a plastic stick in less time than it takes to brush your teeth.

I note the starting time on my watch, and then very deliberately look out the window. Across the parking lot is the dormitory where I lost my virginity. Beyond the dorm is the old science building where I spent most of my waking hours—studying invertebrate zoology, comparative anatomy, organic chemistry. Somewhere in there was the embryology lab where I once successfully transplanted the wing bud of a chick embryo. It was strange really—to have begun one's sexual life in the midst of an intense intellectual immersion into reproductive biology. I had spent my days poring over micrographs of fetal cross sections, completely humbled by the operatic beauty of it all, and my nights in sticky dormitory couplings, actively trying to prevent sperm and egg from finding each other. This all took place in an age that now seems so fleeting one almost doubts it ever really existed: the handful of years between *Roe v. Wade* in 1973 and the advent of AIDS in the early 1980s, that brief time when sex did not hold between its teeth the red rose of either ruin or death. Now I have returned—married, contraceptively unprotected, and twice as old as I was when I became semiskilled at prenatal chicken surgery.

The snow falls harder. Already the quadrangle's sward of brown grass is buried.

Am I pregnant? It is an old, old question. How many women have asked it before me? How many women right now are standing at windows waiting for urine-soaked sticks to turn color? Some are praying not to see lines. Some are trying to will them into existence. *Am I pregnant?* At this particular moment I'm not sure what answer I'm hoping for. Mostly I'm unnerved by the ease of the experiment I'm conducting, as though such a venerable and terrifying question should demand an animal sacrifice, or at least intricate and difficult operations. I reread the instruction sheet. I notice it refers to the plastic stick as "the wand."

I guess that about a minute has passed. Two more to go. To avoid looking at my watch, I decide to think about the menstrual cycle. Reviewing the inside of the human body is a habit of mine, my own private form of meditation. Once, I stayed in a London hotel that became the unintended site of a terrorist attack. While being assembled, a bomb exploded in a room across the courtyard from my own, killing its makers and a sleeping woman next door. In the days that followed, I traced over and over in my mind's eye the passage of venous and arterial blood through the heart's four chambers. It was a way of slowing down my own heart—and not replaying the image of windows shattering.

So, the menstrual cycle.

At the end of a period, the lining of the uterus is thin and bare— like a layer of silt left behind after flood waters have receded. The ovaries, too, are smooth and quiet. Then, high in the brain, the pituitary gland begins to drizzle into the bloodstream a substance called follicle stimulating hormone. True to its name, the hormone awakens in one or the other ovary a whole choir of follicles. Like bubbles, they rise to the surface in unison. Each one is a sack that holds a single human egg. Typically, only one follicle will ultimately surrender its singular possession, but all participate in the task of turning testosterone into estrogen, and it is this collective effort that makes the next step possible.

The assembled estrogen seeps from the follicle-studded surface of the ovary and swirls around in the bloodstream. Some reaches the brain, and, in a second round of call and response, the pituitary gland replies by releasing back into the blood another substance called luteinizing hormone. Like the initial hormone that set the whole process in motion, this, too, is received by the ovary, and it induces one of the swollen follicles to break through the ovarian surface. An egg is delivered out into the headwaters of the fallopian tube. Ovulation. All this in less than two weeks.

The faucet drips. The radiator hisses and bangs into action. I guess that another minute has passed. If I look down at my watch, I'll see "the wand," so I keep my eyes on the falling snow.

It's easy to think of the egg as a little gondola floating serenely down the Venetian canal of the fallopian tube, but this is not quite right. I remember the textbook case of the young woman who lost an ovary and a fallopian tube to surgery. Unfortunately, her remaining ovary and tube were located on opposite sides from each other. To the amazement of all concerned, she got pregnant anyway. Under the influence of estrogen, fallopian tubes move. They stretch, and they bend, and their mouths are actively attracted to ovulating eggs, a drawing power that apparently extends even across the continent of the pelvis. Moreover, once the egg is captured, a fallopian tube has muscles and cilia that ferry it downstream. This is not to say the tube does all the paddling. A living egg denuded of its outer coating will not move. Fallopian transport is a mutual affair, and something in the egg itself assists in the journey. No one knows exactly what.

I wonder what time it is. Down in the parking lot, the last of my students are negotiating their way through rows of cars. But I am not ready yet to consult the plastic oracle on the sink.

During the next three or four days, the floodplain of the uterus is completely transformed. Its flat endometrial lining rises and thickens. Spiral arteries coil through it like snakes. The deeper layers swell with starch-filled glands, and the surface crawls with immune cells. The elixir responsible for this luxuriant growth is the hormone progesterone, which trickles into the bloodstream from the ovarian follicle that released the ovulated egg. Once its solo performance is over, the emptied-out follicle does not sit down with the rest of the choir. Instead, it balls up, turns yellow, and begins secreting hormones. Called the corpus luteum, it is this new gland that turns the interior landscape of the uterus into a lush marshland.

Now we come to the crossroads, the crux of the matter, the source of my lady-or-the-tiger inquiry. An ovulated, unfertilized human egg has a lifespan of just twelve to twenty-four hours. Forty-eight hours, tops. If it dies a maiden, its journey ends. The yellow moon of the corpus luteum soon wanes. As progesterone levels fall, the root ends of the spiral arteries constrict, and the whole endometrium blanches with the loss of blood flow. The starchy pools evaporate. The curly stalks of the spiral arteries senesce. White blood cells infiltrate. All that is left is the denouement of menstruation: the base of the spiral arteries reopens and a surge of fresh blood carries the dying tissue away. In the last twenty-five years I've already gone through several hundred rounds of flooding and renewal. The almanac of the uterus is steadying.

If, on the other hand, something else has happened during the trip down the tunnel—that subject of seventh-grade film strips and intense theological argument—then our story changes. If a living zygote emerges from the far end of the fallopian tube, then the rest of my life is going to be very different.

When an egg is fertilized by a sperm in the upper reaches of the fallopian tube, the first cell division happens in about twelve hours. Four days later, as it bobs out into the womb's delta, there are fifty-eight cells, arranged in a cluster like a mulberry. At this point, a bubble of fluid begins to fill one side of the ball of multiplying cells, and the outermost cells on the other side fuse together. Between the two is a teardrop of cells destined to become the embryo. The bubble is the amnion, the fused part the placenta. One week after the egg's successful affair with the sperm, the whole unit sinks into the endometrial marsh in a process called implantation. The fused cells push long, amoeba-like fingers deep into the uterine lining while secreting digestive enzymes that facilitate its burial. In response, the tips of the spiral arteries break open and spurt like geysers. Thus, life begins in a pool of blood.

Twelve days after conception—that's about where I would be now, if indeed I am there at all—the uterine lining has already grown over the point of entry, and the embryonic placenta has sent siphoning hoses into the bloody lagoons beneath. Equally important, it has begun the manufacture of a hormone called human chorionic gonadotropin—HCG—which spills into the mother's capillaries and circulates until it reaches the ovaries. HCG stops the menstrual cycle at summer solstice. It does so by commuting the monthly death sentence of the corpus luteum. Estrogen and progesterone therefore keep flowing from the ovary in ever larger quantities. The uterine lining is not shed but becomes ever more overgrown. More and more spiral arteries wind upward and break open to feed the new life buried there. Immune cells surround it and offer their protection.

HCG is the hormone that pregnancy kits attempt to detect. If it is present in blood, it is present in urine. If it is present in urine, it can be poured over plastic sticks embedded with antibodies. If the antibodies have been extracted from mice previously exposed to the hormones of pregnant women, then they will bind to the HCG in the urine. If the antibodies can be made to change color once they are so bound, then pregnancy is made visible. If I am pregnant, then I should be able to see it. Now.

I look at my watch. Five minutes! I look down at the stick. Two lavender lines. Unmistakable. Now there are two of us. And I am late for class.

2

Hunger Moon

FEBRUARY

*T*he season's only snowfall melts and then freezes, cruelly, into pleated sheets of ice that last for weeks. Bundled up, I carry my secret with me, imagining the baby (the baby!) as a lavender thread caught within a plush red carpet. The pregnancy seems unreal. I still look the same, feel the same, eat, sleep, and think the same. Like everyone who is not pregnant, I skate gingerly across the ice, head down, arms out, in my daily circuits to class, library, home, and back. Except that I am overcome with a new sense of urgency. I begin reading embryology texts again. I also collect a few popular guidebooks for pregnant women.

I quickly learn that embryologists and obstetricians speak two different languages and utilize two different calendars for chronicling the passage of unfolding events. One is a fortnight ahead of the other. The embryological timetable uses the moment of fertilization as its starting point. This seems sensible, and it is the system I am used to. By the embryologists' accounting, a human pregnancy is thirty-eight weeks long. More or less.

The obstetricians, however, begin the clock with the first day of the woman's last menstrual period. By their method, gestation is an even forty weeks. Their argument for adding two weeks to the beginning of pregnancy is that the fertilization is an unknowable point in time, whereas the onset of menstruation is subject to data collection—either because it has been dutifully recorded in a woman's week-at-a-glance appointment book or because it can be deduced with a little reflection: "Let's see. I was just stepping onto the subway platform when I realized my period had started. That was the day I had planned to go Christmas shopping, so it must have been Monday, the twenty-first." The assumption is that menstruation, on average, precedes ovulation and therefore conception by fourteen days. This is not an unreasonable system either. In fact, it's very practical. Using the obstetrical calendar, a date of birth can be quickly predicted by subtracting three months from the date of last menstruation and adding seven days.

The problem with the obstetrical method is that it pretends a woman is pregnant two weeks before the egg boat has even left the ovarian dock. This is the fiction the whole system hangs on. The surreal result is that a newly pregnant woman is fast-forwarded in time: one short week after a missed menstrual period she is said to be five weeks pregnant.

For a while, I walk around translating the obstetrical calendar into the embryological one I am familiar with. The obstetrician I choose from the Yellow Pages of the phone book is first interested in seeing me when I am about eight weeks pregnant—by which he means six weeks since I actually became pregnant. The pregnancy advice books note that morning sickness often sets in at six weeks, by which they mean four weeks. Finally, I give in and adopt the new, accelerated way of marking time. In some ways, it more closely mirrors the experience of pregnancy discovery. Learning I am pregnant is like crossing the International Date Line. All of a sudden, time skips forward.

Jeff feels the new time sense, too—ever since the afternoon two weeks ago when I handed him the tiny wand, tattooed with its pair of colored lines. Standing in his sculpture studio, he took it and turned it over slowly.

"Is it a thermometer?"

I shook my head.

"Is it . . . a clock?"

This was a response I hadn't expected.

"Yes, in a way." I laughed, sure I had misled him. But objects are his medium. He wasn't thrown off by my words. He looked again.

"Are you pregnant? Does this say you're pregnant?"

I nodded furiously, and then we were hugging and laughing. And then I cried, and Jeff held his head in his hands. And then we walked home in the snow with the cars crunching slowly by us, and began to make dinner in an already darkening kitchen, and by the time we had finished, it was truly dark and we sat together quietly like that for a long time, feeling the hours of the short winter days flying by us and pressing behind us at the same time.

Two weeks later, we are flipping pages in our date books and comparing our various plans for art shows, book projects, travel, teaching commitments. My due date is October 2. We pencil it in our calendars as though it were some kind of deadline for a grant application.

"You know, it's only a guess. It could be four weeks early. It could be two weeks late."

"I know."

"Only twelve percent of women actually give birth on their due dates."

"Really?"

Silence.

"Let's just take things one step at a time. That's what you always say, right?"

"I know."

Silence.

"Do you think I should cancel my trip to Toronto?"

"Why? It's only a few weeks from now."

"It's expensive."

Future time increasingly seems like some kind of finite resource, like coal or aluminum ore, that must be inventoried, processed, allocated, bankrolled. This kind of stocktaking is new for us. I wonder if all adults who are parents think this way.

I start paying attention to the silver maples outside the windows of the faculty guest house where we are living. *Acer saccharinum.* It's a fast-growing tree. Homeowners plant them when they want shade in a hurry, but their crowns are brittle and come down quickly in windstorms. Against a gray February sky, their bare, pointy branches are pencil sketches of themselves. In early spring, pom-poms of tiny flowers will open from lateral buds and shower sidewalks and car windshields with chartreuse confetti. Soon after, deeply cut, silvery white leaves will unfurl. Then the helicopters of winged seeds will whirl down and lie topsy turvy in the summer grass. Finally, the leaves will roll up into dry, papery tubes and these too will float down so they can be raked into heaps of ashy lace. But before these leaves fall—if all goes well—I will have a baby. October 2.

I peer more closely at the hunched-up leaf buds paired along the twigs, barely visible, barely there at all. In February, October does not seem possible. Nothing except February seems possible in February—not the wind travels of pollen, not the making of seed helicopters from flower tassels, not the appearance of fancy leaves from the sides of cold twigs, not the formation of babies from menstrual blood.

Organogenesis is the formation of body parts. It takes place in the month between weeks six and ten, as the obstetricians date it. By the time it is over, the embryo is the length of a paper clip, and, by definition, all the organs and structures of the body are present in "a grossly recognizable form." At week eleven of pregnancy, no further assembly is required: the embryo is knighted a fetus and simply grows bigger until it is ready for birth, when it weighs about the same as a gallon of milk.

Of all the biological processes I've ever studied—from photosynthesis to echolocation—organogenesis is, hands down, the most fantastical. Sometimes it seems like a magic show. At other times it's like origami, the formation of elegant structures from the folding of flat sheets. It also involves cellular wanderings worthy of Odysseus. No single metaphor can describe it. It certainly isn't like taking a lump of clay and molding a little head from one end and legs and feet from the other.

The events of weeks four and five prepare the way.[1] While still sinking down into the uterine lining, the inner cell mass flattens out into a bilaminar, or two-layered, disc. The edges grow out and begin to curve around in opposite directions until the disc is surrounded by two slightly flattened balls. Then it gets complicated. An opaque line begins to form down the middle of the disc's top

---

[1] From here forward, I use the obstetrical calendar when I refer to the human pregnancy timeline.

layer. At one end of the line, a bump rises up like a miniature volcano with a tiny crater at its summit. This line is called the primitive streak, the bump is called the primitive node, and its crater the primitive pit. These are temporary landmarks in a protean landscape. It is the task of these three structures to send moving cells in the right direction. The primitive streak is a kind of cave door that opens into a hidden space between the two cell layers. In a great exodus, cells from the top layer stream through the streak and fan out. Now there are three layers. By the end of week five, its work finished, the primitive streak is already fading from sight. With this, organogenesis commences.

The disc's three layers are the original tribes of Israel. All body parts originate from one of them, but it is not always obvious which organ comes from which. For example, it makes a certain amount of sense that hair should derive from the outer layer (ectoderm), muscles from the middle layer (mesoderm), and the bowel from the inner one (endoderm). But why should the vagina trace its ancestry back to the mesoderm while the more external bladder originates from the endoderm? Or why should the brain, like the skin, arise from cells in the ectoderm? Trying to decode these aspects of embryology once brought me to the brink of despair.

The trick to understanding how it all comes to be is to trace the lineage of each tissue layer from start to finish. This is like learning all the begats of St. Matthew: the ectoderm gives rise to the primordial epithelium, which gives rise to the proctodeal epithelium, which gives rise to the stomodeal epithelium, which gives rise to the enamel of the teeth. With each generation, the structures change shape and get more elaborate. Cylinders form as the ends of flat sheets grow together. At one point, the whole embryo folds laterally. Organogenesis begins with three flat layers and, one week later, produces a coiled, segmented object that looks like an architectural detail on the end of a stair banister. Three weeks and a few more folds later, a "grossly recognizable" human being resides in the wetlands of the uterus.

What seems like sleight-of-hand work is actually governed by two key embryological principles. One is migration. The other is induction.

Migration means that the cells of the developing embryo don't just grow and divide. They actually break free, sprout snail-like feet, and walk over the bodies of their neighbors before settling down elsewhere—often in some distant locale. The pilgrimage through the primitive streak is only the first of many migrations. In male embryos, primordial sperm cells form out in the yolk sac and sojourn through the gut for a while before finally colonizing what eventually will become the testicle. Eventually, these cells move out of the body cavity a second time when the testicles themselves descend into the scrotum.

No important journey ends without profoundly changing the one who undertakes it. Induction is this change, and it happens when migrating immature cells—so-called stem cells—meet others along the way. Through these various encounters, stem cells differentiate: they evolve from unspecialized tissues into definitive organs and structures. By the time the migrants settle down again, they have acquired an identity; in that time-honored tradition of youthful wandering, they have found themselves. For example, when certain cells on the top layer of the bilaminar disc pour through the primitive streak and flow out beneath, they brush by cells on the bottom layer. This contact induces the middle-layer cells to turn into blood vessels. If the two layers do not touch, these vessels never form.

This kind of transformation comes at a price. Once the fate of a cell is fixed, it loses the ability to play any other role. A blood vessel cannot then become a tendon or lymph duct—even if it is touched by cells inducing it to do so. Embryologists talk about embryonic stem cells passing through "restriction points" as they migrate. During these moments, whole strings of genes are turned off, leaving only the few needed for a cell's new, more specialized life. Certain genes elsewhere in the embryonic landscape direct all these cellular blackouts through a series of chemical cues called signaling episodes. One key gene involved in a lot of this work is called, whimsically enough, sonic hedgehog. From its perch in the cells near the primitive node, sonic hedgehog directs the development of body parts such as the brain, intestines, and limbs.

It's easiest to see how induction works when something goes wrong. Consider DiGeorge syndrome. People afflicted with it are born with malformed hearts. They also have immune deficiencies, low blood calcium, oddly shaped heads, and cleft palates. None of these problems seems to be related to any of the others, but in fact all the defects arise in tissues that derive from one source known as cardiac neural crest cells. On a particular day during organogenesis, members of this clan are supposed to emerge from a fold of neural tissue and shape the great blood vessels leaving the heart. Other neural crest cells stray into the various arches above the heart, where they participate in the formation of the facial bones and two different glands in the neck, the parathyroid and the thymus glands. The first regulates calcium levels, and the second bears the responsibility for turning immature immune cells into a well-regulated militia. The meanderings of cardiac neural crest cells are ultimately directed by a piece of DNA that lies on chromosome 22. If this chunk is missing, the result is DiGeorge syndrome, with all its disparate anomalies. For want of a nail a kingdom is lost.

Because rare problems offer such important clues to normal development, embryology textbooks are full of pictures that pregnant women shouldn't look at. I do because I am seeking images to make the early weeks of pregnancy seem real and because the language of embryology has a heroic, epic resonance. I feel a little like a migrating embryonic cell myself, sent out on a journey that seems not entirely of my own choosing or under my own direction—even though this is a long-hoped-for pregnancy. I suspect I will be changed by it, that some new identity is forthcoming. Restriction points lie ahead.

At the end of week six, my pregnancy becomes empirical. I wake up nauseated. The rest of the month is a return to childhood.

It all starts with my toothbrush, which suddenly seems too large for my mouth. It keeps making me gag. I buy a little baby toothbrush festooned with sparkles and cartoon characters. For a few days, this seems to solve the problem. Then I notice I have too much spit in my mouth. Excess saliva is an official symptom of pregnancy. It's called ptyalism. I learn this not from my embryology textbooks but from one of the popular week-by-week guidebooks for pregnant women, which I mostly avoid because their medical illustrations are terrible and their gushy, overly reassuring tones annoy me.

Swallowing the saliva makes me queasy, so I start looking for discreet places to spit during my morning walk to campus. Behind the retaining wall on the quad. Into the frozen flower beds near the English House. I haven't spit in public since about third grade. My aim was better then.

By week seven, spitting advances to throwing up. I spent a lot of my childhood vomiting, both because I suffered from terrible motion sickness and because I was the daughter of a public schoolteacher, which meant that entire summers were spent in the backseat of a car, driving from one national park to another. Athletic humiliation could also provoke nausea. During the school year, most of my vomiting was done on the high-gloss floorboards of the gymnasium. The whistle was blown, the wretched game was stopped, the janitor was summoned, and some kind of pink, fruity-smelling sawdust was sprinkled over the frothy puddle while I stared, mortified, at my canvas shoes. I was less inclined to vomit in class, where I tended to excel, except for one time in second grade when I threw up on the boy who sat directly in front of me. I was sent home with the flu. He went on to become popular in high school. For four long years, he greeted me in the hallway with feigned retching and the hissed warning, "Don't puke, Steingraber."

It's a refrain I now repeat on the way home from class. Spitting on the university landscaping is one thing. Vomiting is another. Usually I make it back to the guest house. As soon as I see the sink in the bathroom, I let go. It becomes a conditioned response. If I lie down and avoid going into the bathroom, I don't vomit. The problem is that I have to pee all the time now. This is because rising levels of progesterone have softened the muscles of the pelvic floor, allowing the uterus to slump onto the bladder. I have to pee, ergo, I have to throw up.

I descend further into childhood. Progesterone also slows metabolism. I am tired. I go to bed at nine. I take naps. I wake up cranky and shuffle out to the dinner table. My husband sets a toasted cheese sandwich before me. It's what I have requested, but I look at it suspiciously.

"You cut it wrong," I hear myself say. "And it's the wrong bread."

I can't explain what's happening to me. The way food looks suddenly determines whether or not I can swallow it. Other rules follow: I can eat cold bananas but not the ones stored at room temperature. I would like eggs for breakfast, but only if they are very hot and if the yolks are hard but not broken. I can drink water between meals but not during. I discover that most of my favorite foods—beans, salads, tofu, vegetables—are yucky. I stare glumly at my plate a lot in a way I remember doing when I was about three, my parents cajoling, "But you *like* chop suey! You've always liked chop suey!"

I leave behind the high-art world of embryology and begin reading about morning sickness. It turns out I am in good company. More than three quarters of U.S. women suffer from nausea in the second month of pregnancy, and slightly more than half experience vomiting. I'm in the sizable minority—25 percent—who throw up daily. Nausea in pregnancy is not limited by region, lifestyle, race, or class. Women of the hunting-gathering !Kung people of Botswana complain of it as do Japanese, Arab, and European women and mothers-to-be up and down the Americas. In South Africa, surveys of pregnant women found similar incidence rates among whites and blacks. Among indigenous societies, the data show no relationship between morning sickness and agricultural practices, work habits, social structure, community size, or settlement patterns.

Neither is morning sickness a recent phenomenon. The earliest description is inscribed on papyrus and goes back four millennia. Aristotle commented on it, as did the Roman physician Soranus, who advocated dry foods, weak wine, massage, and carriage rides to ease the misery. I am impressed with the compassion that the ancients extended the sufferers of morning sickness. (Which, by the way, is not limited to the morning but is often most intense upon waking. To this I can attest.) Early in the twentieth century, attitudes grew more surly. The absence of any adequate medical explanation for morning sickness—and the fact that some women are spared it altogether—allowed psychological theories of causation to flourish and mercy for the afflicted to wane. In one hospital in the 1930s, pregnant women prone to sickness were confined to bed and forbidden visitors and vomit bowls until they showed improvement. As further incentive for recovery, the nurses who cared for them were instructed to refrain from changing their sheets promptly. Throughout the century, morning sickness was variously blamed on neurosis, an unconscious desire for abortion, a rejection of motherhood, a scheme to avoid housework, and sexual dysfunction.

The most astonishing article I come across was published in 1946 by a Scottish physician who claimed there was a relationship between morning sickness and "excessive mother attachment."

This discovery had other corollaries: "A study of the emotional state of these patients ... revealed a common feature—i.e. sexual relationship with the husband gave rise to disgust. ... I have confirmed the findings in many hundreds of women. In doing so I noted that a high proportion of them at marriage were unduly attached to their mothers."

Removal of the pregnant woman from the proximity of her mother was the proposed cure. I wondered how anyone could ever concoct such a hypothesis until I ran across a recent article in the nursing literature that reported on successful coping strategies in women with severe pregnancy sickness: "Most women reduced their social commitments during the early months of pregnancy, *becoming much more dependent on their mothers* and close friends for help in meal preparation and child care" (my emphasis).

To wit: Pregnant women who throw up a lot seek the help of their mothers. Perhaps the good doctor had simply confused effect with cause. In any case, further study has uncovered no correlation between the way a woman feels about sexual reproduction and her frequency of nausea and vomiting. For that matter, severity of morning sickness does not vary with marital status, number of previous pregnancies, employment, or habitation—although it may be more common in urban areas than rural and it is definitely more common in women whose mothers also suffered from it. Another reason to call Mom.

So what does cause morning sickness? The always-reassuring pregnancy advice books delight in reporting that no one really knows, but those who suffer should take heart: nausea is a sign of a healthy pregnancy. This, indeed, appears to be the case. Women with severe morning sickness have fewer miscarriages, stillbirths, and premature deliveries, and their babies are at lower risk for heart defects. I *am* reassured—even though I am bothered by the mystery surrounding this ailment. Why should something experienced by the majority of the world's women be impervious to medical explanation?

Part of the reason is that sorry little research has been devoted to its study. I gather together a comprehensive file on the topic, and the resulting stack of books and journal articles from the medical literature takes up scant room on my desk. What we know for sure is that pregnant women with nausea have unusual electrical patterns flickering across the surfaces of their stomachs. Normally, the stomach goes through a sequence of electrical oscillations called the slow wave, which causes gentle contractions. Disturbing the speed of the slow wave has long been known to cause nausea and vomiting. Recent studies show that sufferers of morning sickness have slow wave rhythms that are either faster or slower than normal. Either way, contractions stop, and this morning's breakfast threatens to reappear.

But what causes slow-wave disruption? Most investigators believe it must be a hormone. HCG from the placenta is the one most often picked out of a lineup of suspects. Several pieces of circumstantial evidence implicate it. High blood levels of HCG are known to cause nausea. And women pregnant with twins, who have higher circulating HCG levels, often have more intense morning sickness. Most damningly, the rise and fall of blood HCG levels track closely the trajectory of nausea and vomiting during pregnancy, with its initiation at six weeks, its peak at nine weeks, and its eventual waning at around fourteen weeks. And yet, certain cancers known to elevate HCG to very high levels do not induce nausea and vomiting.

This inconsistency is pointed out by researchers who finger progesterone or estrogen as the likely culprit. During pregnancy, blood levels of both are kicked up to unprecedented levels by the intrepid corpus luteum, the ovarian gland that oversees pregnancy until the placenta is ready to take over. Moreover, nearly all women who experience nausea while on the Pill, which is a mix of estrogen and progesterone, will also get nauseated during pregnancy. Also, progesterone and estrogen given together to nonpregnant women alter gastric slow wave and induce nausea. On the other hand, estrogen and progesterone levels remain high throughout pregnancy while nausea almost always subsides by the fourth month. Moreover, there is no correlation between blood levels of these hormones and severity of sickness. Do we pregnant women simply adjust to rising hormone levels? Do we all simply have different thresholds? Or is yet some other unidentified agent responsible?

There is no shortage of candidates. Early pregnancy is associated with altered thyroid functioning. Thyroxine may therefore play a role. Hormones that prepare the breast for lactation also rise dramatically during this time, as do an assortment of growth factors with names like activin and inhibin. Perhaps one of these is the true agent. The ways in which hormones are carried in the blood—some are escorted by proteins and others circulate freely—also shift during pregnancy. Perhaps it's not any one hormone per se that is responsible but changing methods of transport. Perhaps the brain is involved: one pair of researchers has nominated the structure in the back of the brain stem called the area postrema as the place to look for the source of pregnancy sickness. This low-hanging knob serves as a kind of toxic detector, functioning in taste aversions and palatability decisions. One grand unifying hypothesis posits a hormonal conspiracy: estrogen and progesterone act on the area postrema while HCG disrupts the muscular contractions of the gut, thereby sending vomiting signals to a digestive system already primed by nausea.

In short, no one knows the cause of morning sickness because few have looked, and those who have looked have lifted their hands in surrender pretty swiftly when the answer proved elusive. I am therefore happy to discover two woman researchers who are working on the question, from two very different ends of it. One is a dietician, the other an evolutionary biologist. Their work forms the only two books on the topic that I can find in print. Miriam Erick, the dietician, cares for pregnant women in Boston who have been hospitalized with hyperemesis gravidarum, a rare but extreme form of morning sickness that can be life threatening. (Hyperemesis, or violent, prolonged vomiting, was rumored to have killed Charlotte Brontë, the author of *Jane Eyre*.) Erick's job is to find something these women can eat. Her starting point is their encounters with various food items. Margie Profet, by contrast, is a MacArthur Award–winning scholar who toils in the lofty confines of Harvard and Berkeley, far from the bedside vomit bucket. Profet's approach is conceptual, and her starting point is Darwin.

Erick has collected a lot of careful observations that warrant further study. First of all, she notes that there is no one food that nauseated pregnant women seek out: solutions are highly individual. Indeed, relief is often found in novel, highly flavored foods rather than in retreat to familiar, bland ones. If there is any single food strongly favored by sick pregnant women, Erick reports, it is tomatoes. I am relieved just reading this. The standard advice to eat crackers, sip ginger ale, and seek out tasteless foods is not working for me at all. Morning sickness is not like having stomach flu or a hangover. It is connected to a deep kind of hunger. Not eating at all, or nibbling on sick-person food, intensifies the misery. A kind of civil war rages: the thought of food is revolting, but only food—and lots of it—has the power to quell the revulsion. And what I want is not my usual whole-grain vegetarian fare but pork chops and cole slaw, two things that have not graced my plate for twenty years or more. This is not to say I crave these dishes; they are simply among the few foods I can imagine being able to chew and swallow. I throw up a bowl of cream-of-wheat and then wolf down a plateful of raw cabbage with mayonnaise and feel better. Pizza is also high on my list—perhaps by virtue of the tomato sauce. Erick's observation also explains why some surveys find that pregnant women with nausea shun meat while others report actively seeking it out.

Erick has documented one other intriguing pattern: nausea in pregnancy is triggered more often by smell than by taste. This probably explains why I can eat refrigerated bananas but not the more aromatic ones from the fruit bowl. Pregnancy enhances the ability to smell; some evidence suggests that estrogen is responsible. Moreover, studies from the space program (where nausea is a huge threat to the success of some very expensive missions) indicate that vomiting can be induced by electrical stimulation of the olfactory tubercle. In the search for causes to morning sickness, these seem like important clues.

As for me, the world has indeed become a very smelly place. I've always wondered about animals whose senses are keener than ours. Now I've become one. This is not necessarily a pleasure. Most of the human world smells downright nasty. I'm aware of paint fumes inside the kitchen cupboards. Some kind of swamplike odor rises from the bathtub. Vapor trails of deodorant and aftershave follow people down the sidewalk. Car exhaust is unspeakable. Finally, I learn to eat dinner in the bedroom, the least smelly room of the house, and the number of meals lost to the bathroom sink declines. Jeff, the short-order cook, breathes a sigh of relief.

In contrast to Miriam Erick and the immediacy of her work, Margie Profet takes a much longer view. Profet is less interested in what biologists call proximate causes and more interested in the ultimate ones. That is to say, all possible immediate triggers to vomiting aside, why would a hormonally reactive digestive system have evolved in the first place? Her hypothesis is that morning sickness is an adaptation to protect embryos during organogenesis. Nausea and vomiting, Profet argues, ensure that food-borne toxins do not reach the womb while that most delicate of human operas runs its course. It is a bold proposition.

The toxins that concern her most are the natural ones found in plants. Plants originally evolved these to deflect the advances of plant-eating insects and other herbivores, and they are very effective. They continue to be found, albeit in small amounts, in many domesticated vegetables and spices consumed by humans: potatoes, cabbage, mustard, pepper, etc. To make her case that these substances could harm the embryo, Profet points to several pieces of evidence. First, the period of morning sickness overlaps almost exactly the period of organogenesis, which is the phase of prenatal life most vulnerable to toxic threats. Second, as previously noted, women with morning sickness have better pregnancy outcomes. Third, the food items most repulsive to pregnant women, so she claims, are strongly flavored vegetables, highly spiced foods, and other items chock full of chemical repellants, such as coffee beans. Fourth, vomiting in humans is long known to function as a poison response mechanism. On this last point, Profet is assuredly correct. This is why cancer patients vomit in response to chemotherapy and radiation. Both are poisons. When the body detects their presence, it employs the only means it has to remove them, however inappropriate. One vomiting expert defines the subject of his study, emesis, as "the reversal of a mistake."

On the other hand, several predictions that follow from Profet's hypothesis are not really borne out in real life. Vegetables high in naturally occurring toxins are the strong-tasting and bitter ones, such as kale, cabbage, and brussels sprouts. And yet these are exactly the ones that appear to prevent health problems, such as cancer and some birth defects. Whether this is because the vitamins, minerals, and other beneficial chemicals they carry with them outweigh the effects of the toxins or because we have evolved effective detoxifying mechanisms to render them harmless is not yet clear. One recent study that tested Profet's hypothesis found no link between food intake of bitter vegetables and vomiting in newly pregnant women. More important, it found no connection between eating vegetables high in natural toxins and adverse pregnancy outcomes. In other words, women with morning sickness did not avoid these vegetables more than women without, and eating them did not appear to harm their babies. However, this is the first study of its kind to test Profet's ideas. The jury is still out.

There are other problems, too. Profet's second claim—that pregnant women tend to shun strongly flavored plants and spices—is not consistent with Erick's observations. That fruit most well tolerated by pregnant women, the tomato, for example, is a member of the nightshade family, which includes all kinds of truly deadly species. And how to explain my predilection for cole slaw? Furthermore, if vomiting is a means to avoid plant toxins, then we should see its presence in other pregnant animals—and more often in herbivores than carnivores. But there is no evidence for pregnancy sickness in other species. Horses are known to be incapable of vomiting, as are rats, mice, and rabbits. And animals that do vomit—primates, cats, dogs, ferrets, shrews—are mostly meat eaters.

A recent revision of Profet's hypothesis therefore posits that although morning sickness may indeed serve an evolutionary function, its original purpose may have lain not only in creating aversions to plant toxins but also in helping women avoid spoiled animal products, which teem with pathogens and parasites. Such dangers would have been particularly acute prior to widespread refrigeration. Claiming that aversions to meat, poultry, and eggs are at least as common as vegetable aversions during pregnancy, these researchers investigated the few traditional societies in which morning sickness has never been reported. They found that these cultures were significantly less likely to rely on animal products as dietary staples than traditional societies in which morning sickness is common.

Finally, although there is no doubt that vomiting is a poison control mechanism, humans also exercise this reflex in response to other kinds of problems. On the official list of factors known to cause vomiting are anxiety, horrific sights, and extreme pain. Furthermore, food aversions are only one of the triggers of nausea in pregnancy. Research shows that any type of sensory stimuli can provoke it, including bright colors, motion, and unpleasant noises.

At the end of the month we pay our first visit to the obstetrician. Behind the reception desk, a collage of newborn-baby photos papers an entire wall. They surprise me, and I realize I haven't yet connected my own pregnancy with childbirth yet. In the waiting room, I fill out a long medical questionnaire and watch all the other pregnant women as they are put through their paces: into the bathroom for a urine sample, then up on the scale, then a blood pressure check, then back to an examination room. Then it's my turn. In spite of the morning sickness—or maybe because of all the eating I do to submerge it—I have gained four pounds. Jeff joins me for the exam. He sits on a stool near the door as I climb up onto the table's crackly paper. Naked under an open-backed gown, I should be cold, but I feel humid and tropical. The doctor walks in. He is a big man with a kind of chummy intensity reminiscent of political candidates. He talks first and listens second. He sits with his legs sprawled apart and gestures broadly in a way that makes him take up even more space than his large frame already requires. His nurses and other patients call him by his first name—as in Dr. Dan. I consider introducing myself as Dr. Sandra but refrain. He explains everything thoroughly enough, and I decide I can work with him. Since we'll be back in Boston by month six, I don't have to imagine Dr. Dan actually delivering the baby.

As the pièce de résistance at the end of the visit, he places an ultrasound Doppler transducer on my belly and turns up the dial on the amplifier hanging from his belt.

"You're thin. We might be able to pick up a heartbeat."

He moves the probe over my skin slowly and tips his head to one side, as if trying to tune in a distant radio station. We hear static and then a deep pulsing that we're told is the sound of my own blood flow. Then nothing but static again. Jeff and I look at each other. Suddenly, there is a quicker, higher note behind the sonic thumps and whooshes.

"There it is."

We all listen. It sounds like someone applauding underwater.

The heart is the first organ to develop. It begins pumping blood twenty-two days after conception—week five by the obstetrical calendar. We are hearing a heart that has been beating for three weeks.

"Sounds like a boy to me," says Dr. Dan.

"Are you kidding or do you know something I don't?"

"Well, I have a fifty percent chance of being right, don't I?"

I don't usually appreciate wisecracks during medical exams. However, they are almost always a good sign. It's when doctors get quiet and tight-lipped that I worry.

At home I crawl into bed. Jeff climbs in after me and we burrow under the covers. The window is open to keep cold, scentless air flowing in.

"Look," Jeff says. "You can see the sunset reflected in the chapel windows across the alley."

"The days are getting longer."

Earlier this week, Jeff arranged the bedroom furniture according to the Chinese principles of feng-shui in the half-serious hope that external harmony might quiet my inner disequilibrium. The new view alone makes it worthwhile. I am becoming dependent on him in ways I hadn't anticipated and can barely acknowledge. The triumph of a few weeks ago has yielded to a peculiar invalidism.

"I can smell your skin."

"Uh-oh."

"No, it's okay. You know, I'm a damn bloodhound now. If you run away, I can track you down by your scent trail."

"What does it feel like?"

"Right now I feel okay. I need to eat soon, though."

"No, I mean, what does it feel like to be pregnant?"

I laugh. "I thought you wanted the nausea report." I think awhile. "It feels like a desire to hibernate."

I unzip my jeans, and Jeff lays his hand on my belly. We listen, as though the embryonic heartbeat might suddenly become audible again through his palm.

"It sounded strong, didn't it?" he says. "It sounded determined."

Jeff is the intuitive one. His perceptions are data I've learned to take seriously.

"I feel softer somehow. Like the edges of me are blurring."

"Your skin is changing," he replies. "It feels more rubbery."

He moves his hand over my pelvis and into the curved space between hip and rib. In moments like these I remember I'm married to a sculptor. I reach over the bed and grab the embryology atlas lying on the floor and flip to the section on organogenesis. We look together for a while at the diagrams and electron-scanning micrographs. Two days after the heart starts beating, the eyes begin to take shape. Two days after that, limb buds sprout from the shoulders. The next day, the neural tube closes to become the spinal cord. And the day after that, rudiments of the legs and feet appear.

"No wonder you want the outside world still and quiet," Jeff says.

"What do you think about when you look at pictures like these?"

"They remind me of a performance art piece I did for the Cambridge River Festival. The one that involved a marching Sousa band."

We lie together until the chapel windows are drained of color. Jeff gets up to start dinner. I'm half sleeping when a series of images plays through my mind's eye: a marching band takes the field. Some of the players stop, turn, and walk in different directions. Out of a series of straight lines, a snake emerges with a flickering tongue. Then the snake disperses and reassembles as a flock of birds. And then the birds turn into falling maple leaves. October.

3

Sap Moon

MARCH

Something in the season begins to loosen. The change is almost imperceptible. The scenery is the same—brown stubble and black scribbly branches—but the lighting is different. Less glistening, more mushiness. Cue the wind.

At eleven weeks pregnant, I'm either feeling slightly better or else I've simply adjusted to the misery. In either case, the rattling of windows is making me restless, so I fill my pockets with cheese as a hedge against nausea and drive old Route 66 nine miles southwest to Funk's Grove. At sixteen hundred acres, it is the largest stand of uncut timber left in central Illinois. Funk's Grove is a preserve in the old, feudal sense of the word. A century and a half ago, the original Funk patriarchs laid in a fortune by selling seed to local farmers, and they set this land aside for their own personal idylls. Their latter-day descendants have been generous about allowing the public into the grove. Many generations of biology students have been brought here to learn a thing or two about tree identification and forest ecosystems. I was one.

During my senior year of college, an enthusiastic new ecology professor lured me out of the laboratory and into the field, where the ability to run experiments is a function of air currents and weather, of time of day and season. One of my first studies was interrupted by the fact that my eyelashes froze together in a blizzard. Another ended when my notebook sank into a stand of cattails. I fell in love with field work right away—as much because of its precariousness as in spite of it. I liked the way the ability to collect data was dependent on ancient skills: how to set traps in the dark; how to tie knots in the rain; how to identify trees by their bark, mammals by their tracks, birds by their song. Inspired by Funk's Grove, I left the lab bench for the woods and never looked back.

It's too raw today to hike my favorite part of the refuge—the prairie savanna where thick, wide-armed bur oaks stand among acres of windblown grass like the original giants of the earth. So I head for the shelter of maples, which crowd together near Timber Creek. It's syrup season. The larger trees are tapped for sap collection, some outfitted with old-fashioned metal buckets and others with a complex arrangement of plastic bags and tubing. I wander among the buckets for a while, listening for the *plink-plink* of dripping sap.

Plant physiologists still can't explain why maple sap runs in the spring. It's a mystery that secretly pleases me. All trees stockpile sugar during the winter, and in most species simple capillary action can account for its ascent from roots to branches in the early spring. This is the same adhesive force that draws a drop of water through a paper napkin. But this principle cannot account for the ten to twelve gallons of 4 percent sucrose solution that your average sugar maple can pull up its trunk and pour into a bucket during the month of March. Injure any other tree, and sap will merely ooze from the wound. But the complex hydraulics of maples somehow generates an interior force that exceeds the outside air pressure. Sap spurts from every gash and broken branch.

I lean against the trunk of a small untapped tree, nibble on a few cheese cubes, and try to imagine what is going on inside the bark. Way above my head, the wind in the crowns sounds like an enormous exhaust fan, but here below the air is quiet. The sun comes out for a moment, and before another sheet of clouds can cover it back over, the shadows of waving branches dance on the furrowed trunks and the mats of slick leaves.

My botanical reverie soon turns obstetrical. In fact, the internal anatomy of a human placenta closely resembles a maple grove: the long columns of cells sent out by the embryo into the uterine lining during the first few weeks of pregnancy quickly branch and branch again until, by the third month of pregnancy, the treetops of an entire forest press up against the deepest layers of the womb. Meanwhile, the open taps of the uterus's spiral arteries send jets of blood spurting between these arboreal structures.

As the mother's blood trickles down through the canopy of placental branches all kinds of important transactions take place. Most notably, carbon dioxide and metabolic wastes are swapped for oxygen, water, minerals, antibodies, and nutrients. This is the same process by which the blood inside our own capillaries is cleansed and refueled but with one major difference: rather than relying on simple diffusion, the placenta actively pumps much of what it needs out of the percolating raindrops of maternal blood. In this way, the fetus is guaranteed a steady supply of needed materials even if the mother's blood levels of, say, calcium or iodine are unusually low or high. The placenta does rely on passive diffusion to bring in oxygen. This is why oxygen levels in umbilical-cord blood dip when pregnant women are exposed to tobacco smoke. Many larger molecules transported into the placenta are picked apart before they are allowed to cross the border between mother and child. Some proteins, for example, are disassembled and carried over brick by amino-acid brick. Then they are rebuilt on the other side.

Thus resupplied with food and oxygen, fetal blood inside the placental branches flows into the umbilical cord and into the belly of the fetus. In the other direction, the placenta sends out fetal waste, but this is not all. It also pours a host of hormones and other chemical signals into the free-flowing fountains of maternal blood. These are then carried into the mother's body. By the third month of pregnancy, they initiate inconspicuous but fundamental changes. Some of them alter metabolism and tinker with cardiac functioning. Some of them quietly redirect blood flow. (Eventually, the uterus will receive fifty times more blood than it did before pregnancy, and the pregnant woman's total blood volume will increase by a third.) One placental hormone begins preparing the breast for lactation. Another shuts down the ovary's corpus luteum; beginning in the third month, the placenta takes over progesterone production. Still other placental hormones alter the structure of the mother's own hormones so they come to serve slightly different purposes. In all cases, a pregnant woman aids and abets her own infiltration. It is she who provides the cholesterol that the placenta then rearranges into various steroid hormones. These are then released back into her bloodstream to trigger the above-mentioned changes.

The result is that I feel subtly hijacked. There are a few visible changes. Although my uterus is still contained within the bony cradle of the pelvis, my belly is thickening and softening, as though I were subsisting on a diet of coconuts and avocados. Also, my nipples are darker, bumpier, and when touched, feel electrically charged. Then there are the hidden changes. The pace and depth of my breathing feels different. And I'm aware of the way my pulse rate changes when I stand up, as though my heart were receiving messages of a slightly altered frequency. My balance is off. All these changes can be explained by placental hormones. One of them, for example, loosens joints in preparation for childbirth. This probably accounts for the slight wobble I feel in my hips as I walk.

There are a number of things that cannot yet be explained. One is how the placenta avoids tripping the silent alarm that alerts the mother's immune system to the presence of an intruder. The placenta is made up of the cells of two individuals—indeed, it is the only mammalian organ with this characteristic. In that sense, it is like the lichen growing here in the furrows of maple bark. Part fungus, part algae, lichens represent a symbiosis so complete that the two organisms are, for all intents and purpose, one creature. Likewise, a placenta is an intertwining of mother and child in the closest kind of embrace biologically possible. Yet, because the child's portion of the placenta is made up of cells genetically different from those of the mother, it should be identified as non-self by the mother's body and rejected, like any other implanted tissue. Why it is not is a question earnestly pursued. Both cancer researchers and those who oversee organ donations have a stake in the answer. Invasive tumors can also evade immune detection. We wish they couldn't. Grafts and other transplants cannot elude surveillance. We wish they could. Deciphering the placenta's relationship with the maternal immune system may help solve both these problems.

The other mystery is why placentas of different species all look so different. Those who study comparative anatomy marvel at how variable this organ is. Even closely related mammals can have placentas of wildly dissimilar anatomies. This observation is unexpected because most structures vital for survival are modified slowly throughout the Sturm und Drang of natural selection. Once a workable placenta evolved, its basic form should have been conserved. And yet, the Rhesus monkey, which also experiences a twenty-eight-day menstrual cycle, has a placenta that rests lightly on the surface of the uterine lining, never burying itself into the underlying tissues. Furthermore, it is heart-shaped. Other monkey species—along with horses, pigs, and sloths—have diffuse placentae in which the entire fetal pouch is attached to the uterine wall in a kind of theater-in-the-round arrangement. By contrast, a pregnant cat, dog, or elephant nurtures its babies with a band that encircles the gestational sac like a seat belt. Sheep and cows have tufted placentas. Humans have simple, round placentas whose point of attachment is restricted to one area of the uterine lining. So do apes, armadillos, hamsters, and vampire bats.

By month three of pregnancy, a human placenta is two inches in diameter. The attached umbilical cord is about four inches long. It will eventually grow into a curly, twenty-two-inch-long, half-inch-wide rope. The placenta will expand into a disc that is eight inches wide and an inch thick and weighs slightly more than a pound—about the size and shape of a single-layer cake. In all species, the placenta is expelled with the fetus during birth. We are the only mammal that does not eat it.

The placenta is a biological mystery. It is an evolutionary shape-shifter. It dodges the mother's immune system while immunologically guarding the fetus. It is the flat cake that feeds us all. It is another brain that is slowly overriding my own. It is a blood-drenched forest. It is the sapwood of pregnancy.

At least three places in the human body possess an ability to block harmful substances from entering areas particularly sensitive to toxins. One is in the brain. One is in the testicle. One is in the placenta. These barriers are all functional rather than anatomical. That is, no special wall, ditch, moat, or partition stands between, say, brain cells and the capillaries that feed them. There are only the usual cell membranes, but these membranes are specially equipped with ion pumps and other subcellular gadgets that allow them to exert some control over which blood-borne molecules are allowed to pass through them.

The placental barrier is located in the skin of the placental branches. It consists of a four-layer, semipermeable membrane interposed between maternal and fetal circulation. When we say something *crosses* the placenta, we mean it passes through this membrane. Inside a placenta are only capillary-filled fetal branches soaked by spumes of mother's blood. That's it. The placental barrier does an admirable job of keeping out bacteria, which are usually too large to pass into the placental branches. Those that do slip by are swiftly dispatched by special immune agents called Hofbauer cells. Also, certain adrenal hormones not needed by the developing fetus are deactivated by placental enzymes.

When it comes to toxic chemicals, however, the placenta is not really a barrier at all. Chemical substances carried in the mother's circulation are sorted by the placenta primarily on the basis of molecular weight, electrical charge, and lipid solubility. In other words, small, neutrally charged molecules that readily dissolve in fat are afforded free passage regardless of their capacity for harm.

Consider pesticides. Those with low molecular weights cross the placenta without restriction. For them, there is no barrier. Pesticides made of bigger, heavier molecules are partly metabolized by the placenta's enzymes before they pass through, but sometimes this transformation makes them *more* toxic, placing the fetus at even greater risk. Or consider mercury, that meddling destroyer of brain tissue. When mercury is attached to carbon, it is called methylmercury. Even if the mother's blood is contaminated with only trace amounts of methylmercury, the placenta will still actively pump it into the fetal capillaries as though it were a precious molecule of calcium or iodine. As the pregnancy continues, the mercury levels in umbilical cord blood will eventually surpass their levels in the mother's blood. In the case of methylmercury, the placenta functions more like a magnifying glass than a barrier.

More profoundly, chemicals don't even have to cross the placenta to cause harm. Some lodge in the placenta and create injury there. For example, nicotine damages the placenta's amino acid transport system, which is used to ferry proteins from the mother's blood into the baby's. This helps explain why the babies of smoking mothers weigh an average of seven ounces less at birth. (Nicotine also passes through the placenta and into the body of the fetus.) Similarly, the industrial pollutants called PCBs alter the placenta's blood vessels in ways that reduce their flow, and the heavy metal nickel, a component of car exhaust, interferes with the placenta's ability to make and release hormones. In short, the placenta not only fails to keep the fetus out of harm's way, it cannot even prevent itself from being damaged. Like any other living tissue, it is fragile.

So where did the idea of an impermeable, all-protecting placental barrier come from?

Not from the ancients, certainly. Aristotle and Hippocrates both thought that the placenta was the place where the mother's blood was funneled directly into the fetal umbilical cord. So did Thomas of Aquinas in the twelfth century. All of them were wrong, of course, but their mistake led to the mostly correct assumption that whatever passes into the mother's body passes also through the placenta. Even in ancient Carthage, newlyweds were forbidden alcohol to prevent damage to wedding-night conceptions. Then, in the fifteenth century, Leonardo da Vinci was among the first anatomists to observe that the blood of the mother and baby do not seem to commingle. Years later, this suspicion was confirmed in a ghastly experiment that involved the injection of melted wax into the uterine artery of a dying pregnant woman. A postmortem examination showed no wax in the fetal tissues. The death of this unfortunate mother gave birth to the placental barrier concept.

Ann Dally, a medical historian, chronicles the misbegotten belief in the impermeable placenta further. By the mid-nineteenth century, the Victorians' veneration of pregnancy reinforced the notion that the placenta was an unbreachable bulwark, even though by now there was plenty of evidence to the contrary. For many decades, teratologists (those who study birth defects) had been publishing reports on congenital malformations induced in animals by environmental substances. But these studies were not thought relevant to humans or were dismissed because the evidence did not fit prevailing ideas. This kind of denial continued into the twentieth century. By the 1950s, an extensive body of literature documented that fetuses could be harmed by a variety of events experienced by their mothers, such as malnutrition and exposure to x-rays, pharmaceuticals, and certain chemicals. And yet, as Dally recalls from her own experience in medical school, "Medical students were taught that the human placenta gave perfect protection to the fetus and was impervious to toxic substances. . . . There seems to have been an attitude of mind that idealized the womb and placenta and ignored most of the extensive existing evidence of fetal damage through environmental influences."

The idea of the impermeable placenta has had a long and ignominious life. Many thousands of women and infants have been harmed because of it. In fact, its ghost still lingers in present-day policies on toxic chemicals; typically, environmental regulators do not consider transplacental effects when setting limits on human exposures. This is maddening because at least four different transplacental tragedies played themselves out in the twentieth century, any one of which should have been sufficient to drive a stake through the heart of the barrier myth forever. The first involved a virus. The second involved a drug. The third involved waste materials from a plastics factory in a Japanese fishing village. And the fourth involved a hormone. Their names resonate like the names of famous battlefields: Rubella. Thalidomide. Minamata. Diethylstilbestrol.

It was not an embryologist who discovered that rubella—German measles—could cross the placenta and maim a human embryo in the early weeks of pregnancy. Nor was it a teratologist. It was an ophthalmologist in Sydney, Australia, heartsick over a run of babies born with congenital cataracts. Perhaps because he was a physician and not a lab researcher, Dr. N. McAlister Gregg's 1941 report rocked the world of medicine.

Gregg did some careful sleuthing. He noticed the children brought to him for surgery shared similar birthdays, even though their birthplaces were far-flung. In addition to their sightless, milky eyes, they also shared other problems: heart defects, feeding problems, failure to thrive, a susceptibility to sudden death. He then realized that the early period of their gestations corresponded to the peak of a widespread outbreak of German measles in 1940. During that summer, military camps dotted the countryside and served as breeding grounds for a variety of infectious illnesses, which subsequently spread to civilians.

A rubella–birth defect connection seemed improbable. Unlike other forms of measles, rubella is usually a mild disease. But a conversation between two mothers in his own waiting room started him wondering whether the illness might have another personality inside the womb. Both women recounted having had rubella early in their pregnancies. So Gregg began interviewing the other mothers of his tiny patients. Of seventy-eight mothers, all but ten could recall a bout with rubella in the summer of 1940. He probed further. Even among those who couldn't confirm having suffered from German measles, it was an outstanding possibility. ("[T]he mother stated that she was kept so busy looking after her ten children that she could not recollect any details of her own health beyond the fact that she was ill at about the sixth week of pregnancy when one of the other children died suddenly from whooping cough. Even though she was ill, she was unable to go to bed.") Gregg correctly reasoned that fetal exposure to rubella during the time when the eye is forming causes "derangement" of the tissues. As a result, the lens—that little football-shaped prism behind the pupil that focuses incoming light—turns white or smoky instead of becoming transparent. In addition, rubella interferes with cardiac and brain development. It also causes profound deafness.

In 1964, twenty-three years after the publication of Gregg's landmark paper, a global rubella epidemic erupted that would fill schools for the deaf and blind for years to come. More than 20,000 children were maimed by congenital rubella in the United States alone. Desperate mothers sought legal abortions in Japan, petitioned courts to have them here, or turned to illegal abortionists. Finally, in 1969, the first vaccine was marketed. It was a triumph for public health. Now, thirty years later, rubella is all but unknown. In fact, it has become such a vague and obscure threat that many mothers hesitate to vaccinate their own children against it. The course of the disease being so mild, they wonder why they should bother, forgetting that the point of rubella vaccination is not to spare their children the discomfort of German measles but to prevent them from spreading the virus to newly pregnant women, in whom infection is devastating. We inoculate our babies to keep other babies from ruin.

It occurs to me that Jeff and I are probably among the last generation of prospective parents with firsthand memories of the disease. Jeff's mother contracted rubella shortly after becoming pregnant for the fifth time. On the advice of her physician—and with his discreet assistance—she ended the pregnancy. "I looked like a strawberry," she recalls. "And I had four other children to think about."

To me, rubella is the boy in my Sunday school class who wore thick glasses and hearing aids and laughed at the wrong times. He was always going to the hospital for various operations. Once he demanded loudly to know whether I was wearing a Kotex, and I complained about him to my mother. She told me about pregnancy and rubella. *Rubella*. It seemed too beautiful a word to explain what was wrong with Stevie.

Now I call Mom to ask her again about rubella. Did I ever receive the vaccination? She doesn't remember.

"It went on the market in 1969. I would have been nine or ten."

"Whenever the vaccine became available in our area, you had it. I would have made sure of that."

"Well, maybe I didn't need to. If I'd already had German measles, I mean."

"No, you never had rubella."

My mother trained as a microbiologist. I believe her. Anyway, I am asking for reasons of pure curiosity, not out of fear. The blood draw taken at my first prenatal visit shows that I'm immune to rubella. On some ordinary day that neither my mother nor I can remember, I must have been vaccinated against it. Better than a placental barrier, I have antibodies. And all of us pregnant women who were vaccinated against rubella as young girls have an eye doctor who listened carefully to mothers to thank for that.

Dr. Gregg's 1941 study, humbly published in the *Transactions of the Ophthalmological Society of Australia*, has been hailed as the first to document a causal link between structural human birth defects and environmental factors. Maybe it was, but reading it more than a half century later, I'm more impressed with the part of his message that was ignored. In his paper Gregg warns not only about infectious agents like rubella but about other "toxic influences . . . known to be transmissible transplacentally." If a virus could cross the placenta and wreak havoc on embryos, then so, potentially, could other materials. To bolster his case, he goes on to mention studies—already published in the medical literature of the time— that implicated a variety of substances. Had the entire scope of Gregg's warning been heeded, subsequent epidemics of birth defects might well have been avoided.

Like those created by thalidomide.

Sitting at my desk, I have to take a deep breath before opening the books on this topic. I am not a believer in maternal impressions—the old mystical idea that seeing a spotted fish will cause my baby to have birthmarks or that unhappy encounters with one-legged men will make for lameness. Nonetheless, pregnancy has made me superstitious. My aversion to pictures of damaged children is as strong as my aversion to root vegetables. And I already know that the damage created by the sedative drug called thalidomide is as stark as it comes: babies born with missing ears and lobster-claw hands. Babies with toes growing directly out of their hips. Babies born with only heads and oval, limbless trunks.

But more powerful than my desire to turn away from these images is the need to explore them. I'm inspired here by the underworld investigator in Adrienne Rich's famous poem "Diving into the Wreck": a woman diver descends alone into the black ocean to find a sunken ship, "to see the damage that was done / and the treasures that prevail. . . . / the wreck and not the story of the wreck / the thing itself and not the myth." I am a pregnant biologist searching for the voices of mothers and scientists. I want to hear the warnings both heeded and unheeded. I want to know about the lives blasted and the battles fought. I want to find the treasures that prevail. So I open the books and dive in.

Thalidomide is the generic name of a drug first synthesized in Germany in 1953. It proved ineffective for its intended purpose as an anticonvulsant. But then, in 1958, thalidomide was repackaged as a sedative and vigorously marketed, praised by its makers as unusually safe: it didn't cause hangovers and suicide by overdose was impossible. Physicians soon discovered that it worked to quell morning sickness, and this quality became part of its advertised appeal. Had I been a pregnant mother in 1958, I would undoubtedly have welcomed a prescription.

As we all know now, thalidomide was safe for neither fetuses nor adults. Before it was finally withdrawn from European and Canadian markets a few years later, at least 8,000 children had been born with malformations of the kind that mothers fear most. Thalidomide's signature birth defect was "reduction limb deficit," dwarfed or missing arms and legs, especially one wrenching variation on the theme called "phocomelia," in which the limbs resemble tiny flippers. The damage was more than physical. The birth of these babies wrecked marriages, impoverished families, and crushed mothers under the weight of relentless guilt. In addition to outright deformities, thalidomide also triggered countless miscarriages and stillbirths, and it often brought on nerve damage in nonpregnant adult users. This is how the U.S. Food and Drug Administration recently described the manufacturer's original claims for the drug: "It was promoted by its maker as being nontoxic, with no side effects, and completely safe for pregnant women. Not one of these statements was true. In addition to the effect on the fetus, in adults it caused peripheral neuritis, a painful numbing of the hands and feet that is often irreversible. . . . There were scientific tests, that, had they been conducted, might have shown thalidomide to be unsafe. The drug companies involved, however, did not perform those tests."

The tests necessary to prove the maiming powers of thalidomide were in fact performed—but as a vast, unintentional experiment on humans than ran almost four years. In the fall of 1961, a scientist published a paper that implicated thalidomide as the cause of phocomelia in Germany. Almost simultaneously, an Australian obstetrician, William McBride, published a letter in the leading British medical journal, *The Lancet*, asking whether any other physicians had noticed an epidemic of strange limb deformities in babies born to mothers who had been prescribed thalidomide during early pregnancy. Like the rubella report of his compatriot two decades earlier, McBride's letter broke a dam of silence. Similar reports began streaming in from around the world, and the drug was swiftly withdrawn from the European market.

How did thalidomide come to be sold to pregnant women in forty-eight countries without any advance demonstration of its safety? The popular mythology is that there were no reasons to suspect it was unsafe. No reasons to do more testing. But this is only a half truth. Simple naïveté cannot explain why the drug continued to be marketed in Canada after it was already banned in Europe. Moreover, as Ann Dally points out, uncomfortable inklings of evidence for harm had emerged even before the drug went to market in Europe, but they were disregarded. Indeed, there was enough preliminary evidence for Frances Kelsey, an FDA physician, to be persuaded to deny thalidomide entry into the United States. And thereby hangs a tale.

In 1960, a Cincinnati pharmaceutical company filed an application to make and distribute the drug here. The marketing department had grand plans: thalidomide would be sold as an over-the-counter remedy for all kinds of human ailments. These included not only insomnia and morning sickness but also anorexia, premature ejaculation, asthma, alcoholism, and "poor schoolwork." The job of evaluating the safety and effectiveness of thalidomide fell to Kelsey, who had worked for the FDA for only a month. Approval was expected to be swift. But in the data provided her by the manufacturer, Kelsey saw warning signs. She slowed down the application process by asking hard questions: Why did the drug cause tingling in the hands and feet of some adult users? How did it affect metabolism? And how exactly did it behave in pregnant women? The company had insufficient answers, so she delayed approval, quickly developing a reputation among drug companies as an obstructionist bureaucrat.

What made Frances Kelsey see signs of toxicity where others saw none? In hindsight, she has said that her sense of caution emerged from her previous work on malaria. She remembered how human embryos lacked the ability to metabolize the antimalarial drug quinine in the same way that adults could. Could the same be true for thalidomide? She also *remembered the story of rubella.* So she kept asking the applicant for more data until, finally, the reports from Germany and England broke and "approval became unthinkable." In 1962, Dr. Kelsey received an award for distinguished service from President Kennedy. It occurs to me that thousands of us middle-aged Americans unknowingly owe our undeformed limbs to this woman, who believed the placenta was permeable when others did not.

What are the other submerged lessons we need to recover from the thalidomide disaster? It seems to me there are at least two:

If our goal is to protect human embryos, we cannot afford to wait until we understand everything about how a chemical might inflict its damage.

Scientists finally learned the mechanism by which thalidomide harms babies in 1991—thirty years after it was pulled off the market. As it turns out, this drug stops blood vessel formation and slows the production of certain proteins when it travels to the fetal side of the placenta. This discovery finally solves the mystery of how thalidomide erases fetal limbs, but its solution—however interesting scientifically—was not necessary to protect public health. Frances Kelsey acted in advance of this knowledge.

The timing of fetal exposure is at least as important as the dose.

The story of thalidomide troubles a fusty but deeply cherished principle of toxicology: the old notion that the dose makes the poison. According to this precept, the higher the teratogenic exposure, the more severe the birth defect. With thalidomide, however, the day the exposure occurred was as important as the amount of exposure in determining damage. The critical window of vulnerability for thalidomide turns out to be very specific: namely, 35 to 50 days after the last menstrual period. These days represent the most intense period of organogenesis. The wide variety of defects exhibited by the thalidomide babies was a simple matter of the calendar. Embryos develop from the head down and from the center out. Thus, pills taken between days 35 and 37 resulted in babies with no ears, whereas pills taken between days 39 and 41 resulted in no arms. Days 41 to 43, no uterus. Days 45 to 47, no leg bones. Days 47 to 49, deformed thumbs.

A cold rain pelts the windows. I'm back in bed again. Good sleeping weather, I tell myself. Any excuse will do.

The sound of a key turning in a lock: Jeff's home from the studio. I can hear him on the landing stripping off his paint-spattered work clothes. The door bangs a second time: he's letting the dog out. The sound of ripping envelopes: he's sitting naked on the stairs reading the mail. Now he's walking quietly from room to room, looking to see if I'm home yet. The bathroom is the first place he checks. But I haven't thrown up for days now. The bedroom is his second guess.

"There you are. I should have known."

"You must be freezing. Get in here with me. Just don't jiggle the mattress."

Jeff topples slow-motion onto the bed like a wounded King Kong falling from the top of the Empire State Building, a stunt that makes me laugh uncontrollably. We snuggle into the covers. Still not used to my mushy belly, I feel self-conscious. If the second month of pregnancy is a return to childhood, the third month is the reinstatement of puberty.

"I feel weird and . . . thick."

"I think you are weird and . . . beautiful."

Ah, the husbands of women in their first trimesters. How effusively admiring they must be.

"So tell me what's going on in there now." Jeff rests his hand above my pubic bone.

"Compared to last month, it's just details. The fingernails are growing in. The ears are moving up. The eyes get shifted toward the center of the face. Oh, and the genitals are forming, too."

"How big is it now?"

" 'At the end of the third month, a human fetus is supposed to be about two and a half inches.' " I'm quoting from one of the obstetrical texts.

Jeff measures this out on the back of his hand. His forearms and wrists strike me as miraculously lovely. I can't shake the images of reduction limb deficits.

"What do you remember about thalidomide?" I ask Jeff.

"Thalidomide babies . . . babies with flippers. I remember seeing their photographs when I was a kid."

"According to this survey I found, two thirds of those under forty-five years old don't recognize the word."

"Really? I remember thalidomide."

"Do you remember Minamata?"

"No."

"It happened at about the same time. Do you remember a famous photograph of a Japanese mother bathing her paralyzed daughter?"

"The one by Smith? The photographer for *Life*?"

"Yes."

"It was black and white and darkly lit. It was composed like Michelangelo's *Pietà*, but it was also a baptism. That's what I remember."

The next day in the library, I look for W. Eugene Smith's 1975 photo essay, *Minamata: Words and Photos*, which he coauthored with his Japanese wife. The picture that Jeff can recall so clearly is spread across two pages. The lines are stark and classical. In the manner of Mary cradling the crucified body of Christ, a naked mother holds the body of her half-grown daughter in a Japanese bath. The mother's upturned hand, which lifts the girl's legs, is balanced by the daughter's downturned hand, which just brushes the water's surface. The mother looks at her daughter with adoration. The daughter's eyes are rolled skyward—as if to God—but there is no light of awareness in them. Suddenly, the viewer sees how the fingers touching the water are unnaturally bent, as are the rail-thin legs, and how in the center of the girl's naked chest, which floats in the center of the photograph itself, there is a deep hole that is not a wound but some kind of terrible malformation.

The daughter's name is Tomoko. She was born in 1956 and died two years after her portrait stunned the world, in 1977.

Minamata is an ancient city along the Shiranui Sea in southern Japan. Since feudal times it has been a fishing community, but now Minamata is mostly known as the birthplace of Minamata disease, which is not a disease at all but simply another name for methylmercury poisoning.

Mercury is an ancient element. Called quicksilver by Aristotle, it was named after the speedy planet by sixth-century alchemists who thought it possessed the power to turn base metals into gold. They were wrong. But mercury does have the power to speed up certain chemical reactions. Which is how the city Minamata and the element mercury came to have a common destiny.

In the 1930s and '40s, a factory in Minamata called Chisso began manufacturing acetaldehyde and vinyl chloride—both ingredients in plastics. To do so, it used metallic mercury as a catalyst, which was then dumped into the wastewater that entered Minamata Bay. In the spring of 1956, a five-year-old girl was brought to the factory hospital because her speech was slurred and her gait unsteady. Not long after, her younger sister began exhibiting the same symptoms. Then four of her neighbors became delirious and started to stagger drunkenly. The director of the hospital, Dr. Hajime Hosokawa, was alarmed. He reported to the authorities that "an unclarified disease of the central nervous system has broken out." Because of the clustering of affected families, Dr. Hosokawa assumed he was dealing with a contagious illness—thus the label "Minamata disease." An investigation soon uncovered fifty more cases.

But three clues emerged that argued against an infectious cause. Cats living in the homes of stricken families had mysteriously died. The affected families almost always had ties to the fishing industry. And the homes of the additional fifty cases were scattered over a wide area and not confined to any one neighborhood. What united the victims was a strikingly similar progression of maladies. First the hands and feet began to tingle. Then there was difficulty holding chopsticks. Words became "entangled and knotted" in the mouth. Eventually, hearing was muffled, and a black curtain fell over part of the visual field. In some there was restlessness and a tendency toward shouting. Finally general paralysis set in, the hands became gnarled, swallowing became difficult, and death soon followed.

Once the investigation was under way, observations previously reported but subsequently dismissed suddenly took on new meaning. For six years or more, fishermen had complained about dead seaweed and empty clam and oyster shells. There had been other ominous sightings, too. Floating fish. Seabirds that dropped from the sky while in flight. Paralyzed octopus. Dogs, pigs, and cats that were seen to whirl about violently and then die. Looking at all the evidence together—both medical and environmental—the study group issued a report in the fall of 1956 concluding, correctly, that Minamata disease was not an infectious illness after all but was a form of heavy metal poisoning caused from eating fish and shellfish from the bay. Some kind of heavy metal was getting into the waters of the bay, and the evidence pointed to Chisso.

The release of this report revealing the cause of the mysterious disease should have marked the end of a terrible story. Instead, it was only the beginning. The local government opposed the study group's principal recommendation—a ban on fishing in the bay. At the same time, Chisso, the only possible culprit, refused to change its practices. Instead, it hired experts to refute the evidence and insist there was no proof to implicate the company's actions as the reason for the problem. Meanwhile, a university research team announced it would study the problem further.

At the end of almost four more years of study, this is what the research team found: That cats fed fish from Minamata Bay developed symptoms of Minamata disease. That cats fed methylmercury developed the same symptoms. That the Bay was highly contaminated with methylmercury. That the livers and kidneys of human victims who died of Minamata disease contained high levels of methylmercury. That the hair of living Minamata victims contained high levels of methylmercury. That workers exposed to methylmercury in a British factory had very similar symptoms to the people of Minamata.

Chisso responded that it used only metallic mercury, not methylmercury, and therefore its wastewater could not be the source of the problem. What Chisso did not say was that its own hospital director, the same Dr. Hosokawa who had first noticed the problem, had in 1959 induced Minamata disease in cats fed Chisso factory sludge. This information Chisso executives kept to themselves. Dr. Hosokawa—unlike Dr. Gregg or Dr. Kelsey before him—kept quiet, too.

During those same four years that the research team toiled on and the company doctor held his tongue, the following events happened in Minamata: Chisso diverted some of its wastewater into a nearby river and spread the contamination further. Increasing numbers of babies began to be born in Minamata with what appeared to be cerebral palsy. And the local government began advising abortions for all pregnant women whose hair levels of methylmercury exceeded fifty parts per million.

The babies with cerebral palsy turned out to have congenital Minamata disease. Although they had never eaten fish from the bay, their mothers all had. Some of these babies were also blind or deaf. Some had unusually small heads and deformed teeth. Some had tremors and were prone to convulsions. Autopsy reports showed that those born with Minamata disease had more extensive brain damage than those who contracted the disease after birth. Not counting these congenital cases, 29 percent of the children born in the most contaminated areas between 1955 and 1959 showed signs of mental deficiencies.

Then, in 1962, someone found a forgotten bottle of Chisso wastewater sludge sitting on a laboratory shelf, and researchers uncovered the critical missing link in their painstakingly constructed chain of evidence. The contents of the bottle tested positive for methylmercury. This finding proved beyond a doubt what many suspected all along: that the factory's waste disposal practices were somehow converting elemental mercury, a weaker poison, into organic mercury, a formidable one. But if the research team supposed that demonstration of absolute proof would trigger action, the joke was on them. Chisso blithely went on dumping methylmercury for six more years, stopping only in 1968 when its method of making plastic materials became outmoded and new technology was introduced.

In the end, it was citizen activism and photography, and not the slow accumulation of scientific knowledge, that awakened awareness about the ecology of methylmercury. In 1969, twenty-nine families filed a lawsuit against Chisso on behalf of the dead, dying, and critically ill. Other families appealed to the government for action. Still others began direct negotiations with the company, staging sit-ins outside its Tokyo offices. Protesters there were arrested and beaten, including Smith himself, who was on hand to document their activities. His photographs went out anyway, including one that shows Tomoko being presented before a table of dark-suited officials from Chisso, while petitioners demanded that the men look at her and touch her body. Her face wears the same fixed expression it did in the bath.

In March 1973, the Kumamoto District Court ruled in favor of the families. It noted in its verdict that Chisso had failed both in its obligation to confirm safety "through researches and study" and in its obligation to provide preventive measures "if a case should arise where there be some doubts as to safety." In the final analysis, the court ruled, "no plant can be permitted to infringe on and run at the sacrifice of the lives and the health of the regional residents."

In 1998, I found a translated thesis in the library containing interviews with some of the original Minamata activists. Conducted many years after the trial's conclusion and the payment of indemnity, they express continuing desire for a more profound kind of resolution. One said, "[W]e most ardently long to have the sea and the mountains returned to us as they were before pollution. Money is a nuisance, a troublemaker in the family and in the village. . . . The other world in which we used to live should be brought back to us here and now. Our hope, a very slight hope, is to bring the sea back . . . and an even slighter hope is to return to us our healthy bodies of bygone days."

The most recent forecast is that mercury concentrations in the bay are expected to decline to background levels by the year 2011—more than a half century after Dr. Hosokawa first gave a name to Minamata disease and then fell silent. Fish and shellfish in Minamata Bay were declared safe for consumption in 1997.

What is the best way to honor the life of Tomoko? This is a hard question to answer. The tools of biological research failed to keep Tomoko from harm, and yet much knowledge was learned during all the years of denial and delay, knowledge that still seems important. Perhaps it can yet be acted upon to protect future children. If so, the insights that can be retrieved from the wreckage of the Minamata disaster are these:

Nature is an alchemist.

During the industrial process, the metallic mercury that Chisso used as a chemical catalyst was transformed, in an unintended side reaction, into the potent fetal toxicant called methylmercury. It was this qualitatively stronger poison that then flowed into the bay. We now know that the world's oldest living species—methylating bacteria—also perform this transformation. Since the beginning of life itself, these organisms have subsisted in the oxygenless bottoms of ponds, rivers, and oceans, quietly converting sulfate into sulfide. When presented with a molecule of mercury, they use their singular talent to convert it into methylmercury by combining the free metal with carbon. Thus, whenever metallic mercury is released into an aquatic ecosystem, its power to do harm will intensify through a chemical reaction we do not and cannot control.

Unintended consequences are not always unpredictable consequences.

Even though the environment will have its own way with elements like mercury, certain ecological laws still abide. Central among these is the principle of biomagnification, which refers to the fact that a persistent poison concentrates as it moves up the food chain. Organisms at the top invariably end up with the most poison. In water, toxic substances can concentrate to extraordinary levels because food chains are longer than they are on land. (The buoyancy of water allows aquatic organisms to survive on comparatively fewer calories than their gravity-bound, terrestrial counterparts. Because they spend less energy holding themselves up, the transfer of energy from one link of the chain to the next is more efficient. With less energy lost between links, more links can be added.) In the case of Minamata, mercury levels in the flesh of the fishes hauled onto the decks of the fishing boats were more than a million times higher than that of the water they swam in. In other words, when Chisso drizzled methylmercury into the bay, it came back to land one million times greater in concentration. As a general rule, whenever persistent pollutants are released into the environment at large, people who eat a lot of fish or other aquatic animals will receive the highest exposures.

Of all members of a human population, fetuses are most vulnerable to toxic harm.

As we have seen, the placenta can magnify levels of toxic chemicals even further. In addition, developing organs are more sensitive to damage than adult ones. The window of greatest vulnerability for methylmercury exposure is between months four and six of pregnancy—considerably later than that for rubella or thalidomide. This is the period of brain cell migration. Just as a spider can lower itself from the ceiling by reeling out a single strand of silk, a fetal brain cell moves from the center of the brain out to its surface by rappelling along the length of its own axonal fiber. Eventually, the brain is filled with such spider cells and the webs of neuronal connections they subsequently spin. Methylmercury interferes with this movement from center to surface. Once the critical period for brain cell migration passes by, it does not come again.

Threshold levels of toxic chemicals may not exist for fetuses.

The image of the toxic threshold is as deeply imprinted in the collective psyche as that of the placental barrier. It is equally hard to surrender. Like the belief in placental barriers, belief in thresholds promises protection from harm. As long as exposures to a particular poison remain below the calculated limit, so runs the thinking, risk will be negligible. It's a seductive presumption, and, as ideas go, it has had a long, venerable life. The concept of thresholds is a direct outgrowth of the medieval postulate that the dose makes the poison.

New research from Minamata challenges the existence of fetal thresholds for mercury. During the original investigations of Minamata victims of congenital poisoning, no one thought to ask the question, "What is the least amount of mercury that can cause harm?" Sadly, at last count, only forty-seven of the congenital victims remain alive, and teasing apart their prenatal mercury exposures from postnatal ones would be difficult at this point. However, many families in Minamata follow a poignant tradition: when a child is born, a piece of its umbilical cord is carefully wrapped in gauze and saved in a small wooden box. Families recently agreed to share the contents of these boxes with researchers, who were thereby able to measure the actual prenatal exposures received by these individuals, including those no longer living. Published in 1998, the study found that the cord tissue of children born with congenital Minamata disease contained significantly higher levels of methylmercury than did the cords of healthy children. Furthermore, mentally retarded children without identified Minamata disease had cord levels of methylmercury in between these two other groups. In other words, even far below the threshold level needed to cause the constellation of symptoms we label as a known disorder, brain damage still occurred.

The full moon arrives on the thirteenth of the month, a Friday, just as I am crossing the threshold between the first and second trimesters of pregnancy. Trimesters correspond to no real developmental events. Obstetricians, however, find the division of pregnancy into equal thirds convenient, as do pregnancy guidebooks. Expectations of weight gain, possible complications, various diagnostic tasks—these are all described and parceled out by trimesters. However contrived, they are still the three seasons of pregnancy. Often, the guidebooks say tantalizingly, a woman chooses to announce her pregnancy at the end of her first trimester.

Also approaching, as Jeff reminds me, is the Ides of March. In the Roman calendar, all months had Ides, which represented their midpoint and were supposed to coincide with the full moon. They conveniently partitioned a month into two equal halves. Meetings—including Caesar's fateful one with Brutus and Cassius—were often scheduled during the Ides. *Ides* is Latin for "divide." I take a look again at the play *Julius Caesar*, so full of speech and argument. In Shakespeare's telling, I report back to Jeff, the Ides were a time of public announcements.

But Jeff and I have kept our secret for what seems like so long that the knowledge of the baby has become like the baby itself: buried in a place beyond language, scheming, and confession. I've adjusted to the duplicity of public professor and private mother so completely that I hesitate to disturb the silence about the baby, as though to do so would disturb the baby's own silence. Since no one has thought to yet ask me if I am pregnant, I have not had to lie.

And then the filmmaker Judith Helfand arrives from New York to stay in our guest house and show her latest film, *A Healthy Baby Girl*, on campus. Helfand is the W. Eugene Smith of diethylstilbestrol, DES, the hormone once given to pregnant women to prevent miscarriages that is now known to cause cancer and infertility in their daughters. Like Smith, she has documented the damage done by a transplacental chemical exposure, the denials of the responsible industries, the citizen activism that followed, and the cycles of guilt and shame that can blow apart relationships within affected families. The difference is that Judith turns the camera around. She is herself a DES daughter, and before she screens her film she will stand at a podium and describe to students her own losses to this drug. They include her uterus, cervix, and the top third of her vagina. They also include her dreams of having a baby.

In early December, shortly before moving back to Illinois and a month before I became pregnant, I spent a night at Judith's apartment on Manhattan's Riverside Drive.

"This is the house my uterus bought," she remarked wryly as we rode up the elevator, referring to the lawsuit against the drug company that was settled in her favor.

Even without the camera on, Judith practices and encourages autobiography, constantly exploring the power within acts of personal disclosure. She is also one of the most attentive listeners I have ever met. Perhaps this is why, at 2 A.M., we were still at her kitchen table eating eggs and fruit, and I found myself describing my own desire to have a baby, as well as my fear, based on several consecutive months of sex and menstrual cycles, that I wouldn't be able to.

"Wait," she said, rising from the table, "Just wait."

I misunderstood, thinking she was simply advising patience. But then she began rummaging in boxes stacked near the bookshelves in the next room.

"I think it will happen for you. But wait. Just wait a minute."

She returned with a Hebrew book of prayers and a small painted figure, which she held up to the light.

"It's a mezuzah," she explained, a Jewish talisman intended as a sign of faith.

Judith instructed me to attach it to the entryway of my house or to any location that marks a division between public and private, outer and inner. *Mezuzah* is Hebrew for "doorpost." This particular one was unusual, even subversive, she continued, because it was shaped like the torso of a woman's body. A typical mezuzah stays far away from graven imagery. Whatever their outward shape, every mezuzah contains a handwritten scroll of scriptural verses. These passages are from Deuteronomy—a book of what we called the Old Testament in Methodist Bible school, which the Jews know as the Torah—and are Moses' words about sacred obligations. Moses makes reference to the seasons, to planting and harvesting, to rain, grass, cattle, and corn.

"As you go in and out of your house, just let her remind you of the sacredness of ordinary life," Judith said, as she wrapped the mezuzah in cloth and pressed it into my hand.

I in turn wrapped it inside a pair of socks and packed it in my suitcase, where it stayed until we moved to Illinois and Jeff affixed it to the doorpost of our bedroom.

So perhaps it is not such a surprise that as we walk out of the faculty cafeteria and into a March windstorm, heading for the university auditorium where she will show her film, she stops suddenly and puts a hand on my arm.

"Sandra, are you pregnant?" She holds me in a fierce gaze.

"Yes," I finally say, laughing. "Three months. I got pregnant as soon as we moved here."

Then we are both laughing, her black hair blowing between us, wet leaves flying around us. And in that moment I have never felt closer to or more divided from another woman.

During the next few days, I will watch *A Healthy Baby Girl* at least three more times, as I shepherd Judith to history classes, nursing classes, biology classes, where she is a scheduled speaker. But even during this first viewing, the story is familiar.

During some parts of the movie I feel I am watching the thalidomide tragedy unfold all over again—only this time without Frances Kelsey. The drug DES was first synthesized in the 1930s. Although its chemical structure looked very different from that of estrogen, it proved an uncanny mimic. It also fattened livestock and poultry. In 1941, DES was marketed as both a feed additive and as a treatment for menopausal symptoms, vaginitis, and gonorrhea. It was also used to suppress milk production in mothers who chose to bottle-feed their babies. A few years later, the FDA approved DES prescriptions for pregnant women. The belief was that miscarriages were triggered by hormonal imbalances, a problem that could be fixed by administering ever larger doses of synthetic estrogen throughout all three trimesters of pregnancy. More than a half century later, an investigation by the National Academy of Science would delicately call this line of reasoning "a rationale difficult to reconstruct."

That is to say, it made no sense. No animal studies even suggested DES had the ability to prevent miscarriage. In fact, they all hinted at its other ominous powers. One study from the 1930s found that DES caused breast cancer in mice, while another reported deformities in the reproductive organs of offspring of mice that received DES. A couple of well-designed human studies in the 1950s found that DES actually *increased* the risk of miscarriage. Nevertheless, obstetricians continued to see the drug as a kind of all-purpose charm against the evil eye and went on prescribing it for another dozen years. All told, between 1947 and 1971, DES was manufactured by more than two hundred different drug companies and prescribed to about 4 million women in the United States alone. As we now know, it did not prevent a single miscarriage.

The next chapter of the DES story reiterates the rubella story. In the late 1960s, a cluster of rare cancers baffled the medical staff at Massachusetts General Hospital in Boston. Within three years, seven young women were diagnosed there with clear cell cancer of the vagina, a disease almost unheard of in women under seventy. Finally, a doctor who listened to mothers figured out the cause. One mother mentioned to the gynecologist treating her daughter that she had been prescribed DES while pregnant. He then remembered to ask the question of his next patient's mother. She had taken DES in pregnancy as well. So had five other mothers. In 1971, Dr. Arthur Herbst and his colleagues presented a paper connecting prenatal DES exposure to cervico-vaginal clear cell adenocarcinoma. This announcement marked the end of DES prescriptions to pregnant women and the beginning of a flurry of data collection.

Once the scales fell from the eyes of the medical community, all kinds of additional problems became apparent. Mothers who took DES during pregnancy were found to have increased rates of breast cancer. Their sons and daughters were shown to suffer from unusually high rates of immune system disorders. Many also have reproductive tract abnormalities. In the sons, these include undescended testicles and hypospadias (in which the urethra opens along the underside of the penis instead of at the tip). In the daughters, these include strangely shaped uteruses, which place them at high risk for infertility, tubal pregnancies, or preterm labor. In all, more than 1,500 papers have been authored on the consequences of prenatal exposure to DES.

Once again, timing of exposure proved as important as dose. We now know that prenatal exposure to DES on certain key days of pregnancy suppresses the activity of a gene called Wnt7a. However unassuming its name, this gene is responsible for directing the migration of cells destined to become reproductive tissue. Some of the malformations created by the disabling of this gene are as dramatic as those created by rubella or thalidomide, but, of course, the damage is not visible from the outside of the body. *No arms* registers an immediate reaction in the delivery room. But a two-horned uterus will likely not get discovered for years.

When the lights come up after the film, Judith describes how she recuperated from her hysterectomy in her old childhood bedroom where her mother, twenty-five years earlier, had brought her home as a newborn. The intrusive presence of the camera in this tiny room reminded her that the private problems caused by chemicals like DES are also public issues.

"Toxic exposure affects the most private parts of our lives. It forces us to give language to things we otherwise might not talk about in public—body parts, intimate relationships, the future we want to take for granted."

On the day Judith leaves for New York, she asks me to take her to "a sacred place." We drive to Funk's Grove. This time I continue past the sugarbush and into the drier upland oak-hickory stand where the trees are cathedral-sized. Within the stand is a clearing that has been turned into an outdoor chapel, with fallen logs as pews and a great stump for a pulpit. We continue past these trees and walk deeper into the forest. Judith is way ahead of me, and I watch her touching the shaggy bark of the hickories and looking at the patterns of light in the branches above.

Her visit has brought a question into sharp focus for me. How can I reconcile my old identity as a biologist with my new one as expectant mother? Mothers always want to know what they can do to protect their babies. I certainly do. Biologists are always calling for more research. I do this, too. However self-serving, the biologists' appeal for further study is a truthful acknowledgement of how little we really know about living systems. This is why a recent monograph on the human placenta begins with the humble admission, "Only one thing is evident: what we know is only a tiny part of what we need to know."

And yet the history of the placenta is also a story about failing to pay attention to the knowledge we already had—by ignoring it outright; by dismissing its relevance; by equating the call for more research with adjournment of action. Even the rubella discovery of Dr. N. McAlister Gregg, who is now lionized as a hero of public health, was initially met with cool requests for more data. In a paper published in 1944, researchers reviewed his evidence for transplacental rubella infection and concluded, "Although the possibility remains he cannot yet be said to have proved his case." Such skepticism prevents scientists from making claims they must later retract. But in this case, as in those of methylmercury and DES, forbearance may in fact have prevented prevention. An effective rubella vaccine came too late for those blinded and deafened by the 1964 epidemic.

Now that I've explored the wreckages of pregnancies past, where do I want to locate myself along the line between knowledge and action? What are my sacred obligations?

I sit down under a hackberry tree, letting the whole length of my back slide down its warty bark. Judith is inspecting a huge white oak. She has an ear pressed against its trunk. In this protected grove, where I once awoke to biology, I am reminded that the open doorway between the outside world and the womb is a wondrous and mysterious threshold. It should not enter our awareness only when poisons flow through it.

4

Egg Moon

APRIL

*I*n early April the silver maples are knobby with buds, and I quit sleeping. The robins wake me first, singing their slurred triplets over and over into the gray air. Then come the cardinals with their loud and liquid phrases, which, as a world-weary teenager, I heard as insightful commentary: *To wit, to wit, to wit: What cheer? What cheer? To wit: What cheer?* Finally, the mourning doves begin their soft question—*I love who? who? who?*—just as light fills the window.

Of these three species, I consider doves the real harbingers of spring. Their flocks arrive sometime in early March. So do the robins, but some of them stay the winter as well; members of their ranks can be seen parading around front lawns on the occasional warm day in January. The corn-crunching cardinals are bona fide all-season residents, although, ecologically speaking, they arrived only recently, having extended their range into Illinois about a hundred years ago—just in time to be appointed the official state bird. Illinois is also the winter home for a few species that, weeks from now, will migrate farther north. The studious little insect eater called the brown creeper is one of these. Creepers are bark-colored and mostly silent, but they can be identified easily by their work habits. They spiral methodically up the trunk of a tree, stopping to chisel spider eggs out of the crevices. When they get to the top branches, they fly down to the base of the next tree and spiral up again. It goes on like this all day—fly down, spiral up, fly down, spiral up. One has been foraging all winter in the scrim of trees that lines the alleyway. Nuthatches also pry insects out of tree bark but bring a whole different approach to the task. They race upside down while laughing weirdly to themselves. They, too, will soon be leaving for points north.

One morning, in the middle of a predawn testimony to the mirthfulness of robins, I hear fluttering right outside the bedroom window. I lift the blind, expecting to see either a creeper or a nuthatch. Instead, a trio of tiny olive-green birds stares back at me. One hops closer, blinks, then bobs his head, the top of which is painted bright pink.

"Well, who are you?"

As if in answer, the bold one bows to show me again his splendid little cap. Then more fluttering and prancing around at the ends of the maple branches. Then all are gone. I know I won't sleep again until I can identify them, so I pull back the blankets and pad out to my study. Somewhere in the stack of boxes on the far wall is my bird book. As I pull boxes down to find it, I'm aware of my belly—harder now and rounder, not just thicker. The window on this side of the house is still dark enough to be a mirror, and in it, backlit by the light behind me, I can see an obviously pregnant body through the thin white cotton of my nightgown.

"Who are you?" I ask for the second time before sunrise.

I make a good guess with the boxes, and find my grubby field guide wedged between two stacks of textbooks. I start flipping through the section on songbirds. It doesn't take long. There is only one olive bird with a pink spot on its head, and it is famous for fluttering around at the ends of twigs: the ruby-crowned kinglet.

The next morning there is a new song in the mix—a thin little violin voice calling *Old Sam Peabody, Peabody. . .* , with a plaintive fade-out at the end, as if further searching would be futile. This is a white-throated sparrow, a bird I know by heart. I peer out the window to see if I can locate it. Instead, I find the maple branches full of kinglets. Dozens of them, all tipping their caps and bouncing on the bud-swollen twigs.

There is the white-throat song again, even closer. And then again. *Old Sam Peabody, Peabody. . .* But I can't find the singer. Among the flashes of pink and green I'm looking for inconspicuous black and brown feathers, a gray breast, a white throat. Nowhere.

"What have you done with Mr. Peabody?" I ask accusingly of the kinglets, but if they know anything, they're not talking.

The next morning I wake at 3 A.M., absolutely convinced I hear a veery singing. I lie in the darkness—yet undisturbed by robins—listening for it again. Nothing. Finally, I pad back to my study to check the bird guide. The veery, like the robin, is a thrush. Its call is officially characterized as "a descending flute-like song," but that description does not come close to capturing its otherworldliness. The first time I heard it, in a Minnesota pine forest, I froze to the spot. The veery's song is a wild, electronic, downward spiral of notes. "The song that will be playing when the alien spaceships land" would be a more apt description. According to the book, it's not possible that I have just heard a veery. Its earliest known arrival date in central Illinois is April 20, two weeks from now. Also, it's a bird of deep woods, not backyards. Also, it doesn't sing in the dead of night. I must have been dreaming.

I climb back into bed but can't sleep. In the fourteenth week of pregnancy, I've entered a new phase. Torpor has given way to a state of high alertness. I'm more watchful, and my sense of hearing seems to have become more acute, too. With my new powers of perception, I try listening for the sound of songbirds migrating. This isn't as far-fetched as it sounds. Serious bird scholars often go out on damp spring nights and listen for the faint *chip-chip-chip* of birds calling to each other as they pass by, a thousand feet overhead. Master birders can identify species just by the pitch and timbre of these distant flight notes. I'm nowhere near that good, but I try to imagine them out there anyway—warblers, flycatchers, thrushes, hummingbirds—following the Mississippi Flyway north. Some of them are crossing the Gulf of Mexico tonight. Some are over Arkansas. Some are directly over my roof. Some are still in the mangrove swamps of the Caribbean and the mountaintops of El Salvador, waiting for a tailwind, judging the cloud cover.

A lot of mystery still surrounds the migration of songbirds. For one thing, they only travel at night. For another, most are too small to wear radio transmitters. Therefore, most of what we know about their spring and fall travels comes from radar, which can only track groups, not individuals. Before radar, researchers estimated the intensity of songbird migration by moon watching. This was a quaint but highly skilled practice that involved counting the number of birds seen flying across the face of the full moon. It required clear skies, a telescope, and elaborate calculations to account for angles of entry, altitude, and percentage of night sky occupied by the moon. Moonwatchers made fantastical claims: 200 bird silhouettes crossing the lunar window in an hour meant that 3 million migrants had passed by during that hour. Which meant that *billions* of birds were on the move during particular nights of the year. There was a lot of skepticism about these extrapolations until they were confirmed by radar operators.

I must have dozed off because I suddenly become aware of robins caroling. And then *Sam Peabody, Old Sam. . .* I creep to the window ledge and let my eyes adjust to the dimness. Empty branches. No sign of the kinglets today, and no white-throated sparrows. Either I'm a truly incompetent birder or the tree itself is singing.

Jeff stirs in the bed.

"Sandra, what are you doing up? Are you worried about something?"

"Hang on a minute."

Silence. More robins.

"Sandra? Honey?"

"Shh. Just listen with me."

Old Sam Peabody. . .

"Did you hear that? I think we're having a son."

On the night of the full moon, I am fifteen weeks pregnant and in Boston, having flown here for an amniocentesis. This was a huge decision—whether to have the test at all, and if so, where. Actually, the where question was easier to answer. My so-called health maintenance organization refuses to pay for nonemergency health care outside Massachusetts. And I am living five states away for an interval of time—five months—long enough to require routine prenatal care but not long enough to win local health insurance coverage. The result is that buying a plane ticket to see an HMO-approved gynecologist in Boston is cheaper than paying Dr. Dan to do an amniocentesis in Bloomington. Since I'm fond of my Boston gynecologist—who is my age and gender and is not predisposed to exam table jokes—this situation is something of a relief. But it does mean that I face the procedure alone. Buying another ticket for Jeff, on top of paying Dr. Dan for monthly checkups, is not in our budget.

The question of whether to do it at all is more complicated.

Amniotic fluid is the oceanlike substance unborn babies float in. It offers fetuses buoyancy, protection from trauma, and oxygen. Like semen, amniotic fluid is made up of two basic elements: living cells and the liquid they're suspended in. In this case, the cells represent sloughed-off fetal skin tissue. Amniocentesis means puncturing a pregnant uterus and aspirating about 30 milliliters—one shot glass full—of amniotic fluid, which is then sent to a genetics lab for examination. The cells it contains are grown in tissue culture to increase their numbers and then inspected for chromosomal defects. This takes about ten days.

In the meantime, the liquid fraction is run through a gauntlet of tests that can reveal the presence of other abnormalities. For example, alpha-fetoprotein is a substance produced by the fetal liver. No one knows what function it serves; the liver stops making it soon after birth. Alpha-fetoprotein is normally present in amniotic fluid at low levels. If, however, the sheet of tissue that rolls up to form the brain and spinal cord does not seal correctly, this protein will pour out of the abnormal opening. Thus, high levels of alpha-fetoprotein in amniotic fluid can indicate the presence of a neural tube defect, such as spina bifida, in which a portion of the spinal cord is herniated—protrudes through the skin.

By examining both the liquid and the cells, amniocentesis can potentially uncover hundreds of different congenital problems. Extracting this fluid from the belly of a pregnant woman is not, however, without its dangers. In the pamphlets handed out to expectant mothers considering the test, the risk is described as "small but real." Specifically, amniocentesis triggers miscarriage in about one in every 200 women. Except that the pamphlets don't usually serve up the statistic that way. What they usually say is that amniocentesis increases the chance of miscarriage by 0.5 percent. This number represents an average, calculated from the statistics on pregnancy outcomes gathered from clinics and hospitals across the country. Presumably, some individual practitioners have higher rates and some lower rates. When I questioned Dr. Dan about his own fetal death rate following amniocentesis, he answered with a story: A pregnant mom came to an amnio appointment and then changed her mind on the table. The next day the mom miscarried. Had she actually gone through with it, she would have blamed the procedure for the loss of her baby, right? The Parable of the Fickle Mom had a legendary feel to it. I was not reassured.

What drives most women to accept the small-but-real risk of amniocentesis is fear of Down syndrome. This fear is long-standing and is carried in the very name of the disorder. John Down was a medical supervisor at the Earlswood Asylum for Idiots in England. In the mid-nineteenth century, he categorized mentally deficient patients according to their resemblance to non-European nationalities—as though the retarded were members of other races. Some, he said, looked Ethiopian, others Mongolian. A century later, in 1958, a French geneticist determined that Down's so-called Mongols have forty-seven chromosomes—one more than the usual. These are the people we now say have Down syndrome, which is the most common chromosomal abnormality that can be detected prenatally.

Because the odds of bearing such a baby rise steadily with maternal age, genetic counselors offer pregnant mothers a simple risk-benefit analysis to guide their decision-making: After age thirty-five, the chance of carrying a child with Down syndrome equals or exceeds the chance of a procedure-induced miscarriage (0.5 percent); therefore amniocentesis is prudent and justifiable. Before age thirty-five, the risks are reversed, and therefore the test is not recommended. All things being equal. On average.

The logic is impressive, cool, irrefutable. But I, who am a good three years beyond the age where the equation is equally balanced, keep falling through trapdoors when I try to follow the path where that logic leads. Beneath its smooth surface lie a number of vexing paradoxes that won't go away. Vexing Paradox Number One: I am searching for something (genetic abnormalities) that I don't want to find. Vexing Paradox Number Two: Wrestling with the decision of whether to have amniocentesis has both drawn me closer to the baby and distanced me from it. That is to say, I now care so deeply about this pregnancy that I want to stop caring deeply until I get the results back. And most obviously, Vexing Paradox Number Three: In the desire for an undamaged baby I am subjecting the baby to danger.

"Parents must weigh the potential value of the knowledge gained . . . against the small risk of damaging what is in all probability a normal fetus." This is how a medical encyclopedia boils down the amniocentesis dilemma. I imagine calmly loading the bricks of knowledge on one side of a scale and then rolling the horrible possibility of killing the baby up onto the other side and then stepping back to see which way the bar tips. It's an arresting image. And as several smart critics of amniocentesis have pointed out, the knowledge gained is not always so clearly a benefit—even for those who believe that aborting a damaged fetus is morally justifiable. For example, amniocentesis can tell you that your child has a rare chromosomal abnormality about which little or nothing is known. Then what? The sociologist Barbara Katz Rothman calls this kind of information "incapacitating knowledge." She also asks whether courage might lie in daring to leave some questions unanswered.

And yet I have decided to go ahead with it. In the end, knowing simply seemed better than not knowing. In this, I feel less akin to Eve in the Garden than to a Boy Scout troop in the woods. Be prepared—it seems as good a guiding principle as any.

Rayna Rapp, a medical anthropologist, studies pregnant mothers like me who consent to amniocentesis, as well as those who refuse it. She has found that women's decision-making is influenced as much by extenuating circumstance and personal conviction as by statistical charts. Some women decline it because they are repelled by the idea of offering their baby up for genetic quality control. Some women accept it because they fear the lifelong care of a disabled child would eventually fall to another beloved child of theirs. Some decline it because they have already struggled with years of infertility and want nothing more to do with reproductive interventions. Some accept it because it seems to offer some measure of control over their future. In many ways, I am typical of those who consent: I am white, college educated, and lacking in strong religious ties or extended kinships.

Two other big facts of my life are relevant here. I am a cancer survivor. And I am an adoptee.

Having been diagnosed with cancer—in my case, bladder cancer at age twenty—means a couple of things in this context. First, like a bride jilted at the altar, I've been badly betrayed—not only by my own runaway cells but by those who issue medical reassurances along the lines of "don't worry, the odds of there being any sort of problem here are negligible." Twenty-year-old women are not supposed to get bladder cancer. I did. Other women might dismiss the possibility that their babies could be afflicted by rare but devastating problems. I don't. Second, like a defendant biding his time while the jury deliberates, I'm used to waiting for medical verdicts. Many women who have undergone amniocentesis report how amazingly stressful are the days spent anticipating the phone call from the genetics lab. I, who have waited for biopsy reports during Christmas holidays, final exam weeks, and summer vacations, will not be amazed.

The adoption piece is more bewildering. It has existed in my life before memory, before language, before thought. Unlike the experience of cancer, it's hard to judge its psychic effects, although now that I am pregnant, I find myself wondering about it more. Thinking about my adoption is like looking at faraway stars. It makes me feel small and vaguely sad. Being adopted and pregnant also presents some large, practical problems. The primary one is that I have no information about my family medical history. In most states of the union, including Illinois, adoption records are still sealed by law. This fact comes as a great surprise to many folks because the enforced secrecy around adoption seems so anachronistic. (Records were originally sealed in the 1930s and '40s to protect adopted people from discrimination based on their illegitimate and, it was thought, shameful conceptions.) But the truth is that I am still barred access to my original birth certificate. The adoption agency that handled my case is more sympathetic than most to the abridged civil rights of adult adoptees, but sympathy cannot answer the questions the genetic counselor had for me—any Down syndrome in my family tree? Cystic fibrosis? Tay-Sachs disease? Thalassemia? Spina bifida? Mental retardation? I feel myself lost, without a genetic compass to navigate by. Meanwhile, the advocates of amniocentesis, who would have us believe in the primacy of DNA, are largely silent about the situation in which most adopted people in the United States find themselves. The only reference to adoption that I can find in all the guidebooks for prenatal screening is a single passing mention: "Most patients who were adopted pose a medical history problem for the field of genetics"—as though the source of all the trouble is adopted people themselves and not the state-sanctioned ignorance we're forced to live with.

I agree to submit my baby's chromosomes for analysis in part because I know nothing about my own. Indeed, the first information I learn about my unborn child will be exactly the kind of information

I lack about myself. Of what value is this knowledge? I've absolutely no idea.

Jeff and I have sublet our apartment while we're away in Illinois, so I spend the night before the test on the couch of Ellen Crowley, a cancer activist and friend who lives in the tiniest possible condominium at the toniest possible address in Boston's Back Bay. It's a warm, clear night, and even at midnight the traffic outside on Beacon Street shows no sign of letting up. My appointment tomorrow is at eight. Ellen has a mammogram scheduled at about the same time—same hospital, different floor. We're both hoping for good news. Before retiring for the night, Ellen offers me a Valium, which I laughingly refuse, so she plies me instead with satin sheets, a goosedown comforter, and an oversized feather pillow.

I fall asleep thinking about songbirds. They have three different compass systems embedded in their heads. One allows them to navigate by the sun, another by the stars, and the third by the earth's magnetic field. Sometimes they get lost anyway. At about 3 A.M. I wake up to the sound of a veery singing . . . but then realize it's just a car alarm in the distance. I decide that none of my reasons for having this test makes sense.

A few hours later, in a small, darkly lit room in the sonography unit at Beth Israel Hospital, I'm met by another friend, Janaki Blum, who is also a biologist, also a new mother, and who underwent amniocentesis herself a year earlier. Taking Jeff's place, Janaki will watch, make mental notes, and hold my hand as the needle goes in. Suddenly the tiny room fills up with women. My gynecologist—now obstetrician—walks in and greets me warmly. The technician and the chief sonographer take their places and begin flipping switches and unwrapping the assembled objects. The mood is buoyant.

They begin quickly. The dome of my belly is bared to the ultrasound probe, which looks like the kind of spoon that you eat Japanese soup with. The probe locates a pocket of fluid safely away from the body of the fetus. The needle slides in about two inches below my naval. A second later, as it passes through the uterus, I feel a sharp cramp, as during menstruation.

"Normal," my obstetrician says, breezily.

Muscles do this when they are stuck with needles.

Everyone else is watching this moment on the screen of the ultrasound monitor. I am not. I am thinking very hard and very deliberately about hummingbirds.

The nests of hummingbirds are constructed of spider webs and dandelion down. They are lined with lichens and moss. They usually contain two eggs.

I glance down briefly. The syringe is half full of fluid already.

The eggs are the size of peas. When baby hummingbirds hatch, they are said to resemble wet bumblebees. "Normal" is a very nice word.

The first syringe is replaced by a second.

Hummingbirds fly over the Gulf of Mexico from the Yucatan in a single night. It's a distance of 500 miles. Some of them probably came across last night—assuming the high-pressure system over New England extends all the way down there.

The second syringe seems to be taking longer to fill up.

In truth, I don't like hummingbirds. Up close, they're too impossibly small, with too much nervous, insect-like whirring. Still, the entire gulf in a single flight is impressive.

The needle is out. We're done. The mood is still upbeat. The obstetrician hands the pair of vials to the technician who holds them up to the light like glasses of fine wine.

"Nice color," she says. "Do you want to hold them?"

And she passes the vials, hot as blood, into my hands. The fluid inside is pale gold. It seems to glow.

"It's like liquid amber!" I sputter. "Like an amber jewel!" It occurs to me that amniotic fluid might be the loveliest substance I have ever seen.

The obstetrician touches my arm. "That's baby pee," she says, smiling. "We like it yellow. It's a sign of good kidney functioning."

I look at the vials again.

Oh. Right.

Amniotic fluid is a mixed drink, with contributions from both baby and mother. Some proportion of amniotic fluid is secreted by the lining of the amniotic sac itself, and some of it is blood serum from the mother, which passes freely through this lining. And some of it is baby pee. We know this because fetuses without kidneys (who can survive only until birth) are surrounded by too little amniotic fluid. But what goes around comes around. Fetal urine itself is distilled from amniotic fluid, which is continuously sipped and swallowed by the baby. Amniotic fluid also soaks right through the skin because the outer waterproofing layer doesn't form until week twenty. The fetus also inhales it during rehearsals for breathing. In these ways, amniotic fluid bathes the inside as well as the outside of the developing body.

Amniotic fluid is a biological mystery. It is bacteriostatic, meaning that bacteria will not grow when cultured in it, so amniotic fluid undoubtedly helps keep the womb a sterile place. But what it does once it seeps inside of the fetus—through the mouth, through the lungs, through the skin—is not at all clear. Some researchers suspect it plays an integral role in establishing the fetal immune system. As it washes through, amniotic fluid exposes the respiratory and gastrointestinal tracts to various immunological factors. This contact may recruit the mucous lining of these sites for future work in immunity.

Whatever its internal activity, amniotic fluid eventually reenters the womb as urine. Here it is absorbed back into the body of the mother and replaced by fresh fluid, in a ceaseless cycle of emptying and refilling. This process speeds up as pregnancy progresses. By the third trimester, amniotic fluid will turn over every three hours. By birth, every hour. But at fifteen weeks, the baby and I require twenty-four hours to replace the volume of fluid just removed.

The obstetrician is finishing up. She reminds me to drink plenty of water today.

Drink plenty of water. Before it is baby pee, amniotic fluid is water. I drink water, and it becomes blood plasma, which suffuses through the amniotic sac and surrounds the baby—who also drinks it.

And what is it before that? Before it is drinking water, amniotic fluid is the creeks and rivers that fill reservoirs. It is the underground water that fills wells. And before it is creeks and rivers and groundwater, amniotic fluid is rain. When I hold in my hands a tube of my own amniotic fluid, I am holding a tube full of raindrops. Amniotic fluid is also the juice of oranges that I had for breakfast, and the milk that I poured over my cereal, and the honey I stirred into my tea. It is inside the green cells of spinach leaves and the damp flesh of apples. It is the yolk of an egg. When I look at amniotic fluid, I am looking at rain falling on orange groves. I am looking at melon fields, potatoes in wet earth, frost on pasture grasses. The blood of cows and chickens is in this tube. The nectar gathered by bees and hummingbirds is in this tube. Whatever is inside hummingbird eggs is also inside my womb. Whatever is in the world's water is here in my hands.

So caught up am I with the ancestry of amniotic fluid that I almost forget to look at the ultrasound monitor, where, in a kind of silent movie, the baby is swimming around, sans needle. The technician is explaining that she has two ongoing purposes here—to see how the fetus has reacted to the procedure and to take some measurements.

A sonogram is a picture made of echoes. More specifically, obstetrical ultrasound bounces high-frequency sound waves against the body of a living fetus and then converts the returned energy into electrical signals, which are visually displayed on a computer monitor. To untrained eyes like mine, ultrasound images look more like the markings on the Shroud of Turin than medical illustration. I see only faint patterns of light and shadow where the technician points out various fetal structures—bladder, aorta, femur, face. Although happily nodding in response, I am more interested in watching the technician's face—is she relieved? concerned? bored? unsure?—than the baby's. I know plenty of women who experience their fetal sonograms as an ecstatic event—they come back marveling about the beating heart, the waving limbs—but I bring a whole different set of associations to the sonography table. I've lain in this semidarkened room before, for the purpose of being scanned for signs of tumor. On those days, the only heart beating was the one pounding against my own rib cage. On those days, I hoped to see nothing. I have to remind myself that the discovery of a growth in my abdomen is *not a bad thing* this time.

Obstetrical ultrasound is a modification of military technology designed to detect submerged enemy warships. Just as radar was turned from aircraft detection to the surveillance of migratory birds, sonar has been adapted to the detection and diagnosis of submerged fetuses. Ultrasound is useful for finding prenatal problems for which chromosomal anomalies are not responsible—like certain kinds of heart defects. In addition, by measuring the size of the head and the length of the long bones, sonographers can calculate the age of a fetus to within seventy-two hours. In cases where an expectant mother has irregular menstrual cycles, an ultrasound image can recalibrate a due date, avoiding future suspicion of premature or overdue labor.

But ultrasound can also mislead. A six-year study in England found that nearly one third of all birth defects escaped ultrasound detection. Perhaps even more worrisome, in 174 of the more than 33,000 pregnancies followed in this study, ultrasound images revealed an anomaly where there was none. That is to say, 174 babies said by ultrasound to be afflicted with some kind of birth defect were born perfectly healthy and normal. This can only mean that 174 mothers spent countless hours seeking advice from experts, praying for guidance, imagining how their lives were going to change, agonizing about what they did to cause the problem—all for no reason. Whereas amniocentesis gives information that is highly accurate but sometimes lacking in biological context or predictive powers, ultrasound gives meaningful, predictive information based on what the fetus actually looks like—but is occasionally wrong.

Janaki senses that I am not really following the show here. She squeezes my hand.

"Look, Sandra, there is the spine. Can you see it?"

Out of the grainy darkness, a strand of pearls floats into view. Around it an entire human form takes shape. I see a back, an ear, a head. And then the vertebrate body abruptly rolls over, like a sea mammal executing a turn in an aquarium tank. And then two arms fly up in synchrony and come back down and fly up again. A small bird migrating across an open ocean. A white silhouette against the black moon of my own body.

And for the third time this week, I peer into a window, asking, "Who are you?"

Two days later, back in Illinois, I hand Jeff the envelope that the sonographer handed to me as I was buttoning up my coat to leave.

"What's this?"

"Still shots from the ultrasound, but"—I lay my hand over his as he begins to open the flap—"don't be disappointed, Jeff. They look like tabloid photos of Bigfoot."

He pulls out the pair of tiny portraits, printed on slick paper. One is the fetal body in profile. The other is a frontal view of the head. They are even more murky and smudgy than the movie version. I somehow feel the need to apologize.

"If you want, I can show you the structures the sonographer pointed out to me."

But I don't have to. Jeff quickly points them all out to me. The curve of the forehead merits his particular attention. That's when I remember that the early anatomists were all artists.

"When do we find out the results of the other tests?" he asks.

"Ten to twelve days."

"And when do we leave for London?"

"Twelve days."

We both think about this for a while.

"I think it's going to be okay," Jeff says, looking again at the collection of echoes that is the face of his child.

And with this prediction, the days of waiting begin. Twelve days from the one in which I saw my own amniotic fluid, I am scheduled to fly across the Atlantic for a two-week book tour of England and Ireland. On this journey, Jeff comes too. I've been assured that the results of the amniocentesis will be back from the lab before we leave.

Meanwhile, the myrtle warblers arrive in Illinois for a few weeks' stay and flash their yellow rumps in the tree branches, calling *check, check, check*, as though testing microphones. Their busy presence inspires confidence. Myrtles are tough little birds, withstanding late snows in the spring and fueling themselves with poison ivy berries in the fall. Sadly, they are often killed in collisions with broadcast towers. In October 1985, more than 300 myrtle warblers were found dead beneath a television tower in Springfield, Illinois, on a single night. I wonder what will happen to the myrtles as the rage for wireless communication raises more and more of these structures across the prairie. I start keeping an eye on the nighttime weather forecasts, hoping for clear skies. Clouds force migrating birds to fly lower where they sometimes steer toward the tower lights that are intended to warn planes off. For some reason, myrtle warblers are particularly susceptible to these kinds of attractions. Perhaps they mistake towers for stars.

Television and cell-phone systems are not the only hazards. Later in the week, I have lunch with Given Harper, a local biologist who has been studying pesticide contamination of Illinois birds. He's particularly interested in analyzing their tissues for the presence of organochlorine pesticides. These are a family of synthetic chemicals made by joining chlorine atoms with carbon molecules—

an arranged marriage that is unusual in the natural world but easy enough to engineer in a laboratory. DDT is probably the most famous representative. All members of the clan kill pests by chemical electrocution, that is, they poison insect nervous systems. But many chlorinated pesticides also have two other properties once they enter the environment at large. Like mercury, they biomagnify. Like DES, they possess the power to redirect hormonally controlled biological processes.

Harper and his colleagues collected dead songbirds during the spring migration of 1996—many of them tower kills—and analyzed their tissues for the presence of these chemicals. Contamination was ubiquitous. The bodies of more than 90 percent of the seventy-two birds he studied contained at least one such pesticide—and often three or more. The most common pesticides detected were dieldrin, heptachlor, and DDT (or, more precisely, the metabolic breakdown products of these chemicals). In keeping with the principle of biomagnification, birds dining higher up on the food chain—the insect-eating warblers and flycatchers—carried higher burdens of pesticide than the vegetarians, such as grosbeaks and indigo buntings—although these species, too, were contaminated.

Chlorinated pesticides are largely banned for use in the United States and Canada, and have been for decades. It is therefore easy to imagine that migrating birds collect these poisons in their tropical winter homes and then carry them, like unwanted souvenirs, back to their summer cottages up north. But this assumption is troubled by some of Harper's other findings. Illinois bats and nonmigrating resident birds, including the northern cardinal, are also contaminated with DDT. To wit: At least some birds and mammals who live among us are being poisoned right here. This discovery means one of three things. Either chlorinated pesticides are being blown in on the wind from elsewhere, or they have persisted these many years in soil and water and sediments, quietly seeding the food chain. Or perhaps they are still being used in central Illinois in spite of laws to the contrary.

Could locally used pesticides be contributing to the mysterious decline of migrating songbirds? Harper is a careful scientist. It remains to be determined, he says, whether contamination at the levels he is finding interferes with the hatching success of songbirds. And the scientific literature offers few clues. Most studies of pesticides and bird reproduction have focused on species higher up on the food chain—the predatory hawks, falcons, eagles, and cormorants. Most studies of songbird reproduction focus on habitat loss.

On the way out of the cafeteria, Harper identifies some bird calls coming from the shrubbery. This is my chance to brush up.

"By the way, what's the warbler that says *witchity-witchity*? It hangs out by the—"

"Yellowthroat."

"Oh, right. I used to know that. . . You know, there's a white-throated sparrow singing *Sam Peabody* right outside my bedroom window every morning, but I can't ever see it."

"Oh, they're everywhere right now."

After we part company, I keep walking, turning south toward Franklin Park, where the trees are just beginning to flush out and the two old magnolias are already leaning low under the weight of their own blossoming. The day is mild and sunny, and I am itchy in my clothes. I have taken to cross-dressing ever since my discovery that nothing conceals a round belly better than a man's suitcoat made of wool. It works so well that I have begun to suspect this is why they were invented in the first place. I have already gained twenty pounds but am convinced, thanks to Jeff's old herringbone and camel hair blazers, that no one is the wiser. I'm still in my own pants, unzipped and held together at the top by a rubber band laced through the button hole. This can't go on much longer, if only because the weather's getting too warm.

In the park I position myself on a bench near the picnic tables. Determined to find Sam Peabody, I scan the green-tinged branches, looking for a bit of moving bark, listening hard. A long number of minutes passes before I realize that the people picnicking at a nearby table are waving at me and calling hello. Assuming they are students of mine, I look over sheepishly, embarrassed that I've been spotted staring deeply into foliage.

"Hello! Hello!" say the picnickers, beaming and smiling.

They are not my students. Accompanied by two teachers, they are a group of children with Down syndrome. In slow motion, I lift my hand and wave back.

On Friday, one week after amniocentesis, the tattoo beneath my belly button—a pinprick ringed by a small purple bruise—has completely vanished. I decide to call the obstetrician's office in Boston. Just to check in. Just to see.

No, says the receptionist, the results are not back yet. We'll call you just as soon as we hear anything.

I like her voice. Serious, happy to help, call anytime.

I spend the weekend walking the Constitution Trail, a paved north–south path, previously a railroad track, that slices through miles of backyards, loading docks, athletic fields, city parks, and even a patch of prairie grass. Local residents are proud of it, planting flowers along the route. The daffodils are in full bloom, competing with forsythia bushes for brilliance of yellow. The cardinals singing in their branches have never been redder. Nor have the tulips. The puffed-up robins patrolling the newly green grass refuse to be silenced by the gravelly roar of the Rollerbladers. Out of my jacket, I am attracting knowing smiles from mothers pushing strollers. Spring is an out-of-control carnival. I am out-of-control pregnant.

The cells of my baby are growing not only in my body but somewhere in a laboratory in Boston, where they are bathed in a broth made from fetal calves.

Only about 10 percent of the cells captured during amniocentesis are alive, but these can be coaxed to grow and divide if carefully nurtured in an incubator at human body temperature. At some point, usually five to nine days later, these living cells can be harvested for genetic analysis. This involves more than just taking a look through a microscope. Chromosomes normally exist inside cells as slender, loopy threads of DNA that are impossible to study. Only when a cell is preparing to divide (remember mitosis?) are its chromosomes transformed into the stout, rod-shaped bodies that grace the pages of science magazines and biology textbooks. Only in this compressed, contracted state can they be examined. Thus, the fetal cells collected for genetic screening have to be arrested in their growth cycle just at the point where they are about to split in two. Not before. Not after. The chromosomes must also be stained to bring out their individual banding patterns. A geneticist friend of mine claims that a properly stained human chromosome that has been captured in the moments preceding cell division should look like a headless man in a striped prison suit.

A human being is supposed to have forty-six chromosomes. Half of these are inherited from the mother and half from the father.

That is, an egg cell has twenty-three chromosomes, and so does a sperm; when the two become one, the resulting embryo gets the full set of forty-six. Their coming together during fertilization creates chromosomal pairs. The chromosome from the sperm that bears, say, the gene coding for eye color now cohabitates with the corresponding chromosome from the egg, which also carries a gene for eye color—although one might carry instructions for brown eyes, the other, for blue. In other words, each chromosome has a doppelgänger. A twin. A counterpart. Or, to use the language of biology, a homologous copy.

Matching them up is the first task of prenatal genetic screening. This happens in several steps. First, one of the embryo's cells is chosen for analysis. Then its chromosomes are photographed as they lie stained and scattered across the floor of a glass slide like so many shoes. Then the photograph is cut apart. Pairs are identified and brought together. They are then arranged in a grid of orderly rows. (These tasks are now all accomplished by moving images around on a computer screen.) By tradition, chromosomal pairs are displayed in descending order of size. Thus, chromosome pair number one, placed at the top of the first row, is the longest and pair number twenty-two, at bottom right, the shortest. The sex chromosomes are customarily placed at the very end and are thus labeled pair number twenty-three, with XX being the nomenclature reserved for daughters and XY for sons. Finally, the pieces are all pasted back together again to form a new picture, which is called a karyotype. The final result looks a bit like a family portrait in which sets of twins are lined up from biggest to smallest.

At the end of the day, one hopes for a karyotype that shows exactly twenty-three matched pairs. Anything else usually has serious consequences for development. An extra chromosome, for example, is called a trisomy. The classic example is three copies of petite chromosome twenty-one, which results in Down syndrome. But there are others, too. Edwards' syndrome is trisomy eighteen, meaning that the fetus possesses three chromosomes eighteen instead of the usual two. It is often lethal. Trisomies can also affect chromosomes pairs eight, nine, and thirteen as well as the sex chromosomes. All are caused by an error in cell division called nondisjunction, that is, a chromosome's failing to pull apart when it was supposed to during the formation of eggs and sperm. This means that one or the other parent has contributed twenty-four chromosomes to the embryo, rather than the required twenty-three. The developing baby consequently ends up with a total of forty-seven individual chromosomes. Most nondisjunctions originate in the egg, but a small fraction of Down syndrome cases can actually be traced to the sperm. We know that the risk of Down syndrome rises dramatically with the age of the mother. It's not clear whether this is also true for fathers.

Geneticists also use karyotypes to look at other problems. On rare occasions, during the formation of eggs and sperm, a piece of one chromosome breaks off and becomes reattached to the end of another. This is called a translocation. Sometimes a small part of a chromosome is simply missing, an anomaly called a deletion. These can be ferreted out by looking at the patterns of horizontal stripes—the so-called bands—along the arms and legs of specific chromosomes. A standard karyotype has 400 visible bands, each of which contains many hundred genes. Even with recombinant DNA techniques, fluorescent dyes, and computers assisting the work, karyotyping remains a laborious art, dependent on human perception and judgment.

I wonder where in this process my fetal cells are. Still quietly incubating? Or have they already been harvested, stained, and photographed, their chromosomes spread across a computer screen, magnified a thousand times? Perhaps at this very moment, while the Illinois sun slants through ironwood trees and while pigeons clatter under the slats of old train trestles, someone in Boston is sitting down with a fresh cup of coffee to start the sorting and counting. Maybe there is a radio playing in the lab. Maybe the geneticist has noticed something slightly odd and is calling a coworker over to take a look. Maybe the two of them decide it's nothing after all. Maybe the report is already typed up. Maybe everything is just fine.

What's starting to bother me about amniocentesis is not the anxiety it creates (which is considerable) nor the coldheartedness of it (also considerable), but its narrowness of focus. The whole enterprise implies that the future life of a child can be read by counting its chromosomes and scrutinizing their architecture. But the children of Minamata had perfectly normal chromosomes. So presumably did the thousands blinded by rubella and the legless ones exposed to thalidomide. Indeed, the majority of birth defects are not

attributable to inborn genetic errors. And yet we put legions of geneticists to work looking for them, and we ritualize amniocentesis
as a rite of passage for pregnant women, as though chunks of DNA
were the prime movers of life itself. As though pregnancy took
place in a sealed chamber, apart from water cycles and food chains.

What if amniocentesis inquired about environmental problems
as well as a genetic ones? Only one study of environmental contaminants in amniotic fluid has ever been done, and it found detectable
levels of organochlorine pesticides in one third of the thirty samples
of amniotic fluid tested. Of particular concern, say the researchers,
is the discovery of DDT, which was found in concentrations
roughly equivalent to that of the fetus's own sex hormones. Because
DDT is known to interfere with the biochemical pathways that sex
hormones operate along, the question arises as to whether this kind
of contamination can alter the unfolding development of the fetal
reproductive tract. The researchers also found trace levels of PCBs
in some of the samples. These chemicals not only have been linked
to birth defects but also are thought to suppress the immune system. As we have seen, amniotic fluid itself is believed to play a role
in establishing fetal immunity. Are inhaled and swallowed gulps of
PCB-laced amniotic fluid sabotaging this process even as they initiate it? No one knows, but the answer could be relevant to all unborn babies, not just the very few who have inherited the wrong
number of chromosomes.

The chemicals being discovered in human amniotic fluid are,
of course, some of the same ones that my colleague Given Harper
is finding in the tissues of migrating and resident birds. I think back
to my own amniocentesis epiphany. *Whatever is in hummingbird
eggs is also inside my womb. Whatever is inside the world's water is also
here in my hands.*

Monday, day ten. It's very possible the results will arrive today. But
when I get home from my afternoon class, there is no message on
the answering machine. So I call again.

No, I'm sorry, says Cindy, the nice receptionist, with genuine
empathy. They didn't come back today. Don't worry though.

Tuesday, day eleven. I call again.

Oh, hi, Sandra. No, we still haven't heard anything. I know
you're leaving tomorrow. Call us before you head out for the airport.

Wednesday morning, day twelve: No, we don't have the results yet. I don't know why. I'll call down to the lab right now. What time is your flight?

Wednesday afternoon, day twelve, at O'Hare Airport: I'm really sorry. The lab hasn't returned my phone call. I don't know what the problem is. As soon as I hear anything I'll leave a message on your answering machine.

Thursday, day thirteen, from a hotel room in London: No message.

Friday, day fourteen, from a phone booth near Hyde Park: No message.

Friday night, day fourteen, from a phone booth next to a cemetery in Kent: Sandra, this is Cindy. Okay, we've got the results. Everything is fine. The chromosomes are normal. . . . And you're having a little girl.

A blackbird is singing in the medieval churchyard where Jeff and I are dancing.

5

Mother's Moon

MAY

I return to Illinois a few days ahead of the nighthawks. When I finally emerge from jet-lagged stupor, they are already calling *Pete! Pete!* from the evening sky. Night after night, storm fronts move across the prairie, raising a mountain range of thunderheads on the horizon. And in front of them are the nighthawks, glimpsable by lightning strike, swooping around in the downpours as unsheltered and oblivious as Lear. Their eggs are equally naked—laid on bare rooftops without even the protection of nests. Curiously misnamed, nighthawks are cousins to whippoorwills and, like them, have wide, whiskery mouths used for scooping moths out of the night sky. Their May arrival is timed to coincide with the metamorphosis of caterpillars into airborne adults. Nighthawks therefore migrate several weeks after the warblers, who dine on the moths' larval predecessors. With predator and prey now both on the wing, it is the season of flight.

Meanwhile, I undergo a metamorphosis of my own, attributable in no small part to a change in wardrobe. While in Boston last month, I was supplied with sackfuls of maternity outfits by Karol Bennett, a professional soprano who is my most intrepid and glamorous friend. Karol sang concerts in Mongolia during her first trimester, gave recitals in Europe in her second, and performed the lead in *Die Fledermaus* in her third. Predictably, her pregnancy clothes are a departure from modesty and pleated overalls. In the sacks are purple silk and black velvet, dresses of crinkled gauze, a royal blue jacket with jeweled buttons, flowing caftans that slide off their hangers. All accentuate curves instead of hiding them. More moth, less larva. On the first day of the university's intensive four-week May semester, I wear one of Karol's bright, slippery tunics to class, causing the department secretary to cease typing and gape at my stomach, asking "How'd we miss that?" as I walk by.

"I'm pregnant," I announce as other faculty join in staring at the middle of my body. It's one of my more redundant statements, but if anyone inferred it before today, no one lets on.

Emboldened either by the nighthawks or by the drama of my new clothes, I begin to take long walks after dark, sometimes at the height of a storm. Tree branches full of thunder. Earthworms writhing on sidewalks. Storm sewers clogged with flower petals and rushing water. It feels good to let go of the fretfulness of the previous month—which, I now realize, kept me more guarded and secretive than I could admit at the time. Prenatal testing is a ring of fire one passes through in midpregnancy. Now that I am on the far side of it, I am grateful for the few things amniocentesis can say with certainty, although I also see more clearly why one might choose to go around rather than through it.

The most troubling aspects of prenatal testing still seem to me the single-minded search for rare genetic defects and the concomitant disregard of environmental threats to pregnancy. For expectant mothers over thirty-five, the hunt for chromosomal trisomies has become a routine part of prenatal care. But ask if your amniotic fluid contains pesticides, and if, so, how this contamination may affect the development of your baby, and you are likely to be met with blank stares. Genes and environment are two partners in a dance of creation. Now that I have been told the results of my chromosomal analysis are "unremarkable" (a lovelier adjective was never spoken), I decide it is time to investigate the other dancer.

On one of my nightly walks, I notice tiny white flags sprouting on neighborhoods lawns and the university grounds. I bend down to read the message they carry: TREATED WITH PESTICIDES. KEEP OFF. The rain that falls on the grass beneath the flags runs onto the sidewalks and soaks my shoes.

I decide to start with birth defects.

Although it seems heretical to say so, our understanding of birth defects has changed little since ancient times. According to a recent report from Johns Hopkins University, only 20 percent of birth defects have identifiable causes; the vast majority are of unknown origin. Our situation is not so different, then, from that of the Babylonians of 3000 B.C., who also didn't know what caused birth defects but thought the children born with them were messengers. Indeed, the word "monster" means to show or warn. The birth of so-called monsters was not always bad. Some were even deified. For example, the Chaldeans thought male infants born without penises foretold that "the master of the house will be enriched by the harvest of his fields." Typically, however, the birth of infants with misshapen parts has inspired awe and dread, if not outright terror. Historians of embryology point out that many mythological monsters—including mermaids and Cyclopes—are based on careful observations of particular kinds of congenital malformations. Prenatal testing, then, is only the most recent method of divining the future by interpreting signs of human deformity.

With the advent of modern genetics, embryologists turned to theories of inheritance to provide explanations for congenital defects. For the most part these explanations did not hold up under further observation and testing. Nevertheless, the presumption that heredity can account for many birth defects continues to this day, even though there is little evidence to support it. As noted by a recent review of the subject, "The role of genetics is often . . . overstated when the [cause] is actually unknown." In fact, most of what is known about developmental abnormalities points to a much larger role for the environment. For example, even moderate amounts of alcohol can cause mental retardation and a subtle alteration of facial features known as fetal alcohol syndrome. The mother's exposure to cigarette smoke, even passive exposure to secondhand smoke, can lower birth weight. So can lead. "The lesson," concludes the recent Johns Hopkins monograph on human birth defects, "is that the fetus is sensitive to the environment surrounding the mother."

This is not to imply that genes contribute nothing to the process. But what initially looks like inheritance can have environment wrapped around it. For example, if toxic exposures damage the DNA of eggs and sperm, these genetic mutations can potentially become inherited. Environmental insults may also interact with genetic factors that predispose the embryo to birth defects but are not by themselves capable of initiating them. Unfortunately, the nature of the defect doesn't always indicate whether its origin is environmental or genetic. Consider a baby with multiple abnormalities. These might be caused by environmentally damaged tissue that subsequently gives rise to several different organs. Or they could be caused by the inherited mutation of a single gene that regulates the production of a protein needed for the development of these organs. Or some combination of both. The embryological tango between environment and heredity is an intimate one.

One way to gauge the environment's impact on the origin of birth defects is to examine the data from birth defect registries. These consist of coded reports on all birth defects diagnosed in a given population or at a certain hospital over a fixed period of time. Changes in the rate of birth defects can provide clues about their possible causes. For example, a rise in prevalence over time may indicate rising levels of a birth defect–inducing substance in the environment. As important as time trends are geographic patterns: an elevated rate of birth defects in one area may indicate a local exposure to a birth defect–inducing substance. Such substances are called teratogens, a word that carries with it all the anxiety of the ages—from the Greek *teras*: monster. Documenting the rise or fall of birth defects over time or across space is not proof of teratogenic exposure, but it certainly gives us reason to inquire further. According to Richard Clapp, an epidemiologist at Boston University who works daily with this kind of evidence, patterns in registry data "are like red flags saying, 'Dig here.' "

Before I start digging around in the registry data myself, I spend some time looking through pictorial atlases of birth defects. I can't recommend this as an activity for pregnant women. But for me, turning their pages is a kind of meditative preparation for the work ahead.

I begin with the most venerable and definitive treatise of the lot: *Smith's Recognizable Patterns of Human Malformation*, fifth edition. The photo of the author, David Smith, now deceased, is the only picture of a normally formed human in the 857-page collection of black-and-white portraits. Chapter titles include "Facial Defects as Major Feature," "Storage Disorders," and "Senile-Like Appearance." In spite of them, I feel oddly reassured by the visual images categorized here. They are of living people, one or two of whom seem vaguely familiar, like someone I might have seen once on a bus or in a bowling alley. My first reaction is to scan for signs of motherly love—a ribbon in the hair that covers a misproportioned head. I'm most attracted to the pictorial sequences that show the same individual over time. Sometimes, even when the baby picture seems hopeless, the malformation becomes less severe with the passage of years. Sometimes, the final adult picture shows a person who basically looks okay.

Far more disturbing is *Diagnostic Ultrasound of Fetal Abnormalities: Text and Atlas*. Here are babies who look turned inside out; babies who appear trapped inside blocks of ice; babies who resemble gargoyles, or aliens, or Salvador Dali's clocks. The photographs in this book include stillborn fetuses as well as those born alive; often it's hard to distinguish the dead from the living. I look for wristbands and monitors. Some of the babies appear posed as in crucifixion. Some look ashamed. Some defiant. Some appear expressionless because they lack the body parts we associate with human expressions, like mouths.

Finally, there is Bruce Carlson's *Human Embryology and Developmental Biology*. Here I begin to notice how normally formed structures seem miraculous in the context of deformity. As with a photograph of a house that has been hit by a tornado, what fascinates is not so much the lack of a roof but the unbroken vase on the coffee table. So, in the picture labeled "Massive Oopharnygeal Teratoma," I am less struck by the baby's face, which looks like a raft of red balloons, than by the two perfect ears that frame the missing face like tiny seashells.

A sign of life and well-being, fetal movement is usually first detected by pregnant mothers between weeks sixteen and twenty—at about the midpoint of gestation. First-time mothers often experience this event later than those having subsequent pregnancies, probably because they don't know what it's supposed to feel like. Of course, the fetus has been busy for weeks already—spinning, kicking, jabbing, waving, nodding—but, prior to the fourth or fifth month of pregnancy, its movements are not strong enough to trip the mother's nerve endings.

At nineteen weeks, I still can't say I've felt the baby move yet.

At my urging, various other mothers have described the sensation to me, relying on a wide range of romantic metaphors. Like champagne bubbles, says one. Like a butterfly, says another. Like a finger gently tickling you from the inside, says a third. You'll just know when it happens, sighs a fourth, with tears in her eyes.

On Mother's Day, I join my mother, cousins, aunts, and uncles for a potluck in honor of my ninety-three-year-old grandmother, the matriarch of the family. I am nearly the last of her twenty-one grandchildren to reproduce—and certainly the oldest. No one in the family had been breathing down my neck about the long fact of my childlessness, least of all my grandmother, who gave birth to six children in seven years, all before turning thirty. In her view, a problem with reproduction means too many babies, too early, too fast. About pregnancy, she is the least sentimental mother I've ever known.

In a quiet moment, I join her on the couch, where she presents me with a blanket that she crocheted for my unborn daughter . . . in 1977.

"Well, you waited a long time for this one, Grandma," I laugh. "This baby should be in college by now."

"There's nothing wrong with waiting," she replies, patting my hand.

Then I ask her what it feels like when a baby kicks.

"You haven't felt it yet?"

"No."

She is silent for a long time, and I wonder whether she is thinking about something else. Suddenly she jabs me sharply in the ribs with her elbow.

"Something like that," she says.

The information available from U.S. birth defect registries turns out to be astonishingly incomplete. Indeed, the data are so deficient to be almost meaningless for some disorders. This is an amazing discovery. Birth defects are the number one killer of infants in the United States, and, by any count, the prevalence of birth defects remains high despite other improvements in the health of infants and pregnant women, despite increased access to prenatal screening, and despite high rates of abortion when the news from these tests is bad. The crude estimates are these: serious birth defects are diagnosed in 3 to 4 percent of American infants; 120,000 babies are born with major deformities each year; 21 babies die as a result of these defects each day.

The main problem is that there is no national system to track birth defects and report on trends. This was not always the case. In the wake of the thalidomide disaster, several initiatives were put in motion out of a belief that other unidentified teratogens could be threatening babies in utero and that obstetricians needed some recourse besides describing their observations in letters to the editor. Helping to launch the first national registry in 1973 was none less than the medical luminary Dr. Virginia Apgar, famous for developing the scoring method of newborn health so familiar to parents. Operated out of the Centers for Disease Control, the Birth Defects Monitoring Program was intended to serve as the flagship registry in the United States. A few years later, another federally administered registry, the Metropolitan Atlanta Congenital Defects Program, began collecting data as well.

Both registries have failed to match the aspirations of their original advocates. Never comprehensive, the Birth Defects Monitoring Program foundered and was finally dismantled in 1994. At its peak, it tracked only about 35 percent of total U.S. births, and these were not a random sample. Moreover, it did not aggressively pursue information beyond what is found on birth certificates or newborn discharge records. This is a serious shortcoming because some malformations are not evident at birth. Many heart defects, for example, only manifest themselves when babies become physically active. Even when defects are apparent in the delivery room, they are not always recorded on vital statistics records. A 1996 study estimates that only 14 percent of birth defects are accurately reported on birth certificates. The Atlanta registry does actively pursue birth defect diagnoses in children up to twelve months old, but the population it tracks is small in number and not generalizable to the entire United States.

In the absence of a functioning national registry, some state health departments have leapt into the void and set up their own registries. These were evaluated by the Johns Hopkins study and found sorely wanting. Seventeen states have no registries at all, and the ones that do mostly rely on passive reporting by doctors and hospitals, a method of data collection known to lead to under-counts. Only a handful of states actively track birth defects, with registrars visiting hospitals, reviewing records, and following patients after their discharge.

One of these states is California. The California Birth Defects Monitoring Program, founded in 1982, is considered the gold standard of these various registries. Its stated mission is to find the causes of birth defects. One of every seven U.S. births occurs in California, so even though the registry does not cover the entire state, the information it collects constitutes a significant body of data. Its staff pay regular visits to the hospitals within its reporting area and painstakingly pore through medical records. This practice greatly improves the probability of an accurate case count. Of course, the registry's ability to assess the role that environmental contaminants might be playing in the origin of birth defects is limited by the information contained in these records, and hospital personnel seldom ask questions of new parents about their exposures to occupational, household, and environmental chemicals. Thus, the data generated by the registrars are really only clues for further investigation, which might involve intensive interviewing of mothers or collection of blood or urine for chemical analysis.

The follow-up research so far inspired by the California Birth Defects Monitoring Program is impressive—in spite of the fact that the federal funding available for birth defect research is not. For example, interviews with over 2,000 mothers revealed that more than 75 percent of pregnant women have at least one source of exposure to pesticides while pregnant. Elevated risks of particular kinds of birth defects were found among women using pesticides for gardening and for those living within a quarter mile of agricultural crops.

Texas operates another high-quality state registry. Like the now-defunct national program, the Texas registry was started in the aftermath of a birth defect mystery. Between 1989 and 1991, an unusual number of babies in the Brownsville area were born with a condition called anencephaly, which means that some or all of their brains were missing. This kind of defect is usually very rare, yet in 1991 alone, six such babies were born within six weeks of each other—and three of these within thirty-six hours—in a part of southern Texas where pollution regularly wafts over from unregulated industries on the Mexican side of the Rio Grande River. This cluster was first recognized by an obstetrical nurse, but her persistent questions about its possible cause could never be answered, in part because the registry data of the time were lacking or unreliable.

Like spina bifida, anencephaly is a neural tube defect, which means it strikes very early in development. During the first few weeks of pregnancy, as described earlier, a flat length of tissue along the back of the embryo rolls up like a piece of carpet. From the tube so created, the brain and spinal cord will develop. If the middle of the tube fails to curl up all the way, the nerves of the spinal cord are left naked, often becoming knotted, and spina bifida results. If the top end of the tube remains open, the skull and brain cannot form, and anencephaly is the result.

There are reasons to suspect that environmental factors may contribute to this birth defect. About 95 percent of neural tube defects occur in families with no history of the disease. A diet deficient in folate is associated with neural tube defects, and many cases are thought to be preventable by dietary supplements of this B vitamin (provided in the form of folic acid). We also know that the disruption of a particular gene that controls the closure of the neural tube can result in anencephaly. And we know the chances of anencephaly are greater among children of men whose occupations involve handling particular kinds of toxic chemicals. Painters and pesticide applicators are two such occupations. Just how dietary vitamins, genes, and toxic exposures interact to create or mitigate neural tube defects, however, is not clear.

Although both the Texas and California registries now do an admirable job of monitoring neural tube defects, larger geographic comparisons are still difficult to make because registry data are still lacking in so many other states. This same problem compromises the surveillance of most other birth defects. The Johns Hopkins researchers struggled mightily to make sense of the data in the states whose registries at least operate similarly. But they ultimately gave up. Even though some evidence suggested that the rates of certain birth defects are rising, the data were too haphazardly collected to say for sure. For example, the incidence of one kind of cardiac malformation—atrial septal defect, otherwise known as a hole in the heart—more than doubled within the eight-year period 1989–96. But investigators could not eliminate the possibility that this apparent increase simply reflects shifting diagnostic criteria, so poorly organized are the reporting systems.

Late spring in the woods is a time naturalists call the Green Lull. In central Illinois it settles in around the third week of May. Flush with leaves, the forest canopy rustles shut. Little sunlight now reaches the woodland floor, and wildflowers blooming there—spring beauties, trout lilies, bloodroot—wither back into the earth. The flowering trees in the understory—cherry, redbud, dogwood—go to leaf as well. Migrating birds depart for points north. Hidden behind all the new foliage, resident birds are busy nesting. Focused on finding food instead of mates, they sing less.

I choose a new woods to hike in, the bluff- and gorge-filled Merwin Preserve, which is a fifteen-minute drive northeast through some serious corn and soybean fields. I came out here a lot when I was a new cancer patient, mostly to stand on the creaky suspension bridge that sways above the Mackinaw River. It was a perverse ritual. I'm more than slightly unnerved by heights, and the unsteadiness of wooden planks rippling under my feet only added to the anxiety. But in those days, I had bigger things to be afraid of, and scaring myself in the middle of a bobbing bridge was a bit like fighting fire with fire.

On a picture-perfect Sunday afternoon, I bring Jeff out here with me for lunch on the bluffs. Along the floodplains all is lush and uniformly green. Only a few weeks earlier, looking into this little valley was like gazing down at a sunrise. Lavender clouds of bluebells floated under the leafless trees, and just above them hovered yellow clouds of pollinating bees. It was the kind of beauty so intense it was almost painful to look at. Now, deep into the Lull, a calmer aesthetic reigns.

Jeff naps in the grass—no ticks or mosquitoes yet—and I lean against a log and watch light play in the unfurled oak leaves. Even with my eyes closed, I can see the dance of sun and leaf. Which gives me an idea. I pull down my stretch-panel jeans, roll my shirt up my rib cage, and lie back, belly to the sky. In the sunlight, the skin over my abdomen feels taut and tingly. I am a great closed eyelid.

And that's when I feel it for the first time. Like the fluttering of a bird in a cupped hand, only deep inside and down low. Fetal movement. What midwives once called "the quickening."

If there is any one bold, consistent, and statistically trustworthy trend visible in the registry data it is the apparent increase in the rates of hypospadias. Like neural tube defects, hypospadias happens when a strip of flat tissue fails to roll up to form a closed tube. In this case, the tube is the male urethra, which runs down the middle of the penis and so connects the bladder to the outside world. If the urethral tube does not fuse completely, the external opening will emerge somewhere along the shaft of the penis instead of at the tip—or, in severe cases, from the scrotum. (Happily, many such anomalies are repairable with surgery.) Both the Metropolitan Atlanta data as well as that from the Birth Defects Monitoring Program show a doubling of prevalence between 1968 and 1992. In addition, the prevalence of moderate to severe cases has increased, a pattern also mirrored in Europe and Japan. It is unlikely that these trends are the result of better reporting or diagnosis. (The mild form is probably underreported, so these statistics are less reliable.)

The causes of hypospadias, and the reasons for its apparent rise, have not been identified. The leading hypothesis is that environmental contaminants transferred across the placenta may be blocking the biochemical cues that initiate tube formation. (Recall that DES sons are at increased risk for hypospadias.) What is known with certainty is that the formation of the male urethra, which takes place between weeks eleven and fourteen, depends on the secretion of testosterone from the fetus's own developing testicles. Some synthetic compounds widely distributed in the environment possess the ability to interfere with this hormone, as we shall see later on.

Birth defects with more serious health consequences than hypospadias are grossly underrepresented by registry data. This is because many U.S. surveillance systems—even the good ones—only count birth defects among live-born infants. Miscarried and stillborn fetuses are not counted even when they are grossly malformed. The impact of elective abortion is also not considered, even though many parents choose to end pregnancies when a prenatal test reveals a serious birth defect. Most likely to result in a termination of a pregnancy is the discovery of a problem that is sure to result in the baby's death soon after birth. Consider once again that most wretched of birth defects called anencephaly (missing brain and skull). According to U.S. registry data, anencephaly has steadily

declined in prevalence since the 1960s. During this same time, prenatal screening for this defect increased widely (it is easily visible on
ultrasound), as did access to safe, legal abortion. A 1998 study
among women living in Hawaii found that abortion rates following
a prenatal diagnosis of anencephaly exceeded 80 percent. Are fewer
fetuses now afflicted with anencephaly? Or are more and more of
them quietly aborted, never to appear on the list of the malformed?
Under the current system, it is impossible to know.

The same problem haunts the data on spina bifida, whose rates
appear to vary wildly among states. In 1992, the Centers for Disease Control had to admit these geographic patterns were impossible to analyze because the relative impact of prenatal diagnosis was
unknown. (Spina bifida is sometimes lethal, although in some cases
it produces only the mildest forms of disability; severe cases can
lead to paralysis and hydrocephaly—water on the brain. In Hawaii,
the termination rate following a prenatal diagnosis approaches 50
percent.) Not all registries neglect the reality of miscarriages, stillbirths, and abortion, however, and those that consider these factors
make clear how significant their impact is. The Texas, Atlanta, and
Hawaii registries make use of prenatal diagnostic information, as
does the California Birth Defect Monitoring Program. In Hawaii,
including these data increased the calculated rate of certain kinds
of birth defects by more than 50 percent. In California, rates of
anencephaly more than doubled when prenatally diagnosed cases
were included. Similar findings come from France.

With data from U.S. birth defect registries so incomplete, I decide
to ask my question the other way around. What is known about
teratogenic chemicals in the environment? Where are they located,
and who is exposed? The answers are "pathetically little" and "nobody knows." I have reached another impasse.

Most chemicals have not been tested for their ability to have
teratogenic effects. There are now about 85,000 different synthetic
chemicals produced in the United States. About 3,000 of these are
manufactured in quantities of at least one million pounds a year
and are therefore classified as high-production-volume chemicals.
More than three quarters of this group have undergone no screening for possible developmental effects on fetuses and children. And
of the more than 700 high-production-volume chemicals found in

consumer products, for nearly half basic information on developmental toxicity is lacking.

The class of chemicals we know the most about are agricultural pesticides. Because they can linger as residues on food, they are required to undergo more scrupulous evaluation, including tests for fetal toxicity. Those that came on the market before such testing was required, however, were exempt from this kind of analysis and most are still awaiting reevaluation. In the meantime they are allowed to be sold and used freely. These old graybeards include some of the most popular chemicals used in agriculture. The authors of the Johns Hopkins report come to an obvious but heart-stopping conclusion: "[S]ome pesticides currently being used may be developmental toxicants."

A few hundred toxic chemicals manufactured each year in the United States are governed by right-to-know laws, which means that public records are kept on their release into the environment. As currently written, the laws require certain manufacturers and users of such chemicals to report any and all environmental releases—either accidental or routine—to air, water, or soil. The Toxics Release Inventory is the main registry of such events, and it is available to the public through the Environmental Protection Agency. It is hardly comprehensive. Toxic emissions reported to the federal government are thought to account for only about 5 percent of all chemical releases. Nevertheless, the Toxics Release Inventory is the most complete record we have. I take a look at the 1997 data. The list of U.S. toxic releases for that year includes forty-seven different chemicals classified as known or suspected fetal toxicants. The volume released totals 989,700,000 pounds. Chemical manufacturing is the single largest source of these emissions, with paper, metal, rubber, and electric power–generating industries closely following.

I then take a look at the data for Illinois alone, which ranks fourth in the nation for toxic releases. Total of fetal toxicants released in 1997: 39,500,000 pounds. Except in the states of California and New York, right-to-know laws do not govern toxicants used in agriculture. This figure, therefore, does not include pesticides.

At home I try to recreate the conditions out in the forest that convinced the baby to make her presence known to me. I lie down on the bed and loosen my clothes, let my mind wander, visualize flowing water. No stirrings. Well, maybe an occasional . . . blip, but nothing like the beating wings of a bird in flight.

To bring on fetal movement, you should, the pregnancy guidebooks advise, drink a glass of ice water or eat something sugary before lying down. But I don't really want to shock the baby into motion with a cold blast or a surge of glucose. I ask Jeff to join me in the bedroom.

"What are we doing?"

"Well, I thought you could help me get the baby to move again."

"How?"

"I don't know. Maybe sing to her or lay your hand over her."

Jeff looks at me skeptically. I remind him that he once healed my back with a kiss. (This is true. When I met Jeff, I was suffering from a back injury and had just finished five months of physical therapy. The first time he kissed me, it stopped hurting and it has never hurt since.)

"Honey," he says slowly, trying to be nice, trying to be sensitive. "I don't think I have the power to make the baby move. Besides, I'm really busy trying to write the press release for the show, okay?"

Yeah. Sure. Okay.

We are not completely in the dark about the environmental causes of birth defects. Circumventing the mess that is U.S. birth defect registry data, investigations have been launched that address the question from other vantage points. The results of these studies are sometimes conflicting, but a number of patterns exist. Moreover, studies in Europe making use of more trustworthy registries—ones that include, for example, birth defects among stillborn and aborted fetuses—have uncovered trends worth careful consideration. All together, these studies indicate that the environment plays a significant role in shaping prenatal body parts.

One of the most impressive of the European studies comes from Norway, where researchers attempted to sort hereditary from environmental factors. Norway has a very good registry, which can even link records on infants, mothers, and fathers. In a study published in 1994, researchers focused on the phenomenon of recurrent birth defects, that is, the tendency of congenital anomalies to strike more than one child in a family. It is well known that bearing a child with a birth defect raises one's risk of having another child so affected, but is this predisposition due to genetic or environmental factors? To attempt an answer, investigators focused on women whose firstborn child had a birth defect and who then changed either sexual partners or places of residency before becoming pregnant again. If the risk of recurrent birth defects was altered by switching partners, then genetic factors would be implicated. If changes in risk were more closely associated with moving, then blame would more likely rest with the environment. The results were unequivocal: staying in the same house was a much stronger predictor of birth defects in subsequent children than staying with the same partner. "This finding suggests that common household exposures and the natural environment may have a more important role than was previously suggested in causing birth defects," acknowledged the *New England Journal of Medicine* in response to the publication of this study. In its accompanying editorial, the *Journal* contemplated the possibility that perhaps "important environmental teratogens have yet to be discovered."

Still other studies home in on where these teratogens may be lurking. Toxic waste sites appear to be one such place. Studies from Belgium, Denmark, France, Italy, and the United Kingdom all show that the risk of several important defects—especially those of the heart and neural tube—rise significantly if the mother lives within a few miles of a hazardous waste landfill. As the distance between waste site and place of residence increases, the chances of birth defects consistently decreases. These findings are based on data drawn from registries in which maternal age is corrected for and pregnancy terminations included. Because the European data are reasonably reliable, they help substantiate similar findings in the United States. Some of these are based purely on state registry data and some on more thorough studies of individual communities. For example, in California, children born to women who lived within a quarter mile of an untreated toxic waste site were found to have double the risk of neural tube problems and quadruple the risk of heart defects. Similar patterns were seen in New York State. A recent review of both European and U.S. studies coolly concludes that, although some studies showed no significant links, "the weight of evidence points to an association between residential proximity to hazardous waste sites and adverse reproductive outcomes."

One common ingredient at hazardous waste sites is a class of chemicals consistently associated with birth defects: organic solvents. As the name implies, solvents are liquids used to dissolve other substances. Common examples are kerosene, acetone, benzene, xylene, and toluene. Some, like dry-cleaning fluids (perchloroethylene), have chlorine atoms attached to their carbon chains and loops, and these are called chlorinated solvents. Trichloroethylene (TCE) and carbon tetrachloride are other examples. Light, shimmery substances, all solvents turn quickly from liquid into gas, which is one of their functions. In essence, solvents are chemical taxicabs used to ferry other substances to their intended location, which they then, by evaporating, leave there. The liquid fraction of many paints contains solvents, as do glues and adhesives. Solvents are also found in paint thinners and strippers, certain household cleaners, spot removers, and pesticides. Their ethereal personalities make solvents both effective and dangerous. Solvents don't really disappear when they vaporize—they just enter the air, where they can be inhaled. Once inside the lungs, they don't lose their ability to dissolve and be dissolved. They are whisked quickly through the fat-soluble membranes of the respiratory alveoli—and, moments later, through the placenta's delicate tree of blood.

The evidence for a link between solvent exposure and birth defects comes both from the laboratory and from the real world. In experimental animals, many common solvents are dependable teratogens, causing skeletal malformations, small heads, and congenital heart problems. This line of evidence is strong and consistent. But outside animal cages, in everyday human life, exposure to a solvent often includes simultaneous exposures to whatever active ingredients it is carrying, and teasing out its individual effects is difficult. Nevertheless, the human data are compelling. For example, in one area of Tucson where drinking water sources were contaminated with the degreasing agent trichloroethylene, investigators found a threefold increased risk of heart defects among children whose parents had lived there during the first trimester of pregnancy. Tellingly, families who moved into the contaminated zone after the affected wells were closed did not suffer this excess risk.

Similarly, in New York State, elevated risks of congenital brain and spinal cord defects were associated with living near plants that emit solvents.

Many studies of solvents and birth defects have focused on the workplace, where exposures are often higher than at home. Solvents are not just confined to industrial, male-dominated trades. Many women also hold jobs that involve handling them. These include health-care professions, office work, janitorial and housecleaning work, and occupations in printing, graphic design, textiles, hairdressing, and dry cleaning. In Sweden, women working in laboratories had more than the expected number of babies with birth defects. In England and Wales, women doctors working with anesthetic gases while pregnant gave birth to more babies with heart and circulatory problems than other women doctors. In addition, they suffered higher rates of stillbirth. In Montreal, women whose babies were born with malformations reported more exposures to solvents on the job than women whose babies were born healthy.

The results of this study are corroborated by another investigation in which pregnant women were asked about their solvent exposure at work *before* learning whether or not their babies had problems. Then, after their infants were born, information on physical anomalies was gathered. The results were dramatic. Women reporting high exposures early in their pregnancies had thirteen times the risk of birth defects than women of the general population. These included heart valve defects and neural tube problems, such as spina bifida, but also other unusual anomalies: clubfoot, kidney defects, deafness, and abnormally small penises. The women also suffered more miscarriages. These results are also supported by a recent critical analysis that examined all research papers in all languages published between 1966 and 1994 that addressed the issue of organic solvents and pregnancy. The investigators concluded that the maternal exposure to solvents, especially by inhalation, "is associated with an increased risk for major malformations."

Lying on the bed listening to Jeff tap away at the computer in the other room, I realize that part of my eagerness for more fetal movement is so that he and I might, by feeling the baby move together, share the experience of expectant parenthood again. During the first trimester, every meal and snack were points of discussion, and our domestic life revolved around trying to find something that I could eat. Those days are mercifully past, but now I feel on my own, solitary within the middle of my pregnancy.

This feeling of isolation extends to other relationships, too. My childless women friends already seem to see me as a parent, even though I don't know the first thing about diapers or colic or infant car seat regulations. My friends who are mothers, on the other hand, tend to view me as an unknowing ingénue, as though pregnancy were a blissful state of innocence from which I am soon to be rudely expelled. "Just enjoy it while it lasts," they say with a knowing laugh as I describe the various sensations I've been experiencing. None of them seems able to recall with any precision what her second trimester of pregnancy felt like, although they are all too ready to discuss labor and delivery options.

Being pregnant is like walking over a plank-and-cable bridge. Behind me, on one bank, is the tribe of women who are not mothers. They drink wine, stay up late, skip meals, change lovers, study Sanskrit, and write grant proposals for a five-year study of tropical cloud forests. In front of me, on the other bank, is the tribe of mothers. They arrive at meetings late, leave parties early, are badly in need of haircuts, know way too much about the care and feeding of guinea pigs, and have to hang up now. The shore behind me is familiar territory. The shore ahead, terra incognita. But I am neither here nor there. I'm way up on the swaying bridge.

Please, little baby, give me a sign of your presence within me.

Fathers are not exempt from the birth defect lottery either. Most studies of paternal workplace exposures show no association with adverse fetal outcome, but a few important studies do. As mentioned above, babies born to painters have elevated rates of anencephaly. They also suffer more often from heart defects. The sons and daughters of farmers have a tendency toward cleft lips and palates, as do the children of men employed in firefighting. The latter set of studies is particularly convincing because firefighters have known exposures to chemicals that cause birth defects in animals. These exposures have increased over the past several decades in tandem with the accelerating use of synthetic chemicals in construction and home decorating—carpet foams, adhesives in particle board, PVC pipes, and vinyl siding, window blinds, and floor tiles.

Just burning plastic alone gives birth to a slew of noxious chemicals, including dioxin (more on this below).

The international data show a few other trends. A study from the Netherlands found an increased risk of spina bifida when fathers are exposed to welding fumes, cleaning agents, or pesticides. In British Columbia, a study of almost 10,000 sawmill employees with exposures to chlorinated wood preservatives uncovered excess rates of anencephaly, spina bifida, cataracts, and genital anomalies in their offspring.

Down syndrome has been linked with a range of paternal occupations, including janitors, farm workers, metal workers, and mechanics. These associations are biologically plausible because certain chemicals are known to prevent chromosomes from separating properly during cell division, and so-called chromosomal nondisjunction, as we have seen, is the immediate cause of Down syndrome. However, researchers in this study had access only to liveborn cases, and so the results must be viewed with caution. Confounding factors may also exist. It is possible, for example, that fathers employed in these professions tend to live in more highly contaminated neighborhoods than fathers in other lines of work. If so, both parents may be exposed to chromosome-damaging chemicals. Or it could be that fathers contaminate their partners by bringing the residues of toxic chemicals home on work clothes or—in the case of solvents—on their exhaled breath.

The toxicology of semen is an emerging area of study that may eventually shed more light on the question of paternal exposures and birth defects. From what we know already, several pathways of operation exist. Some chemicals injure the DNA strands carried in the heads of sperm cells, while others affect the sperm-producing machinery in the testicles. Some are dissolved in the seminal fluid and swept into the uterine environment with ejaculation. Still others bind to the surface of sperm cells and, like miniature Trojan horses, gain entry into the egg during fertilization. Such substances have the oddly reassuring name "sperm-chaperoned agents."

The long, warm evenings of late May allow Jeff and me to take walks along the Mackinaw after our classes are done for the day. In a few weeks—the short May term over, the grades turned in, the household packed—we will head back to Boston.

Already, I feel the tug of this place. Jeff and I will be leaving just about the time the irises yield the gardens to the peonies. I've always enjoyed that particular change of scenery: irises—modern, dark, asymmetric, elegant—supplanted by those chorus girls of the backyard, the feather boa'd, highly perfumed, overblown peonies. I'll be gone before the meadow roses bloom, before mulberries pelt the grass, before the corn tassels out. Before salvia, dragonflies, jewelweed, chicory, mullein, daylilies, fireflies. It seems an untimely departure.

On the way back home from the woods, we stop in the little town of Hudson to buy treats. While Jeff scours the convenience store shelves for something sweet, yet nutritious, I walk along the sidewalk of the main street in search of flower gardens. Right away I'm surrounded on both sides by white plastic flags: TREATED WITH PESTICIDES. KEEP OFF. The house that sits on this lawn is the village funeral home.

In the mid-1960s, Vietnamese journalists began reporting high numbers of deformities among babies born in rural areas that had been heavily sprayed with herbicides by U.S. troops. The original purpose of this clandestine program was to clear the sides of roads to prevent ambush, and the main tool used to do this was a mix of chemical defoliants called Agent Orange. By 1962, the operation had expanded to include the deliberate spraying of food crops and, later, to carry out the policy called "area denial," that is, the creation of widespread zones of contamination intended to force civilians to relocate. Most famously, defoliants were deployed over forests suspected of hiding guerilla groups. By 1971, 19 million gallons had been sprayed over 14 percent of the land in South Vietnam. Countless acres of crops and forest lay in leafless ruin. Some critics compared the use of Agent Orange in Vietnam to the Romans' salting the land after destroying Carthage.

What finally stopped this campaign is still a matter of debate, but two nails in its coffin were the public disclosure in 1969 that Agent Orange causes birth defects in mice and the congressional hearings that followed this announcement. Of the two herbicidal ingredients that make up Agent Orange, one of them is laced with dioxin, which is inadvertently and unavoidably created during the manufacturing process. Dioxin is an all-purpose villain—able to cause cancer, suppress the immune system, interfere with hormones, and activate liver enzymes. It is also a powerful teratogen. (Dioxin is discussed in detail in Chapter 12.)

It is unclear whether dioxin alone or some mixture of chemicals was responsible for the congenital defects first noted by journalists in babies born at the height of the war, but it is clear that the dioxin exposures continue. For example, in at least one city in the south, Bien Hoa, remarkably high levels of dioxin are found not only in longtime residents but in northern Vietnamese who have recently moved there, in children born years after the spraying stopped, and in those who consume lots of fish. In other words, dioxin left behind from herbicides last applied thirty years ago continues to contaminate this city's inhabitants. The route of these ongoing exposures mostly likely begins with the migration of dioxin from soil into river sediment. From here it moves into fish and then into the people who consume those fish. Similarly, in other heavily sprayed areas of Vietnam dioxin levels remain elevated in soil, fish, meat, human blood, and mother's milk. Unfortunately, a definitive comparison of birth defects in sprayed and unsprayed areas has been hampered by a lack of both research funds and a comprehensive registry. Follow up studies of the American troops, however, reveal that the children of those who served in the sprayed areas of Vietnam have 2.5 times the risk of spina bifida. The Office of Veterans' Affairs now offers compensation for this birth defect.

To remind myself of what exactly happened in Vietnam, I turn to an appendix in my own doctoral dissertation, completed in 1989. It includes a history of herbicide use in Vietnam not because my research had anything to do with the war in Indochina but because my study site in a wilderness area of northern Minnesota had been routinely sprayed by the same mix of herbicides and during the same time period that spraying took place in Vietnam. I was astonished when I made this discovery, which happened by serendipity when the resident park naturalist cleaned out a lot of old files from his office and asked if I wanted them. Within the mildewy boxes were memoranda, maps, minutes of meetings, reports, and unpublished letters that detailed the spraying program, initiated in the 1950s and halted abruptly after the congressional hearings in 1970. As in Vietnam, the original mission was to clear brush away from roads. This goal was expanded to include the creation of brush-free vistas to improve the scenery for tourists and then later to encourage the growth of small pine trees by poisoning the shrubs they compete with. (The defoliants kill only plants with broad leaves, not those with needles. The pines failed to grow anyway.) I was studying the ecological relationship between shrubs and pines, and I thought I was working in a virgin forest shaped only by natural processes. Thus, the contents of these cardboard boxes jeopardized my research project and scientific inquiry in general. My astonishment yielded to fury.

Now, rereading my own words, I have different concerns. I wonder how much dioxin remained in the soil and leaf litter after the spraying was finished. How much was still there when I began tramping around a dozen years later, the egg that became my daughter tucked neatly in my ovary? How much ran into the nearby lakes, whose fish I have eaten? What happened to the helicopter pilot who broadcast Agent Orange over the Minnesota biological station during the tourist off-season? And what of his children?

For that matter, what would it be like to be pregnant in Vietnam, watching leaves shrivel and fall as you feel a baby stirring to life inside you? I imagine the Merwin Preserve with the season run in reverse: green branches turning brown, then barren. New spring leaves pelting the forest floor. The woods left shadowless. The nests of birds suddenly visible, but no birds. A river running naked.

A critical evaluation of the literature on pesticides and birth defects published in 1995 ended this way: "To conclude, the published studies have given some indications of elevated reproductive risk and exposure to pesticides but, all together, the epidemiologic evidence does not allow any clear inference to be drawn."

I basically agree with this statement—it's as true now as then—but would add that the studies needed for the drawing of such inferences have yet to be conducted. For example, I could find no studies that attempted to measure pesticide exposures directly. In other words, the absence of evidence is the consequence of ignorance, not negative results.

Studies published since this review include several worth considering. In Finland—which has a high-quality registry—children born to women employed during their first trimester of pregnancy in agricultural occupations involving pesticides had twice the risk of cleft lips and palates. In Spain, oral clefts were three times more likely among babies born to women similarly employed. In addition, these children had greatly increased risks for multiple anomalies and defects of the nervous system. Also in Spain, the rates of surgical repair for undescended testicles is higher in areas of high pesticide use. These findings are mirrored in Denmark, where the sons of women who worked as professional gardeners in greenhouses, orchards, or nurseries were found to have a significantly increased risk of undescended testicles. Norwegian researchers documented strong associations between spina bifida as well as hydrocephaly and maternal work in orchards or greenhouses. Here in the United States, a study of nearly 700 women in California showed an increased risk of fetal death due to birth defects among babies whose mothers lived near crops where certain pesticides were sprayed. The largest risks were found among pregnant women exposed during the critical first trimester and among those who lived in the same square mile where pesticides were used.

The most thorough U.S. study to date is a 1996 investigation of birth defects in Minnesota. Conducted by Dr. Vincent Garry at the University of Minnesota medical school, this study has several interlocking parts, each of which bolsters the other.

Garry first examined birth defects among the children of registered pesticide applicators (such as farmers) in western Minnesota, which is the prime agricultural area of the state. He found levels elevated above the general population's. This finding is consistent with those of previous studies. More surprising is what he found next. When Garry looked closely at birth defect rates within the general population, he found a clear geographical pattern: nonfarming families living in the western half of the state were 85 percent more likely to have a baby with birth defects than nonfarming families living in the eastern half. In other words, living out among fields of corn, beans, wheat, and sugar beets raises the risk of birth defects even if one is not working in them.

Next, he looked at the seasonality of these defects. In western Minnesota, children conceived in the spring, when pesticide use is highest, were significantly more likely to have birth defects than those conceived at other times of the year. This pattern held true both for the families of pesticide applicators as well as for the general population. No such seasonal pattern was seen in the east.

Finally, Garry compared the type of defects seen in excess—missing or abnormally shortened fingers, toes, arms, or legs (called limb-reduction deficits) and malformations of the urinary and genital tracts—to those reported in other studies of farming communities in Iowa, Nebraska, and Colorado where the same pesticides are used. There was much overlap. In Iowa, for example, these same birth defects, as well as congenital heart problems, were elevated in communities served by a drinking water reservoir that had been contaminated with the herbicide atrazine. Atrazine, on the market since 1959 and banned for use in much of Europe, is the most popular pesticide used in the United States.

One of my last tasks before leaving Illinois is to cancel my subscription for bottled-water delivery. All spring, the blue five-gallon jugs lined our stairwell in mute testimony to my distrust of the local water supply. I am not proud of this. I have always been a big advocate of tap water—not because I think it harmless but because the idea of purchasing water extracted from some remote watershed and then hauled halfway around the world bothers me. Drinking bottled water relieves people of their concern about ecological threats to the river they live by or to the basins of groundwater they live over. It's the same kind of thinking that leads some to the complacent conclusion that if things on earth get bad enough, well, we'll just blast off to a space station somewhere else.

Besides, the sense of safety offered by bottled water is a mirage. It turns out that breathing, not drinking, constitutes our main route of exposure to volatile pollutants in tap water, such as solvents, pesticides, and byproducts of water chlorination. As soon as the toilet is flushed or the faucet turned on—or the bathtub, the shower, the humidifier, the washing machine—these contaminants leave the water and enter the air. A recent study shows that the most efficient way of exposing yourself to chemical contaminants in tap water is to turn on a dishwasher. (This surprises you?) Drink a bottle of French water and then step into the shower for ten minutes, and you've just received the exposure equivalent of drinking a half gallon of tap water. We enjoy the most intimate of relationships with our public drinking water, whether we want to or not.

That said, I have all these gallons of bottled water—supposedly drawn from a deep-well aquifer an hour south of here—on my stairs. About them I can say only this: pregnancy is a brief period of time, and whatever contaminants are in these bottles are assuredly less than what is found, during this month of planting and spraying, in the reservoirs north of here.

Here in Bloomington, drinking water is drawn from two artificial lakes, both created by the damming of creeks. These wind through a watershed of more than 43,000 acres, 85 percent of which are fields of corn and soybean. A few weeks ago, I drove out to each of these lakes, stared out at their surfaces, walked along their banks—swallows winging by—and thought about the communion I share with them, my womb an inland ocean with its population of one. I commend this kind of exploration to everyone, but especially to pregnant women.

I also took a look at the data on the local drinking water. In 1996–97, two pesticides were detectable in Bloomington's tap water—atrazine and alachlor. Neither exceeded its legal maximum contaminant levels, meaning that the water was not in violation of the law. This fact did not reassure me. Compliance is based on the average of four quarterly test results; springtime spikes in excess of the maximum contaminant levels are not considered a legal transgression. But embryological development does not honor averages. Nor are the standards set with fetuses in mind. Furthermore, Bloomington's nitrate levels did violate the legal standards for several years running (1990–93). Nitrates—almost certainly from fertilizer runoff—bind with hemoglobin and diminish its ability to carry oxygen. A published review of the topic admits that the health risk of drinking nitrate-contaminated water "is poorly understood." A recent study of amphibian reproduction found that nitrate levels well below the legal limits for tap water caused developmental abnormalities and death among tadpoles. Do I feel comfortable drinking water that may well contain levels of fertilizer sufficient to kill baby frogs? No.

Thus, bottles of water stand on my stairs. But I am not fooling myself. When people ask me if I drink the water here I answer yes. Every time I have soup in the faculty cafeteria. Every time I have a cup of tea with a student. Every time I breathe.

Just as I hang up the phone with the bottled-water company, the civil defense sirens begin wailing. Tornado warning? No, according to the radio, it's just a severe thunderstorm on its way. Jeff is still across campus, busy dismantling the show that he and his students put together. Their show—an assemblage of sculptural objects in a huge old field house—stands just on the other side of a twenty-foot window. A native New Englander, Jeff is terrified of tornadoes. I decide I'd better go find him.

The wind is hot and full of dust when I first walk outside, one of Karol's dresses swirling between my bare legs. The rain starts just as I reach the parking lot. By the time I get to the field house door, I'm drenched.

Jeff is up on a scaffolding, taking apart a giant pillar made of gauze. He smiles and waves.

"I thought you might be worried about the sirens," I call up.

He gestures to a radio perched on an upended plaster bucket. "I've been listening. The storm sounds like it's going around us. Why don't you stay, though? I'll come down."

Jeff has pizza. I stay.

The group show, "Trophies," is an exploration of athleticism. Everything is on a monumental scale. Besides the Olympic-sized pillars, there are giant balls of bamboo, an altarpiece, and a tower of televisions. There are also sculptures made of old weight machines. Jeff drags one of these over to the great north window so we can sit on a padded bench press and watch the storm come over the athletic field. I'm just about to point out the nighthawks sweeping around above the security lights in the parking lot when I stop in midsentence.

"Is something wrong?" Jeff asks.

"Here," I say, pressing his palm against damp cloth, "put your hand here."

Long pause.

"There!" I say. "Did you feel that?"

Jeff looks puzzled. Then his face lights up.

"She kicked!" he exclaims. "I felt it! Hey, she kicked again! Did *you* feel that? That's what it is, isn't it?"

I say that I guess so. We are in a field house, after all.

6

Rose Moon

JUNE

The farther east we drive, the more off-plumb the roads become. Just beyond Ohio, the great grid that organizes the Midwest starts to unravel. Somewhere among the cow-dotted hills of upstate New York, the four compass points lose their grip on the landscape completely, and I can no longer navigate by which way the shadows point. Even though the highway signs still bear the letters *N, S, E,* or *W* after their numbers, these seem to indicate general trends—not the actual direction one is heading at any given moment. It's as if magnetic north doesn't exist out here, I complain to Jeff, who only laughs in response. Of course, this is the man who never did figure out how to behave at Illinois's ubiquitous four-way stops. ("Everyone else always sits there, so I just go.") Once we cross the Berkshire Mountains, sensible four-ways will be entirely replaced by take-your-life-in-your-hands rotaries, where the junctures of meandering roads are spun into tight circles into which and out of which drivers blindly charge. ("At least," says Jeff, "I know what to do in a rotary. It's all a matter of eye contact.")

Jeff does most of the driving—both because he's not bothered by lack of directionality and because he's not having trouble with round ligament pain. Round ligaments are the bungee cords that anchor the uterus in place. I had never even heard of them until a few weeks ago, when I found myself gasping from a kind of sharp ache that felt as though someone had just snapped a rubber band in my groin. This sensation, classic round ligament pain, often becomes common in the sixth month of pregnancy as the uterus pulls forward. Sudden movements—standing up from a sitting position, uncrossing one's legs, clutching and braking—can aggravate it. So I stretch out in the passenger side and catch up on reading.

Magazines and pamphlets about pregnancy have been piling up by my bed ever since they began arriving unbidden in the mail three months ago. Now I'm curious about what I've been missing. I've also fallen behind in my reading of mother-to-be guidebooks. So I start flipping through the diet tips, the wardrobe hints, the frequently asked questions.

In its narration of life in the womb, the popular literature waxes eloquent over a completely different set of milestones than do the academic texts to which I'm more accustomed. The textbooks devote most of their pages to the complicated early events of organogenesis, with all their origami-like precision. The writing perks up again at the end with the avalanche of hormonal changes that triggers labor and delivery. But the discussion of fetal changes during the second and third trimesters is swift and almost dismissive: growth of body parts, fat deposition, refinement of features. One of these books summarizes the sixth month of human gestation with a pair of sentences that manages to be both blasé and astonishing: "The face and body generally assume the appearance of the infant at birth. Fetuses born from week 25 onwards are generally viable."

By contrast, the popular media pass swiftly over the treacherous early months—except to mention morning sickness and symptoms of imminent miscarriage—and hit their rhetorical stride during the months of mid- and late pregnancy. These periodicals dote lovingly on such achievements as growth of the eyebrows (well developed by month six!), the secretion of waxy *vernix* (protects the skin from chapping), and the growth of *lanugo* (fine downy hair that holds the vernix in place). What mother-to-be can resist these endearing details, this special language, which resembles the vocabulary of a Catholic Mass? ("Vernix" is Latin for varnish, "lanugo," for wool.) From the popular books, I learn that a six-month-old fetus is about thirteen inches long and weighs a little more than a pound. I learn that the top of my uterus has risen above my belly button and that the fetus, now pressed directly against the wall of the uterus, is affected by the womb's various squeezings.

And squeeze it does. The uterine muscles periodically shorten in ways that rehearse the body for labor but do not initiate it. These episodes have their own special name as well: Braxton Hicks contractions. They feel strange—at first, pins and needles tingling and then a sensation of condensing, like snow turning to ice, so that my whole belly is a hard, downward-pressing ball. And then the ice turns back to snow, and the pressure goes away. Normal, the pregnancy guidebooks assure me. Braxton Hicks are perfectly normal.

What the popular books and magazines do not talk much about are environmental issues. Even the March of Dimes publication, *Mama*, which is devoted to the prevention of birth defects, does not mention solvents or pesticides or toxic waste sites or Minamata or Vietnam. There is some kind of disconnect between what we know scientifically and what is presented to pregnant women seeking knowledge about prenatal life. At first, I assumed the silence around environmental threats to pregnancy might be explained by the emerging nature of the evidence. Perhaps the writers of public educational materials choose to present only the dangers for which the data are iron-clad and long-standing. All the books and periodicals include a standard discussion of rubella, for example, and urge pregnant smokers to quit.

But the more I read, the more I realize that scientific certainty is not a consistent criterion by which reproductive dangers are presented to pregnant mothers. For example, pregnant women are urged to drink no alcohol. The guidebooks and magazines are unanimous about this. While fetal alcohol syndrome is a well-described and incontrovertible phenomenon—and new evidence shows that even one good drunk in early pregnancy can affect neurological development—no one knows if an occasional glass of wine is harmful. Nevertheless, caution dictates—and again I wholeheartedly agree—that in the absence of information to the contrary, one should assume no safe threshold level. One of the pregnancy books in my collection, *Life Before Birth*, even quotes Voltaire on this issue: "In ignorance, abstain."

Yet this same principle is not applied to nitrates in tap water. Here we assume we *can* set safe thresholds—in this case ten parts per million—even though these thresholds have never been established for fetuses and even though almost nothing is known about transplacental transfer of nitrates or about how nitrate-inactivated hemoglobin in the mother's blood might interfere with oxygen delivery to the fetus. What's more, we allow 4.5 million Americans to drink water with nitrate levels above this arbitrary limit. Four and a half million people surely includes a lot of pregnant women. We also presume we can set safe limits on pesticide residues, solvents, and chlorination byproducts in drinking water—and yet none of these thresholds has ever been demonstrated to protect against fetal damage. In fact, plenty of evidence exists to the contrary. When it comes to environmental hazards, not only do we dispense with the principle of "In ignorance, abstain," we fail to inform pregnant women that the hazards even exist. The same book that quotes Voltaire on alcohol, recreational drugs, and tobacco contains not a single mention of toxic chemicals in food, air, or water. And the rare book or magazine article that does choose to mention them surrounds the topic with tranquilizing reassurances and downplaying qualifiers.

The more I read, the more contradictions I see. A recent scientific report summarizing the reproductive effects of chemical contaminants in food reaches a strong conclusion: "The evidence is overwhelming: certain persistent toxic substances impair intellectual capacity, change behavior . . . and compromise reproductive capacity. The people most at risk are children, pregnant women, women of childbearing age. . . . Particularly at risk are developing embryos and nursing infants."

By comparison one of the most popular guidebooks to pregnancy opens a discussion of this same topic with a complaint about that kind of bad news: "Reports of hazardous chemicals in just about every item in the American diet are enough to scare the appetite out of anyone. . . . Don't be fanatic. Though trying to avoid theoretical hazards in food is a commendable goal, making your life stressful in order to do so is not."

Of course, the don't-worry-be-happy approach does not apply to smoking and drinking; the authors take a very stern, absolutist position on these topics.

I look over at my driver, who's been singing louder and louder.
"Hey, Jeff?"
"Mmm."

"I'm trying to figure something out."

"What's that?" He turns down the radio.

"Not a single one of these pregnancy magazines encourages mothers to find out what the Toxics Release Inventory shows for their own communities."

"You did it though, right?"

"Yeah, I looked it up on the Internet."

"And?"

"And McLean County is one of the top counties in Illinois for airborne releases of reproductive poisons."

I detail for him the results of my research. The biggest emissions of fetal toxicants are hexane from the soybean processing plant and toluene from the auto plant. My list also includes glycol ethers and xylene. All are solvents.

"Jesus," says Jeff.

"I also found out that the university uses six different pesticides on their grounds and fields. So I looked up their toxicology profiles. Two of them are known to cause birth defects in animals."

"Were these used on the athletic field by my studio? There were always little flags out there."

"I don't know. I'm wondering why our obstetrician never talked with us about these kinds of issues. Or about the problems Bloomington has had with its drinking water. The only thing I can remember him saying was not to eat sushi."

We both laugh. Raw fish is not a common menu item in Illinois diners.

"So what are you trying to figure out?"

"Two things. One, why is there is no public conversation about environmental threats to pregnancy?"

"What's the other thing?"

I quote Voltaire: "In ignorance, abstain." "Why does abstinence in the face of uncertainty apply only to individual behavior? Why doesn't it apply equally to industry or agriculture?"

"Okay, let me think for a minute." Jeff turns the radio back on. And then turns it off again. "I think the questions overlap. Pregnancy and motherhood are private. We still act like pregnant women are not part of the public world. Their bodies look strange. They seem vulnerable. You are not supposed to upset them. If something is scary or stressful, you shouldn't talk about it."

"But pregnant women are constantly being told what to do. No coffee. No alcohol. No sushi. Stay away from cat feces."

"That's still private. Industry and agriculture are political, public. They exist outside one's own body, outside one's own house. You can't do something immediately about them within the time period of a pregnancy. So it seems unmanageable."

"It's pregnant women who have to live with the consequences of public decisions. We're the ones who will be raising the damaged children. If we don't talk about these things because it's too upsetting, how will it ever change?"

Jeff throws me a look.

"You're the writer. Can you find a language to manage it? Break the taboo?"

Now I have to think for a while.

"Jeff, how would you do it? In sculpture, I mean. For example, thirty-four million pounds of reproductive toxicants were released from Illinois industries last year. How would you make that number meaningful to people? How would you show it?"

The car slows as we climb a long hill. The grass blowing along the roadside is as long as horses' tails and is already tasseled with seeds. Somehow summer arrived while I wasn't looking.

"I would cast a lot of human figures—each representing a certain number of pounds of toxic chemicals—and I'd place them standing in a field."

Below us, hayfields stretch out, and rain-wet roses bloom in farmhouse yards. I imagine them out there, an army of silent persons, the weight of their bodies pressing downward, their inanimate presence speaking what we are afraid to say.

Back in our Somerville neighborhood, with its views of Bunker Hill and low-lying, wealthier Cambridge, I forget the expanses of Illinois. Up in our third-floor apartment in this most densely populated city in North America (or so claims the Somerville newspaper on a regular basis), Jeff and I spend a few days bumping into each other and reacquainting ourselves with car alarms and Indian take-out food. In the evenings, we sit out on the balcony and wait for an ocean breeze. The neighbor who shares the balcony with us has planted morning glories and tomatoes, which are already twining up the latticework. In the mornings, I walk the dog to the park, sharing the sidewalk with caravans of strollers pushed by pouty teenagers and muttering grandmothers. I never noticed how many babies lived in my neighborhood. Up and down the block, rhododendrons are blooming in tiny cement yards, and vines of purple wisteria wrap the porches of shingled triple-deckers. Underwear flaps on a hundred clotheslines. From the park's old locust trees hang panicles of fragrant white flowers. It is Somerville's finest season.

With the public library only two blocks away, I resume my research. What interests me now is the sine qua non of pregnancy's sixth month: fetal brain development.

Trying to understand the embryological anatomy of the vertebrate brain nearly unhinged me two decades ago. It was some of the most difficult biology I had ever encountered—and the most beautiful. It was like watching a rose bloom in speeded-up time. Or like spelunking in an uncharted cave. My embryology professor, Dr. Bruce Criley, used to drill us by flashing slides of fetal brain sections on a huge screen while we sat in the darkened lab trying to keep our bearings. "Okay, where are we now?" he would demand, whacking a pointer against an unfamiliar structure. Prosencephalon, rhombencephalon, mesencephalon—ancient-sounding names identified rooms in a continuously morphing cavern.

Both the brain and the spinal cord are made up of the same three layers. The brain then adds a fourth layer when cells migrate from the inside out to form the cortex. It's what happens during and after this migration that is so dazzlingly disorienting. Indeed, in order to explain it all, the language of human brain development borrows its vocabulary from botany, architecture, and geography. There are lumens, islands, aqueducts, and isthmuses. There are ventricles, commissures, and hemispheres. There are roofs and floors, pyramids and pouches. There are furrows called sulci and elevations called gyri. Structures are said to balloon, undulate, condense, fuse, and swell. They pass by, flatten, overgrow, and bury each other. They turn, grow downward, turn again, grow upward.

Some structures are formed from tissues derived from two completely different locations. The pituitary gland, for example, is at the place where an upgrowth from a valley near the mouth meets a downgrowth from the forebrain. Meanwhile, the twelve cranial nerves go forth like apostles to make contact with the far-flung, newly developing eyes, ears, tongue, nose, etc. It was all enough to make us mild-mannered, high-achieving biology majors reel with panic. It also was enough to make us feel, once the lights went on again, that we had just emerged from a secret temple, the likes of which we had never seen before.

On a microscopic scale, the story is a bit simpler—although this may only be because we know so little about what actually goes on at the cellular level. All embryological structures are created through migration. But brain cells travel like spiders, trailing silken threads as they go.

There are two kinds of threads: dendrites and axons. Dendrites are fine and short. They receive messages from other nearby cells. Axons are ropy and long. They send out messages, often over great distances. Of the two, axons develop first. They grow out from the body of the brain cell along a specific pathway and in a specific direction. In this they are guided by proteins called cell adhesion molecules. The dendrites are spun out later. In fact, the peak period of dendrite growth doesn't even begin until late in the third trimester, and it continues until at least a year after birth.

Despite these differences, axons and dendrites have a lot in common. Both types of fibers branch after they elongate so that connections can be made with many other cells. These connecting points—the synapses—continue to increase in number throughout the first two years of life. Both axons and dendrites transmit messages by sending electrochemical signals down their lengths. Sometimes, these signals can also fly between fibers. But in most cases, in order to continue a message from one nerve cell to the next, chemicals have to diffuse across the synaptic space. These are the neurotransmitters, with their role call of familiar names: acetylcholine, dopamine, serotonin.

Fetal brain mysteries abound. Chief among them is the role of the neuroglia, whose name means nerve glue. These are brain cells that do not themselves conduct messages but that apparently exert control over the cells that do. They are far more than glue. In some cases they act as coaches to the neurons' athletes—wrapping their axons in ace-bandage layers of fat and thereby speeding the passage of electricity. They also appear to alter the neurons' diets, for example, by modulating the amount of glucose available. And they provide signals and pathways for migration. In this last capacity, they work in tandem with early-migrating neurons. That is to say, the brain cells that are the first to make the journey to the cortex provide essential cues—along with those of the neuroglia—that help later migrants find their way. But no one knows exactly how these trails are blazed, maps are drawn, and bread crumbs scattered.

Once you understand how the embryonic brain unfolds, chamber after hidden chamber, and how its webs of electricity all get connected up, you can easily see why neurological poisons have such profound effects in utero. Exposures that produce only transient effects in adult brains can lay waste to fetal ones. This happens through a variety of pathways. Neurotoxins can impede synapse formation, disrupt the release of neurotransmitters, or strip off the fatty layers wound around the axons. Neurotoxins can also slow the outward-bound trekking of migrating fetal brain cells. Because the earliest-maturing brain cells erect a kind of scaffolding to help their younger siblings find their way, a single exposure at the onset of migration can irretrievably alter the brain's architecture. A fetus also lacks the efficient detoxification systems that already-born human beings carry around within their livers, kidneys, and lungs. And, until they are six months old, fetuses and infants lack a blood-brain barrier, which prevents many blood-borne toxins from entering the brain's gray matter.

As if all this weren't enough, fetal brains are made even more vulnerable by lack of fat in the fetal body. The brain is 50 percent fat by dry weight, and after birth, body fat competes with the brain in attracting fat-soluble toxic chemicals. But throughout most of pregnancy, the fetus is lean, plumping up only during the last month or so. In fetuses, toxic chemicals that are fat-soluble—and many of them are—do not have other fat depots in which to be sequestered, and so they have disproportionately greater effects on the brains of fetuses than on the brains of the rest of us.

More than half of the top twenty chemicals reported in the 1997 Toxics Release Inventory are known or suspected neurotoxins. These include solvents, heavy metals, and pesticides. And yet our understanding of brain-damaging chemicals is vague and fragmentary. Part of the problem is that animal testing is of limited use in trying to figure out how a human baby might be affected by exposure to a particular neurotoxin. Humans are born at a much earlier stage of fetal brain development than, for example, monkeys. Rhesus monkeys' brains are closer to their final form when they monkeys are born, and the young are upright and walking before they are two months old, whereas the average age of human walking is thirteen months. Certain structures within rodent brains, on the other hand, are less well developed at birth than ours. For example, cells in the human hippocampus, the seat of memory, are finished being produced at the time of birth, whereas in rodents, they are not formed until well into postnatal life. These kinds of differences between species mean that extrapolating from animal studies to humans is tricky. The windows of vulnerability are different. And obviously, conducting controlled experiments on human embryos and fetuses is not permissible.

Unhappily, plenty of human fetuses have been exposed to brain-damaging chemicals anyway—not through controlled experiments but through unintended exposures. There is much we can learn by studying their various deficits. However, this kind of research did not begin in earnest until the last few decades. According to the old thinking, either a chemical killed the fetus or it didn't. Either a chemical could produce an obvious structural deformity like anencephaly (no brain) or it couldn't. Not until the 1960s and '70s did fetal toxicologists recognize that certain low-level exposures can elicit functional abnormalities in the brain. That is, the brain *looks* fine—it has all the necessary structures—but it doesn't *act* fine. Once researchers tested children who had had low-level exposures to toxicants on cognitive and motor performance, subtle problems became apparent. The same was true for animals. As soon as laboratory testing of neurotoxicants was expanded to include not just birth defects but also behavioral problems (learning, memory, reaction time, the ability to run a maze), myriad other problems became evident. In both cases, researchers began to see that toxicants can affect brain functioning at much lower levels of exposure than they had previously imagined.

Unfortunately, this epiphany in brain research happened long after the establishment of environmental regulations governing toxic chemicals. Many of these regulations are based on pre–World War II assumptions about neurological development, not on the findings of recent studies. When it comes to fetal neurotoxicants, instead of following the admonition "In ignorance, abstain," we adhere to the principle "In ignorance and disregarding emerging science, proceed recklessly."

The sixth month of pregnancy is a joyful one. My round belly elicits smiles and happy comments from postal workers, dog walkers, and fellow subway riders, who compete to be the first to surrender a seat to me.

Meanwhile, the random fetal movements of last month have evolved into a predictable and reassuring choreography. And as the weeks go by, I begin to notice something else about the baby's movements: they are often generated *in response* to something that I do. When I take a warm bath, she begins to squirm and shimmy, as if she were bathing as well. When I curl up to Jeff at night, my belly pressing against his back, she kicks—with enough force that Jeff can feel it, too. If I roll over in bed, she sometimes rolls over. If police cars or fire trucks suddenly blare down the street, she becomes very still, and I know I won't hear much from her for a while. I pat my belly and try to comfort her. "It's okay, baby; it's just a siren." In these moments, I realize that I am beginning to perceive her as a sentient being—as a child—and myself more and more as her mother.

At the same time, I can no longer read ahead in the pregnancy books and especially have no tolerance for descriptions of labor and delivery. I turn away from drawings of fetuses descending through fully dilated cervixes, as though merely looking at them could bring on premature labor. Pregnancy has taken on a life of its own. I like holding my baby under my heart, feeding her with my blood. My body has shut tight around her like an oyster clutching a pearl. We are one being in the slow process of becoming two. I can feel her in there—thinking, dreaming, listening, dancing.

A commonly held belief is that natural substances are less toxic to the human body than synthetic ones. Like a lot of folk biology, this idea is both true and misleading at the same time. It all depends on what you mean by "natural."

Consider lead, the element that occupies square number eighty-two in the periodic chart. It is indeed present in the earth's crust. But lead is not really part of nature in the sense that it has no function in the world of living organisms. While abundant in the geological world, it does not naturally inhabit the ecological one. A normal blood lead level in a human being—or any other animal—should be zero. And even in the inanimate world of rocks, the soft, dense, silvery substance we know as lead cannot really be said to exist. Elemental lead has to be roasted and smelted out of other minerals. In this sense, a lead fishing weight is as much a synthetic creation as polyester, plastic wrap, or DDT.

There is no doubt that lead is a remarkable material. Its Latin name *plumbum* (abbreviated Pb by chemists) hints at its usefulness. Think plumbing. Essentially uncorrodible, it has long been used to line water pipes. For the same reason, it has found a place in roofing. Lead salts make excellent pigments, thus lead paint. Tetraethyl lead stops engine knocking, thus leaded gasoline. Lead also has handy electrical properties. Its largest use now is in the manufacture of lead-acid storage batteries, especially the ones used in cars.

Lead is also a formidable destroyer of human brains. This property has been recognized for at least 2,000 years. Once called plumbism, lead poisoning causes capillaries in the brain to erode, resulting in hemorrhage and swelling. Its symptoms include irritability, abdominal spasms, headache, confusion, palsy, and the formation of a black line across the gums. Prenatal transfer of lead across the placenta is also old news. In 1911, women working in the white-lead factories of Newcastle noticed that pregnancy cured plumbism. They were right: by passing lead on to their fetuses, workers lowered their own body burdens and thereby alleviated their symptoms of lead poisoning. Of course, most of their babies died. We now know that lead, once it gains entry into the adult female body, settles into bones and teeth. During the sixth month of pregnancy, when the fetal skeleton hardens, placental hormones free up calcium from the mother's bones and direct it through the placenta. Whatever stores of lead lay in the bones are also mobilized and follow calcium into the fetal body. In this way, a developing baby receives from its mother *her* lifetime lead exposure.

Our understanding about lead's toxicity changed radically in the 1940s. Before then, victims of acute lead poisoning who escaped death were presumed to enjoy a complete recovery. But soon a few observant physicians began to notice that child survivors often suffered from persistent nervous disorders and were failing in school. In the 1960s, behavioral changes were noted in experimental animals exposed to low doses of lead. Then, in the early 1970s, children living near a lead smelter in El Paso, Texas, were found to have lower IQ scores than children living farther away. By the 1980s, studies from around the world documented problems in lead-exposed children who had never exhibited any physical symptoms of acute poisoning. These included short attention spans, aggression, poor language skills, hyperactivity, and delinquency. We now know that lead can decrease mental acuity at levels one sixth those required to trigger physical symptoms. The new thinking is that no safe threshold exists for lead exposure in children or fetuses.

Fetal neurologists have also shed new light on the various ways by which lead wrecks brain development. At levels far lower than required to swell the brain, lead alters the flow of calcium in the synapses, thereby altering neurotransmitter activity. It also prevents dendrites from branching, and it interferes with the wrapping of fat around axons. But it doesn't stop there. Lead affects the adhesion molecules that guide the growth of these axons, thereby altering the architecture of the entire electrical web. It also poisons the energy-generating organelles (mitochondria) within the neuronal bodies and so lowers overall brain metabolism. In laboratory rats, lead inhibits a receptor known to play a key role in learning and memory. The adult brain can fend off some of these problems, thanks both to its blood-brain barrier and to an ability to bind lead to protein and so keep it away from the mitochondria. Fetal brains lack these defenses. This is why early lead exposures have life-changing consequences.

On its surface, the story of lead seems like a story of science triumphing over ignorance. Lead paint was banned in the United States in 1977, the year I graduated from high school, and leaded gas was phased out soon after, finally banned in 1990. With paint and gasoline as the two biggest sources of human lead exposure, the decisions to prohibit—and not just regulate—these products is a shining victory for public health. In their wake, the average blood lead levels in American children have fallen dramatically—75 percent between 1976 and 1991.

But there is another story about lead, told by historians and toxicologists who fought long and hard to banish lead from the human economy. It's a story about the willful suppression of science by industry. It's a story that helps explain why one in twenty American children still suffers from lead poisoning in spite of everything we know. It helps explain why lead, never outlawed for use in cosmetics, can still be found in some lipsticks and hair dyes. And it helps explain why the soil in my neighborhood in Somerville is so full of lead that we are still advised not to grow vegetables in our gardens.

Consider lead paint. Its production was halted in this country in the late 1970s. But in 1925, an international covenant had already banned lead-based paints for interior use in much of the rest of the world. This agreement acknowledged that lead was a neurotoxin and that lead paint in the homes produced lead dust, which is easily ingested when crawling babies put their hands in their mouths or chew on toys. But the United States was not a signatory to this agreement. In fact, the same industry trade group that prevented the United States from adopting the convenant also succeeded in blocking restrictions on lead in plumbing. The lead industry—which owned at least one paint company outright—treated the emerging science on low-level lead poisoning as a public relations problem, dismissing objective research as "anti-lead propaganda."

As has been meticulously documented by two public health historians, Gerald Markowitz and David Rosner, the manufacturers of lead pigments went on the offensive after the 1925 agreement. They reassured the American public that lead fears were unfounded. They even promoted lead paint for use in schools and hospitals. Most wickedly, they employed images of children in advertising. The most famous of these was the Dutch Boy, a cartoon character dreamed up by the National Lead Company. With his requisite haircut, overalls, and wooden shoes, the little Dutch Boy cheerfully sloshed buckets of paint labeled "white lead" in ad campaigns throughout the midcentury. The implicit message was that lead paint was safe for children to handle. The Dutch Boy was even fashioned into souvenir figurines. A 1949 sales manual explained, "The company has never overlooked the opportunity to plant the trademark image in young and receptive minds."

The industry also fought labeling requirements that would warn buyers not to use lead paint on children's toys, furniture, or rooms. Many a nursery was painted with lead by pregnant women eagerly awaiting the birth of their babies. Those questioning the safety of such practices were repeatedly reassured by Lead Industry Associates that a link between lead paint exposure and mental deficiencies had never been proved. And up until the 1970s, this was true—in no small part because the lead industry was the main source of funding for university research on the health effects of lead. Researchers with other opinions and other funding sources were condemned as hysterical and sometimes threatened with legal action. Only when the U.S. government became a major funder of lead research did the case against lead began to mount.

When the truth eventually became undeniable, the industry shifted tactics. Instead of denying lead's powers to damage children's brains, it blamed inner-city poverty and unscrupulous landlords who, the argument went, had allowed paint to peel in their tenement buildings. And the neglected children living there, with nothing better to do, ate it. At one point, recalls a leading toxicologist deeply involved in the lead wars, an industry representative actually suggested that the problem was not that eating lead paint chips made children stupid but rather that stupid children ate paint. All these arguments finally collapsed under the weight of emerging scientific evidence. But decades were wasted in denials, obfuscations, deflections of responsibility, counteraccusations, intimidation of scientists, and attempts to tranquilize a legitimate public concern. The result is that any home built and painted before 1978 probably contains lead paint, and all children and pregnant women living in such buildings continue to face risks from it. And since I live in a century-old building listed on Somerville's historical registry, I am now such a woman. It is a problem that continues to vex landlords and homeowners alike, as removing the lead is expensive and is itself a health menace. It is a problem that could have been solved in 1925.

Now consider leaded gas. In 1922, General Motors discovered that adding lead to gasoline helped alleviate its tendency to "knock," to burn explosively under high compression. Solving this problem meant that automobile engines could be made bigger, and cars could go faster. Ethanol, which can be distilled from corn, also worked well as an antiknock additive but could not be patented and was therefore not as profitable to the oil companies. In 1923 leaded gas went on sale for the first time. This development immediately attracted the attention of public health officials, who raised urgent questions about the effects of broadcasting lead-laced fumes into public air space. At about the same time, serious health problems began afflicting refinery workers whose jobs involved formulating the lead additive. Several died and many others suffered hallucinations. The tetraethyl lead building at one plant was even nicknamed the House of Butterflies because so many employees who worked in it saw imaginary insects crawling on their bodies.

Then a remarkable thing happened. In 1925, a meeting was convened by the U.S. Surgeon General to address the issue of lead dust. And a moratorium was declared. The sale of leaded gas was banned on the grounds that it might well pose a public health menace. It was a perfect expression of the principle "In ignorance, abstain"—what is now popularly called the precautionary principle. Unfortunately for us all, the moratorium did not hold. After the prohibition took effect, the lead industry funded a quick study that showed no problems with lead exposure. Over the objection that lead was a slow, cumulative poison and that such a study could not possibly reveal the kind of human damage researchers were worried about, the ban was subsequently lifted. The production of leaded gas resumed.

It continued for almost seventy years. By the time it was banned again, this time for good, more than 15.4 billion pounds of lead dust had been released into the environment. Much of this has sifted down into the topsoil. As a metal, lead is not biodegradable and is considered absolutely persistent. In other words, it is not going away anytime soon. It is tracked into homes on the bottoms of shoes. It is absorbed from soil into plant roots. This is why, in high-traffic urban areas such as my neighborhood in Somerville, we cannot grow and eat carrots.

The irony of our gardening situation is that lead in gasoline was finally removed on the basis of a landmark 1979 study showing significant IQ changes among first- and second-graders in response to environmental lead exposures. And the children investigated lived here in Somerville.

Should you ever find yourself in Boston, you may wish to pay a visit to the Old North Church in the North End. It's the one-if-by-land-two-if-by-sea church made famous by Paul Revere. If you go, take a look at the pale violet walls inside the sanctuary. Jeff painted them. Well, he and a crew of men that he supervised. Restoration work and decorative painting are specialties of his; these skills have helped to fund a lot of art projects over the years and paid a lot of rent. Elegant old homes up and down Beacon Hill and on Cambridge's Brattle Street contain his handiwork, as do buildings at Harvard University. Jeff is more at ease with a paintbrush and a sander in his hands than anyone else I have ever met, which is one reason (among others) I fell in love with him.

Now we lie awake on a summery night, reggae drifting into the window from the street below, and discuss whether or not he should continue this work. His blood lead levels are more than double that of the average American male. One physician actually congratulated him for this. Given that his line of work puts him in direct contact with old, lead-based paint, she expected they would be much higher. Jeff is very careful. But even when he changes clothes at the job site and leaves his work pants out on our fire escape, he still comes home covered in dust and paint. He's paying the price for reckless decisions made three generations ago.

But we would like to ensure that our daughter doesn't. Almost nothing is known about how lead exposures in fathers affect their unborn children. "Lower lead levels have not been well studied for their possible effects on the male reproductive system or on pregnancy in the partners of exposed males."

In ignorance, abstain. But can we afford to? With a baby coming? In the end, we decide that Jeff should fold his business. And as soon as the baby is crawling, we'll move out of our apartment. We know there is lead paint under the many layers of latex—our landlord has confirmed it—and we know that painting over lead paint is not considered a safe method of containment. We also know that our neighbors around the corner discovered very high lead levels in the soil in their back yard. Nevertheless, a home lead detector kit has revealed no lead on the surface of our interior walls, in the cupboards, or in the dusty corners behind the radiators. For now, we'll stay put. (It's a decision we later come to question. Blood lead levels are measured in micrograms per deciliter of blood. In children, any number below ten micrograms is considered acceptable. However, pediatric researchers have documented impairments in math, reading, and short-term memory at levels down to five. At nine months, our daughter's blood levels were measured at six micrograms.)

"Don't grow our own root vegetables. Quit a job I like. How come we're always the ones that have to do the abstaining?" Jeff wants to know.

And that is my question exactly.

Two doors down from lead, just to the right of gold, occupying spot number eighty in the periodic chart of the elements, is mercury. Its chemical monogram, Hg, is an abbreviation of its older Latin name, *hydargyrum*: liquid silver. It is, in fact, the only metal that is fluid at room temperature. It also expands uniformly in response to increases in temperature, and it does not cling to glass. For all these reasons, mercury has been used in thermometers for hundreds of years.

To the ancient alchemists, lead and mercury were substances of opposing personalities. Lead: dull, sluggish, heavy. Mercury: shiny, quick, changeable. But these contrary materials possess at least two qualities in common. They both blur the distinction between natural and human-made. And they both vandalize fetal brains.

Like lead, mercury is interned deep inside the earth's crust, mostly bound up with other elements. The most common mercurial ore is cinnabar, which is found in relative abundance in Spain and Italy. Unlike lead, the elemental form of mercury exists "naturally," in that it can wend its way up to the surface world of living organisms without any assistance from mining and smelting operations. Slippery and restless, it evaporates out of rock and soil, out of seawater, out of volcanoes and hot springs. As a vapor, mercury can circle the globe for up to a year, eventually coming back down to the earth with rain and snow. This is the wheel of the mercury cycle, as it has been turning for millions of years. The total amount of mercury on the planet remains constant—as an element, it is indestructible—but its exact location is always shifting. As we now know, mercury that drifts into sediment-rich water is quickly transformed by aquatic bacteria into methylmercury. What happens next, however, is a matter of some uncertainty. Apparently, the bacteria release some of this methylmercury back into the water column, where it then adheres to plankton and algal cells, which are subsequently eaten by tiny filter-feeding animals. Alternatively, the bacteria may sequester the heavy metal within their simple one-celled bodies. They are then eaten by various bottom-feeding organisms.

By either pathway or both, mercury, in its more toxic incarnation as methylmercury, is siphoned up the food chain, soon entering the bodies of fishes, and concentrating its poisonous powers more with every link ascended.

Various human activities have greatly speeded up the transfer of mercury from the geological world to the biological one, and this is the unnatural dimension of the situation. As revealed by sediment cores, the concentration of mercury vapor in the atmosphere has more than tripled since preindustrial times. And every year, the amount of airborne mercury increases by another 1 percent. Methylmercury levels are also rising in the flesh of fish-eating birds such as loons, many of which are now suffering impaired reproduction due to mercury toxicity. Some of this is happening because the clear-cutting of forests releases soil-bound mercury into rivers and streams. Some of this is happening because mining companies heat mercury-laced ores to extract gold.

But the biggest single contributor to the accelerating pace of mercury's earth-to-air migration is coal-burning power plants. Like a genie in a bottle, mercury is locked inside subterranean veins of coal, held safely away from living organisms, until it is set loose when this coal is excavated and burned. Mercury releases from U.S. power plants now approach 100,000 pounds each year. More than 6,200 of these pounds, I learn, comes from power plants in my own home state of Illinois, making it the fifth largest contributor of coal-based mercury releases in the nation. The power plant in my own home town—whose stacks I looked at every day of my childhood—is Illinois's third biggest mercury polluter. All by itself, my home county, Tazewell, Illinois, releases 1,146 pounds of mercury into the air each year. To my astonishment, I also learn that there are no laws requiring power plants to control mercury emissions. They are exempt from regulation. I recall knowing this already, but pregnancy makes the knowledge sink deeper. (Two and a half years after my pregnancy's second trimester, on December 14, 2000, the U.S. Environmental Protection Agency announced that it would require reductions of mercury emissions from coal-fired plants. The agency is to propose regulations by 2003, but the new rules are not expected to go into effect until 2004, and compliance is not expected until 2007.)

Mercury vapor also escapes from a multitude of consumer products and industrial operations. Purified mercury is often placed within fragile objects, such as fever thermometers and fluorescent light bulbs, which inevitably break. Some car headlamps contain mercury, as do many electrical switches and thermostats. Sooner or later, almost all of these end up in landfills, junkyards, or incinerators where their core of invisible metallic gas evaporates into the atmosphere. The same electrical properties that make mercury so useful in switches and lighting have also given it a role in the production of chlorine gas, which is created by passing electricity through brine. The resulting chlorine vapor is separated from the alkali (caustic soda) also created during the process by the use of electrolytic cells, which often contain liquid mercury. Afterward, the remaining sludge is dumped, burned, or buried, and all of the mercury it contains slips out into the environment. Because many older chlor-alkali plants rely on these mercury cells, the chlorine industry is the largest consumer of mercury in the United States. However, newer technologies involving synthetic membranes make mercury-filled electrolytic cells unnecessary. (Mercury-dependent chlor-alkali plants are already banned in Japan.)

Even contemporary funeral practices contribute to atmospheric mercury levels. One recent study estimates that a single crematorium releases between two and three pounds of mercury from its stacks each year. These emissions represent vaporized dental amalgam.

There are a few things about prenatal exposure to mercury that science knows with certainty. The mechanism by which this toxin arrests neural development is one of them. Methylmercury halts cell division in the fetal brain by binding directly to chromosomes and interfering with their ability to make copies of themselves. Methylmercury also interferes with the migration of brain cells, especially in the cerebellum, the control center for posture, balance, and muscle coordination. Researchers also know that fetuses receive higher doses than adults because mercury is actively pumped across the placenta. Studies consistently find higher levels of methylmercury in the blood of newborns than in blood samples drawn from their mothers. There is also universal agreement that fish and seafood consumption is by far our most significant route of exposure. All fish contain some amount of mercury, and these levels rise as levels of mercury released into the environment rise. The more fish in the maternal diet, the higher the levels of methylmercury in umbilical cord blood. No one is denying this relationship.

Where arguments fly is over the levels of exposure needed to create lasting and demonstrable harm. This debate has intensified with the recent publication of two exhaustive studies that come to very different conclusions. Both looked at mothers-to-be who ate varying amounts of seafood during their pregnancies. One study was conducted on a group of remote islands clumped between Iceland and Norway in the frigid North Atlantic. The other was carried out on a group of remote islands scattered off the east coast of Africa in the balmy Indian Ocean.

The first investigation, known as the Faroe Islands study, was carried out by a Danish researcher, Philippe Grandjean, and his colleagues. They looked at 1,022 babies born in 1986–87 to women who ate fish and whale meat while pregnant. The main source of mercury in the Faroes is pilot whale, which contains concentrations similar to or higher than those in swordfish. To assess maternal exposure to methylmercury, researchers took a blood sample from the umbilical cord and hair samples from the mothers. True to form, the more seafood consumed, the higher the levels of mercury in the mothers' hair. When they were seven years old, the children were evaluated on their cognitive and motor skills. The results were striking. Researchers found deficiencies in memory, learning, and attention that were proportional to the level of mercury in umbilical cord blood and maternal hair. Thus, the relationship between prenatal mercury exposure and delays in mental development was a dose-dependent one: the more mercury received before birth, the more poorly the child performed on the researchers' tests. To be sure, these children were not actually sick. They were just slower in solving riddles and other puzzles, and they appeared to be behind in their development.

These deficits persisted. In seven-year-old children, each doubling of prenatal mercury exposure corresponded to a delay of one or two months in mental development. Neither mother's age nor education affected the results. Moreover, mercury levels in children's hair were much less useful at predicting problems than were levels in cord blood or their mother's hair. This result suggests that prenatal exposures are a more potent force for dampening intellect than postnatal ones. The study also uncovered cognitive problems at very low exposures—at levels previously considered harmless. As the researchers themselves note, many questions remain to be answered.

Are these delays permanent? Will they worsen with age (as with the Minamata victims), or will they abate? Might other toxic exposures interact with mercury in creating these deficits?

The Faroe Islands study also turned up another unexpected result. As well as exhibiting dose-dependent mental impairment, children with higher prenatal exposures tended to have higher blood pressures. This finding suggests that methylmercury is capable of subtly sabotaging the developing autonomic nervous system, which controls the heart. Since high blood pressure in early childhood can forecast hypertension later in life, it is an important discovery. Once again, childhood exposures appear to be less crucial than those before birth as there was no relationship between child hair levels of mercury and blood pressure in this group of seven-year-olds.

The second study, conducted in the Seychelle Islands by the American researcher Philip Davidson, arrived at completely different results. Using methods similar—but not identical—to those pioneered by Grandjean in the Faroe Islands, Davidson and his team investigated possible associations between mental development in early childhood and maternal-hair mercury concentrations. They found none. "In the population studied, consumption of a diet high in ocean fish appears to pose no threat to developmental outcomes through 66 months [5 1/2 years] of age." This absence of evidence for harm has researchers stumped—especially since it appears to persist at very high mercury concentrations. Indeed, some of the hair mercury levels found among Seychellois mothers approach those found in the 1970s among mothers in Iraq who had unknowingly eaten flour milled from mercury-dressed wheat seeds. Their children developed progressive retardation and paralysis. And yet the children of the Seychelles islanders seem fine so far. Will neurological deficits appear later in life? Or is there something else about their tropical diet that truly mitigates mercury's ravaging effects? Were Davidson's batteries of tests the right tools for unmasking cognitive problems? Or were Grandjean's methods in the Faroe Islands inappropriate? There are not yet answers to these questions.

In the meantime, on Madeira, an island off the coast of Morocco, a team of researchers led by Grandjean has been studying 149 first-graders whose mothers ate varying amounts of deep-sea fish while pregnant. This time, investigators are conducting neurological tests involving sensory perception, which can be more objectively measured than cognitive skills. Once again, maternal-hair mercury is being used to estimate prenatal exposures. So far, researchers have documented abnormalities in auditory and visual latencies among children whose mothers have high hair mercury levels. These kinds of results reflect developmental delays in areas of the brain that control vision and hearing. The Madeira study helps support the results of the Faroe Island study, where the same measurements were carried out with similar outcomes. But the Faroe Islands results are still inconsistent with the results of the Seychelles study, which relied on somewhat different methodologies.

So what is a pregnant woman with cravings for tuna fish to do? No one yet knows how little mercury exposure is required for fetal brain damage. On the other hand, most researchers agree that, whatever the precise figure turns out to be, human harm is being documented at concentrations dangerously close to background levels already found within the general population. Since 1991, the Institute of Medicine, a private nonprofit group that works with the National Academy of Sciences, has advised women even *considering* pregnancy to avoid swordfish altogether, so contaminated is it with methylmercury. The State of Washington and seven other states advise all women of childbearing age, currently pregnant or not, to avoid fresh and frozen tuna altogether and to limit their weekly consumption of canned tuna to no more than six ounces (about one small can). The same recommendations apply to children under six. A report prepared by the Environmental Working Group and the U.S. Public Interest Research Group goes further, arguing that canned tuna should not be eaten by pregnant women more often than once a month.

In July of 2000, the National Academy of Sciences released a report that concluded that *each year* in the United States some *60,000 children* are born at risk for neurodevelopmental problems owing to prenatal exposure to mercury. The risk to women who eat large amounts of seafood during pregnancy, says the report, is "likely to be sufficient to result in an increase in the number of children who have to struggle to keep up in school and who might require remedial classes or special education." These conclusions were underscored a year later by a Centers for Disease Control study. Directly measuring mercury levels in the blood and hair of 700 U.S. women and 300 children, researchers discovered that one in every ten women of childbearing age carries body burdens of mercury approaching those that create risks for giving birth to children with neurological problems. The results of this investigation, which is the first to collect a nationally representative sample of mercury in human blood and hair in the United States, indicate that exposure to mercury is not just limited to large consumers of fish. They indicate that the margin of safety for at least 6 million women of childbearing age—and their children—is razor thin.

When I look into the history of mercury regulation, it very quickly sounds like the story of lead all over again: Industry groups working to downplay the dangers. Regulatory agencies intimidated. Public heath initiatives thwarted. Scientists ignored. Calls for action drowned out by calls for more research. A public confused. It's the same plot, but with a different cast of characters, set fifty years later.

Two different branches of the federal government share responsibility for protecting the public from mercury: the Environmental Protection Agency and the Food and Drug Administration. The EPA, along with the states, is charged with monitoring mercury levels in fish in U.S. rivers and streams. The FDA is responsible for monitoring all fish, both domestic and imported, sold in the marketplace. Neither agency has responded vigorously to the emerging science showing that neurological damage to the fetus is greater at lower mercury levels than previously suspected. Indeed, the maximum allowable levels for mercury in commercially sold fish were set over two decades ago, in 1979, without pregnant women in mind, and when fish consumption was much lower than it is today. And these standards are actually *looser* than those in place three decades ago: in 1969, in response to pressure from the fishing industry, the FDA doubled the amount of mercury allowable in commercially sold fish.

Even if these outdated limits were somehow adequately protective of human fetuses, the FDA, its monitoring program largely dismantled, has done little to enforce them. In 1995, for example, it sampled only thirteen cans of tuna. In 1996, 1997, and 1998, it sampled none. The FDA has also ceased testing shark and swordfish, even though the agency's own limited data show that fully one third of all commercially sold shark and swordfish tested since 1992 exceeded the maximum allowable limits.

Early in 2001, the watchdog magazine *Consumer Reports* released the results of its own fish testing. It found that fully half of all sword-fish purchased in U.S. supermarkets and specialty shops contained concentrations of methylmercury that exceeded the FDA's own action levels. At about the same time, the U.S. General Accounting Office, the research arm of Congress, concluded its own investigation of the FDA's seafood monitoring and enforcement practices. The title of the GAO's 60 page report to the Senate says it all: *Federal Oversight of Seafood Does Not Sufficiently Protect Consumers.*

Bowing to both fishing interests and utility companies, the FDA has also refused to support tighter standards that would set mercury limits in fish at levels more protective of human fetuses. For its part, the EPA does support them—its thresholds for mercury in freshwater fish are several times more stringent than the FDA's—but it has failed to come up with a plan to reduce mercury emissions into the environment. Without such a plan, mercury levels in fish will keep rising, and industry pressure to weaken standards further and turn a blind eye to enforcement will mount. And as long as no one is looking for problems, not surprisingly, none will be found, and no solutions will be demanded.

Frustrated by regulatory impotence, a public watchdog group in Vermont, the Mercury Policy Project, has recently put forth a plan of its own. To any pregnant woman worried about the future intelligence of her child, this proposal sounds remarkably sensible. First, say the authors, mercury-laced trash should be forbidden entry into incinerators and landfills. This means any product containing mercury must be labeled and the manufacturers required to take it back at the end of its life span. Eventually, the manufacture and use of such products needs to be phased out. Fortunately, most mercury-containing products (e.g., thermometers) have substitutes (digital thermometers). Second, the authors of the plan continue boldly, mercury emissions from coal-burning power plants must be curtailed and then ultimately eliminated, a goal that is achievable through a variety of pollution control and preventive strategies. Both of these changes together would reduce mercury pollution by about 85 percent.

By not taking action to remove the sources of mercury from the environment, policy-makers are left with advising pregnant women and nursing mothers—and all females *thinking about* someday becoming pregnant women and nursing mothers—to limit their consumption of fish and seafood. So, for example, on January 12, 2001, the FDA issued new guidelines recommending that pregnant women and women of childbearing age who may become pregnant avoid eating shark, swordfish, king mackerel, and tilefish. (To the disappointment of many consumer advocates, this announcement did not include an advisory about tuna consumption.) Once again, we are the ones pressed into abstention. Earlier, in 1997, forty states released advisories on sport-caught fish in the form of 1,675 separate warnings, which are still in force. The majority of these are directed at children and women of reproductive age, pregnant or not. They caution us to limit or avoid consumption of particular species of fish that have been caught in particular streams, lakes, or coastal waters. This effectively means that any time a woman of childbearing age wants to join in a family fish fry or eat the spoils of her own fishing expedition she must first contact her state environmental agency to find out how many ounces of said fish caught in said location will put her over the recommended limit for mercury exposure, or for some other toxic contaminant. Under these guidelines, certain species of fish are prohibited to women altogether, as are especially large fish of otherwise acceptable species. (The bigger the fish, the more concentrated the poison.)

Advisories are not standardized. Some states are more cautious than others in deciding what risk is acceptable, and their risk analyses are performed on different data sets. This is why the level of mercury considered hazardous in Indiana would not trigger a warning to pregnant women in Illinois. Sometimes different advisories exist for the same species in the same body of water. For example, if you fish in Long Island Sound, the state of New York will provide you with one set of consumption guidelines, the state of Connecticut another.

Obviously, a public health policy that asks expectant mothers to give up certain foods while allowing industries to continue contaminating them is absurd. There is, however, one shred of good news concerning mercury ingestion: Unlike lead, methylmercury persists in human tissue for a matter of months rather than years.

Avoiding fish both during pregnancy and in the year preceding conception is protective against prenatal mercury exposure.

But even if we all planned our motherhoods with this much foresight, an approach to fetal health that relies on nutritional sacrifices by mothers is still unsound. Cutting back on fish is not like forfeiting cigarettes and beer. Fish is good food. It is low in saturated fat and high in protein, vitamin E, and selenium. It is also a leading source of omega–3 fatty acids, which reduce blood pressure and cholesterol. Fish oils also prevent blood platelets from clumping together, which lowers the risk of stroke. For many women, pregnancies and lactation fill significant years of their adult lives. Deciding between protecting their babies' brains and protecting their own cardiovascular health is not a choice they should have to make. And restricting fish consumption is not even an option for some. In many Arctic and Native American communities, fish is the only available protein. Commercial food, when it is available at all, is prohibitively expensive, of insufficient variety, and poor in nutritional value. Studies show that the health of indigenous women often suffers when they bring their dietary habits in line with fish advisories.

Furthermore, the sacrifices required of mothers do not just affect our own bodies. The same nutrients that help lower maternal blood cholesterol also play a critical role in the third trimester of pregnancy when the fetal brain undergoes a growth spurt. During this time, omega–3 fatty acids are mobilized for the proliferation of fetal vascular tissue as well as neural circuitry. Here then is the central irony of our problem: substances present in the flesh of fish promote healthy development of the fetal brain, but we have poisoned the world's fishes with neurotoxic chemicals, so that the same succulent filet that carries fatty acids essential for brain growth also carries an injurious brain poison.

When Jeff and I eloped in the fall of 1996, we had only known each other a few months. Aged forty-two and thirty-seven, we figured we could trust our instincts. When Jeff moved in, he arrived with a number of possessions that surprised me. Chief among them were an enormous pair of rubber waders, a tackle box, and eight fishing rods, a couple of them for fly-fishing; the others were intended for bait-casting or trolling.

Plenty of stories came with the equipment, most of them about Jeff's father, who was an expert fly fisherman. His skills lay not only in the way he tied flies—crafting the illusion of living insects out of feathers, varnish, hooks, and thread—but in the way he could make a handmade fly dance and skitter over the surface of a brook, beckoning a trout below to its last meal. He stored his winning flies—some made of peacock feathers, others as inconspicuous as gnats—on the brim of his fishing hat, a patriarchal icon that has long since been lost. Lost, too, is his wicker creel in which he carried home his catch, wrapped in moss, to be cleaned on the back porch and readied for supper. His tackle box, however, still contains a collection of duck feathers, which he was apparently saving for fly-tying. The man who would have been my father-in-law—a pilot, a Marine, a Madison Avenue ad executive who had majored in music—died from injuries sustained in a skiing accident just as Jeff was beginning college.

In the early 1960s, Jeff, his brother, and his father fished rivers, ponds, and brooks throughout New England, and especially the ones close to their home in Norwalk, Connecticut. Sometimes the three fishermen, up since 4 A.M., were so hungry by midmorning that they cleaned the fish they had already caught and ate them for breakfast. Jeff's father taught his sons how to suspend their catch on green twigs hooked through the gills and hang it over the flames of an open fire. These meals—and all the whispered anticipation in the dark hours leading up to them—are Jeff's fondest childhood memories.

I have a few fishing stories of my own, mostly involving docks on Wisconsin lakes. My father's tackle box was full of bobbers, weights, lures, and spinners—brightly painted fish and frog facsimiles that wiggled as you pulled them through the water. The one that scared me most was the duckling lure: all yellow innocence above and a nest of deadly hooks below. There was also a naked mermaid lure, complete with naked bosoms, her barbed hook hidden among silvery scales.

My sister and I mostly angled for sunfish while Dad cast for bigger prizes farther out. Once, a northern pike—long, heavy, full of teeth—snapped at my line, and I watched in horror as the red and white bobber vanished into the green depths, the reel spinning at a higher and higher pitch as the great fish ran with my line into deep water. The pull was too much. I would either have to let go of the rod or follow it into the middle of the lake.

"Dad! Dad!"

And there he was, my father kneeling behind me, arms reaching around my orange life jacket, his hands on top of my hands, reeling the fish in, playing it out again, reeling it in again.

Now the rivers and lakes of Connecticut are all covered by fish advisories, so contaminated is every single one of them with mercury. So are most of the Wisconsin lakes, where we fished with my father. I wonder how we will explain this situation to our daughter. Will she ever step into her father's waders? Fashion feathers into flies? Learn how to make her grandfather's rod dance in the air? Catch fish for breakfast in the state of Connecticut?

I have a few other questions. In a mercury-poisoned world, what happens to the knowledge that Jeff has, handed down from his father and his father before him, about how to clean and gut a bass? About what kind of water pickerels like to hide in? About how to hang trout over an open fire? One summer in Minnesota, I ran out of money in the middle of my field season. Word got around. Soon, anonymous benefactors began leaving fresh-caught walleye outside my tent. I cooked them in foil over my camp stove. Will my daughter ever enjoy such gifts? The International Joint Commission of the United States and Canada, which manages our border's water systems, recently warned children and women of reproductive age against eating sport-caught fish from any of the Great Lakes, stating categorically that the contaminants they contain pose a threat to their health. It also recommended that the Canadian and U.S. governments immediately issue advisories directly to women that would plainly state that "eating Great Lakes sport fish may lead to birth anomalies and other serious health problems for children and women of childbearing age."

When advisories warn women and children away from fish, more is lost than a good source of omega–3 fatty acids. Whole ways of knowing are lost. I imagine reading to our daughter one of my favorite books as child, *The Runaway Bunny*, first published in 1942, in which a clever mother rabbit remains one step ahead of her baby's attempts to leave home.

"If you run after me," threatens the little bunny in one scene, "I will become a fish in a trout stream and I will swim away from you."

"If you become a fish in a trout stream," replies his sensible mother, "I will become a fisherman and I will fish for you."

The illustration for this page shows the mama bunny in waders, casting a carrot-baited line after her truant offspring. It is the thread that binds mother to child.

If our daughter asks, "What's a trout stream?" what will I say? Will I explain that freshwater trout are now among the most contaminated fish in America, far too poisonous for her to eat? Will I tell her that our government is willing to warn her against eating trout but reluctant to stop the trout from being poisoned in the first place?

I imagine other public scenes. I imagine, for example, thousands of pregnant women marching on Washington, demanding policies that are protective of fetal brain development, that allow us to eat freely up and down the food chain without worry, in keeping with our cultures, our family stories, and our dietary cravings. I imagine us singing new words to an old civil rights song: "We shall not abstain!"

7

Hay Moon

We have come far north. At 11:30 P.M., the hanging basket of pansies outside our guest-house window is still vivid with purple petals. At 3 A.M., when I get up to pee, I can still see them glowing. Evening has turned into morning. As I tuck the curtains around the sill to block out the light, I realize I've never experienced days without darkness between them. Sooner or later, welcomed or unwelcomed, night has always come, like a period at the end of a sentence. But midsummer days in Alaska run on and on, unpunctuated by darkness. The sun circles around the horizon, refusing to set. Softball games and road construction continue around the clock. I sleep badly, as though napping before a bedtime that never comes.

The truly startling thing about pansies in Alaska is their titanic size. One could use them as salad plates. This is not unrelated to the fact that they are radiantly visible in what should be the dead of night. The unending summer daylight encourages the most humble of plants—cabbages and garden flowers—to grow to Alice-in-Wonderland proportions.

Of course, I need only look in the mirror to be reminded how familiar life forms can enlarge to unimagined dimensions. Just at the threshold of my third trimester, I now outweigh my husband. Stepping onto the obstetrician's scale the week before we flew to Anchorage, I watched the nurse adjust the big weight on the lower bar, which could only mean that I'd topped 150 pounds. I had never noticed the lower bar of medical scales; it never applied to me. But I couldn't stop staring as the blocky, black weight settled into its new notch with a loud *ka-chunk*, and the bar still refused to tip until the little square above was slid a long way from the fulcrum.

At about this same time, I noticed I was now bigger in girth than the mannequins in maternity shop windows or the models in the popular pregnancy magazines. Somehow, this, too, came as a shock. Unconsciously, I had taken these images to be the conclusive shape of pregnancy. Now that I had expanded beyond them, I realized that I'd been tricked into seeing the shape of mid-gestation as the finale. Once I figured this out, I could appreciate my new dimensions. My body is no longer represented by advertisers. I am undepicted, on my own, in some wilder territory.

The next morning—or rather, some hours after we closed the curtains and lay down for a while—I learn something else about the shape of late pregnancy. It has the power to change people's minds on all kinds of topics. Including whether or not they should kill you.

Turning left onto a highway south of Anchorage, Jeff fails to see an asphalt-gray Corvette speeding around an oversized SUV whose driver has motioned for us to proceed. Through a series of deft maneuvers on the part of drivers heading in both directions, no one is hit, which seems like some kind of miracle. The Corvette disappears. Jeff continues the turn, waving at those who made room for us to swerve. We drive in silence for a few moments, grateful and terrified at what almost happened. And then we see the same Corvette bombing up behind us, its bumper suddenly inches from ours. Jeff pulls onto the shoulder. So does the Corvette. Its door flies open before the car even stops, and we hear someone yell, "I have a license to carry concealed firearms!"

For some reason, this declaration causes me to open the door of the rental car and step outside. I am acting on pure instinct. My hands upturned in the manner of St. Francis, I begin to talk.

"Thank you so much for not hitting us. We are so sorry. We just arrived in Alaska and we are very sorry. Thank you very much and we are very sorry."

The words come out slowly, as if in a dream. What I notice of the figure running toward me is matted hair, bulging neck veins, military boots, and a surprising number of facial piercings. I don't think to look for weapons. He is screaming epithets as he charges.

"I'm so sorry. Thank you so much for not hitting us. We pulled out in front of you. We really are sorry."

He stops and stares. I keep talking, trying for soothing, reassuring tones. Gradually I become aware that he's not listening at all but, instead, has become transfixed by my enormous belly, which swells out from rib to pubic bone.

I quit talking. The screaming I still hear is the chorus of some death-rock anthem pouring from the Corvette's wide-open door. Its driver continues to examine my stomach. Each of his eyebrows is studded with a row of metal rings.

He shakes his head slowly. Then he starts to cry.

He walks backward toward the Corvette. The door slams. He peels out. I get back in the car.

I'm glad Jeff had the good sense to stay put. We sit quietly for a while.

Finally Jeff says, "You were amazing."

"The funny part is, I didn't do anything."

"But the things you said were amazing."

"He didn't hear me. He just needed to see me."

Jeff rests his head against the steering wheel.

"I'm supposed to protect you and the baby."

"It wouldn't have worked. This time she protected us."

Alaska is the last leg of my lecture tour. I am here at the invitation of citizen groups investigating environmental contamination. In a workshop outside Anchorage, Pamela K. Miller of Alaska Community Action on Toxics passes out color maps of toxic hot spots in the state. It has taken years to bring together data from federal and state right-to-know inventories with information once considered off limits by the military. Alaska is honeycombed with toxic sites, including nine chemical weapons dumps, fifteen radioactive waste sites, six Superfund sites, and 1,668 chemically contaminated areas reported by the Alaska Department of Environmental Conservation. Especially dense with toxic sites is that graceful thread of islands connecting North America to Asia, the Aleutian archipelago. Pam quietly guides us through the patterns of dots and *x*'s and red triangles indicating exactly where these sites are located and how they came to be there. She assumes the same gentle, patient tone of voice that I've heard members of the clergy use when addressing issues surrounded by public denial and private distress.

Of particular interest to Pam and her colleagues is a class of synthetic chemicals that shows up over and over at these sites. These are known as POPs: persistent organic pollutants. They are receiving a lot of attention. Just a few weeks earlier, representatives of the world's nations, under a mandate from the United Nations itself, began negotiating an international treaty to deal with twelve of the most dangerous POPs, with the ultimate hope of abolishing them from the planet altogether. Whatever the outcome, the very existence of the talks is an admission that the dangers posed by these chemicals cannot be contained by all the usual methods of environmental regulation—by filtering, scrubbing, burying, burning, diluting, dredging, storing, exporting, or evaporating them. POPs cannot be effectively managed because by their very nature they are unmanageable substances.

In spite of the happy-sounding acronym—who could fear a substance called a POP?—the name reveals some of the reasons behind these chemicals' apparently unreformable temperament. The middle *O*, for "organic," means that all the members of this family have a carbon skeleton, which also means they tend to be soluble in fat. The only objects in the natural world that contain fat are living organisms. Therefore, when POPs are released in small quantities into the general environment, they become pulled into the oily bodies of plants and animals, where they quickly take up residence. This phenomenon also means that our main route of exposure to POPs is through the food chain—by eating, an activity that is not exactly optional. Certain POPs have chlorine atoms added to their carbon spines, and this makes these POPs even more fat-soluble and therefore more attracted to our bodies. It is no coincidence, then, that all twelve POP chemicals singled out for action by the U.N. treaty negotiators are chlorinated ones.

The first *P*, for "persistent," means that POPs are long-lived. Because few organisms possess the enzymes sufficient to break POPs' molecules apart, they are resistant to degradation. This characteristic has several implications. One is that you accumulate POPs faster than you can excrete them. The older you get, the more POPs you amass. (Excretion depends on enzymatic breakdown into water-soluble components.) And because their life spans often exceed the length of a human generation—twenty to thirty years—POPs are passed from mother to child during pregnancy and breastfeeding. The older the mother, the more POPs her baby receives. The *P* and the *O* together—longevity plus fat-solubility—means POPs biomagnify as they move through the food chain. In aquatic systems, as we have seen, powers of concentration on the journey from plankton to human can reach a millionfold as one link of the food chain feeds the next and the next and the next. Placed at most risk are large predatory animals and human infants, both of whom live at the end of the line.

The last P, "pollutant," means that POPs are toxic. Even in small concentrations, they disrupt a whole slew of normal biological processes in ways that can promote cancer, suppress the immune system, and interfere with brain functioning, fertility, and fetal development. The urgency that drives the international negotiations—and our local workshop here in Alaska—comes from the recent discovery that laboratory animals show harmful effects of exposure at or near levels to which humans in the general population are exposed. This is especially true for embryological effects.

The fact that everyone on earth now carries around POPs in their body fat can only be explained by another characteristic of this chemical tribe: most are semivolatile. Officially, this means that their boiling point exceeds 150° centigrade. (That's 50 degrees higher than the boiling point of water, 100° C.) Practically, this means that POPs evaporate slowly when the weather is warm and condense quickly when temperatures fall. Which means POPs are global travelers: they ride in the wind as an invisible vapor, rising up from the tropical and temperate areas and then precipitating back to earth in cooler zones. Semivolatility plus resistance to atmospheric breakdown means that northern regions are net accumulators of POPs. Indeed, the Arctic serves as their final repository. The obscure quality of semivolatility is what makes POPs a human rights issue worthy of deliberation by the United Nations. No government acting alone can protect its citizens from the harmful effects of POPs. They are poisons that leave nations that use them and enter those that do not. Yet nations have a duty to do no harm to citizens of other countries with which they are not at war.

Who are the POPs exactly? The three most famous members of the clan are the pesticide DDT, the industrial oils called PCBs, and dioxin, the elusive, undesired by-product of waste incineration and certain chlorine-using manufacturing processes. The other nine taken up by the international negotiating committee are aldrin, dieldrin, endrin, chlordane, heptachlor, mirex, toxaphene, hexachlorobenzene, and furans. The good news is that effective replacements are available for many of these products, or are within reach. For example, turnip oil turns out to be a great hydraulic fluid, meaning that PCBs can be retired from hydraulic duty. The main use for chlordane, heptachlor, aldrin, and mirex—all pesticides—is to protect wooden foundations from termite attacks; but stainless-steel mesh can also keep termites at bay. Indeed, most of the chemicals covered by the treaty have already been phased out of use by industrialized nations. The problem is that poor nations lack the resources needed to take similar steps. In both rich and poor nations, POPs already released into the environment disintegrate slowly and travel readily.

The uninvited airborne arrival of POPs into Alaska from Asia, Russia, the lower forty-eight states, and Mexico is a well-known problem to many people at today's workshop. Pam's maps, however, tell of local sources as well. Many of these are long-abandoned military facilities that are located in close proximity to Alaskan native communities and their traditional hunting and fishing grounds. Some of these old military bases are now used as hunting and fishing camps for tourists. At one such former Air Force station, located north of the Brooks Range in northern Alaska, the landfill still brims with PCBs, and the fish downstream show elevated levels of DDT.

Another Arctic source of POPs is the sites making up the Distant Early Warning (DEW) line, established during the Cold War. This line once consisted of sixty-three radar stations strung along the 66th Parallel from Alaska to Greenland. Military personnel assigned to these outposts on the ice-bound land spent their days watching for Soviet attacks from the north. The DEW line now seeds POPs into the surrounding ecosystem from leaking drums and derelict equipment left behind when its facilities were bolted up and forsaken.

There is another source of POPs in inland Alaska, so obvious that no one thought to consider it until very recently: the flesh of migrating salmon. Out in the open ocean, salmon accumulate fat—and therefore POPs—to prepare for the long run through freshwater streams to the spawning lakes at their headwaters. As the journey commences, this fat is burned for fuel, but the indestructible POPs remain in the fishes' bodies. Once their eggs and sperm are shed, the spent salmon die; their carcasses decay and are picked apart by other fish, who then take up the salmon's burden of POPs. Via this bio-transport, salmon can introduce POPs into pristine areas hundreds of miles from crumbling military bases or other dump sites.

A new study of migrating sockeye salmon in Alaska's Copper River shows how this happens. Researchers looked at POP concentrations in grayling, a predatory lake fish that does not migrate but that happily eats salmon eggs when they are available, and in other fish that feed on salmon carcasses. Grayling living in lakes where salmon spawn had more than double the levels of PCBs and DDT than did grayling in a nearby salmon-free lake. In this study, bio-transport had a far bigger influence on POP levels in the lake than long-distance atmospheric input—even though the salmon themselves had levels of pollutants far below those that would trigger a fish advisory.

Alaskans have good reason to worry about POPs: wildlife in other northern areas of the globe, such as Scandinavia, are beginning to exhibit problems that are consistent with what we know about POPs' health effects. One of these is the disruption of sex hormones, which can result in malformed reproductive organs, abnormal mating behaviors, or an inability to maintain pregnancy. Another is disruption of immunity, which can result in death from parasites or infectious diseases that otherwise might be kept in check. Both of these problems are thought to be responsible for population declines among marine mammals in other northern habitats. For example, researchers in England and Wales have discovered an association between PCB levels in porpoises and infectious disease mortality: porpoises that died of infections had significantly higher PCB levels than those that drowned in fishing nets. Highly contaminated Baltic seals frequently have malformed uteruses, and researchers in the Swedish Arctic report increasing numbers of hermaphroditic polar bears, specifically, females with functioning penises. Polar bears, which eat seals, are thought to be the most POP-contaminated species on the planet.

Whether these problems also afflict Alaskan wildlife is not completely clear, but important clues are emerging. Populations of

transient orca whales are declining in the waters off the Kenai Peninsula. When researchers sampled their blubber with biopsy darts,
they found levels of DDT and PCBs comparable to those found in
the beluga whales living in the highly contaminated St. Lawrence
River, a population that has failed to reproduce for decades. It is not
yet known in what geographic region the Alaskan orcas accumulated
their burden of POPs. Some may be of Asian origin; some may be
from local military sites leaking into coastal waters.

The orcas are not the only carriers of high POP concentrations. Sea otters on the Aleutian islands also carry high body burdens of PCBs, and they are disappearing rapidly. Researchers suspect local sources are responsible for at least some of the problem.
Two of the islands in the Aleutian chain are among the most PCB-
contaminated sites in North America—a legacy of their history as
sites for military bases in the war against Japan more than half a
century ago. On three of the islands, blue mussels, a staple in the
otter diet, are likewise contaminated.

All Alaskans wonder what message the polar bears, otters, seals,
and whales have for them, but no one is more concerned than indigenous peoples who rely on fish and wildlife for food. Traditional
Arctic diets, which rely heavily on seal and whale, are highly nutritious and provide all the vitamins and minerals needed for human
health. And yet, ironically, those who consume such diets are
among the most chemically contaminated people on earth. There
are three interlocking reasons for this. One is the slow, inexorable
gravitation of POPs to cold places. From here they cannot evaporate again. The second is the high fat content in the bodies of Arctic animals. Fat draws the condensed, precipitated POPs out of the
annual snow melt and into the food chain. The third is the long
length of the food chains in marine ecosystems. Their many links
allow the forces of biomagnification to work unhindered. (On land,
the food chain has three, or at most four, links, whereas aquatic
systems can easily support food chains of six links or more.)

At the end of the all-day workshop, the sun is still blazing, and I'm
exhausted. I ask Pam a few last questions about her maps and pack up
to leave. On my way out, I'm approached by a woman who has been
watching me intently for some time. It's too late to pretend I haven't

seen her, so I vow to myself to keep the conversation short. She points down at the liter bottle I'm carrying, still half full of water.

"You're not drinking enough," she says, authoritatively.

Before I can formulate a reply, she lets me know that she's a midwife who practices in a small rural clinic nearby. Her name is Yolanda Meza. Many of the mothers whose births she assists are native women, and her concern for their health is the reason she attends presentations on toxic chemical exposures.

"How are you feeling?" Yolanda asks, as though I had just walked into her examination room.

Before I know it, I'm describing to her my recent worry—that I haven't felt a lot of fetal movement. Rather than reassure me that everything is probably fine, she listens closely to my descriptions of when and how the baby usually kicks and then invites me to her office nearby, even though it's after hours and on a weekend.

Thus, Jeff and I follow a battered old car down a series of ever smaller roads flanked by ever larger trees. The Alaskan concept of "nearby," I soon realize, is quite different from my own. At least, I console myself, we won't have to find our way back in the dark. At last we pull into a gravelly turnoff in front of a low, nondescript building. Yolanda unlocks the door, and we all step inside.

Boston's Beth Israel Hospital it is not. Nothing gleams. Cabinets do not open with a neat click. Computer monitors do not fill the desks. Even the telephone is old. The sun-filled room into which Jeff and I are ushered looks like someone's bedroom. No large pieces of equipment fill the corners. Slowly, I become aware of how different a prenatal checkup feels when the trappings of medical technology are removed. Whenever I sit on an examination table with stirrups bolted to one end, I am overwhelmed with anxious passivity, no matter what the occasion. In the presence of plastic tubing and partitioning curtains, I shed my identity and become someone else—a patient who responds obediently but who can't formulate intelligent follow-up questions. But in this room, I am still myself.

"Let's see how she lies," suggests Yolanda after she measures the distance from my pubic bone to the top ledge of my uterus— now nearly as high as my rib cage—and pronounces the distance to be exactly on target for my particular week of pregnancy.

Each fetus has a characteristic "lie," the position it comes to assume in the womb during late pregnancy. Fetal lie is determined by Leopold maneuvers. These involve palpating the uterus in a prescribed, sequential fashion. My obstetrician runs through the Leopold maneuvers as a kind of quick ritual at the beginning of each appointment, chatting with me all the while. I sometimes suspect she is just going through the motions. Yolanda, however, takes much more time with them, and she works in silence. I'm aware that her hands are actually reading my body—and the body within my body. Watching her work is like watching a baker knead dough.

The first maneuver determines which part of the baby is in the fundus, the large upper end of the uterus. It involves palpating the top of the uterus, which feels like a hard, muscular shelf. There is usually one of two possible answers: the head or the bottom. A head feels hard and round; a bottom, softer and less symmetrical. In my case, the answer is the bottom. Which is good.

The second maneuver focuses on the left and right sides of the uterus, to establish which side the baby's back is on, left or right. Yolanda's fingers work up and down my abdomen, pushing one way, pushing another. The back feels like a continuous ridge. The side opposite the back should feel bumpy because it contains a collection of small parts—hands, feet, elbows, knees. The answer today: the right side. This makes sense, as the few kicks and jabs I do feel are most often up under my rib cage on the left.

The third maneuver determines which body part is in the symphysis, the space just above the thick horizontal bar of the pubic bone. Yolanda palpates this area. Once again, the usual answer is either heads or tails. Near to birth, however, as the baby begins to descend deeper into the bony cradle of the pelvis, the answer is sometimes neck or shoulder. As Yolanda's fingers push upward, I feel the baby's entire body shift within me.

"Well, she's definitely head down," she announces definitively. "Here, I'll show you."

She places my fingers on either side of the hard, hair-covered mound under the curve of my belly and asks me to push back and forth, as though passing a ball from one hand to another. I do feel it. A baby's head. Just above my pubic bone, there is a baby's head.

Before I can recover from my astonishment, she places an ultrasound transducer on the lower right side of my belly. Immediately, the sound of a beating heart fills the room. All three of us listen for a few minutes. Yolanda says she is happy with the accelerations in rate that occur from time to time. If I am still worried, or if the baby's movements continue to slow over the next couple of days, I should check into the clinic in Homer, which is the next stop on my tour. Ask for a nonstress test, she says. In the meantime, she continues firmly, drink plenty of water. She then laughingly refuses our attempts to pay her and waves us out the door.

Of the dozen POPs whose fate is being deliberated by the world's nations, the one that has received the most attention from embryologists is the group called PCBs—polychlorinated biphenyls. This is because they injure not only the fetal immune system but also—like lead and mercury—the fetal brain.

PCBs are the mules of the chemical world. Colorless and viscous, they refuse to conduct electricity, to burn, or to alter their behavior in response to changes in pH. Invented in the late 1920s, they quickly made themselves useful in fire extinguishers and as liquid insulators. PCBs were also poured into the ballasts of fluorescent lights and other kinds of equipment where bursting into flames was not a desirable outcome. Their uses expanded to include hydraulic fluid and microscope immersion oil (which allows for brighter, clearer views of some very tiny specimens and to which I have had considerable exposure since childhood). PCBs have also been added to ink, paint, and carbonless copy paper.

Once inside the human body, PCBs continue to resist metabolic transformation and will remain in human fat for twenty-five to seventy-five years. In this they are very different from methylmercury, whose residency lasts a few years at most. As with all POPs, more than 90 percent of our exposure comes from diet, with freshwater fish the source of the highest exposures. Dairy and meat also contribute. Of all mammals, humans are the slowest to excrete and eliminate PCBs, and there is no method known that can speed up this process. Various treatments have been tried, including fasting and saunas; none has worked to lower body burdens. All residents of industrialized countries are now thought to carry some level of PCBs in their tissues.

If PCBs remained as inert inside our bodies as they do inside transformers and capacitors, we would have less to worry about.

But, biologically speaking, they are quite reactive. Just how reactive became apparent in 1968 when PCBs accidentally leaked into cooking oil in Japan. Children born to mothers who consumed the contaminated oil during their pregnancy showed behavioral disorders and were of below normal intelligence. An uncannily similar accident in Taiwan a decade later resulted in almost identical problems: children exposed prenatally showed profound developmental delays and mental deficits. Furthermore, so did children born several years *after* their mothers were exposed. In the wake of these findings, PCB production in the United States ceased in 1976. Although no consumer product now on the market is made with PCBs, much older electrical equipment, especially that in use by industry, still contains this oily fluid. So, of course, does all the scrapped equipment rusting away in landfills and out back on old military bases. Indeed, the quantity of PCBs still in use plus the quantity still languishing in waste dumps exceeds the total amount that has already escaped into the general environment. Without a program to recall and contain them, semivolatile PCBs will continue to insinuate themselves into the food chain for decades to come.

The children in Japan and Taiwan were exposed to impressively high levels of PCBs. Looking at the tragic results, fetal toxicologists began to wonder what effects might exist at background levels, levels found among members of the general population not directly victimized by industrial accidents. Beginning in the late 1970s, a series of studies was launched to investigate this question. The results of these various investigations largely corroborate each other.

One study was conducted in North Carolina. More than 900 pregnant women agreed to participate. When they eventually gave birth, samples of blood were collected from their babies' umbilical cords. Then, at various points in their development, their children were run through a series of psychomotor tests. The results showed a clear correlation between prenatal PCB exposure and poor performance, especially in gross motor function, memory, and visual recognition. The higher the level of PCBs in cord blood, the worse a child's score. After toddlerhood, these deficits disappeared. A significant finding was that a mother's consumption of contaminated fish was strongly predictive of poor early performance by her offspring.

Another study came out of western Michigan. Researchers recruited 200 mothers who, before and during their pregnancies, had eaten fish caught from Lake Michigan. Their children were compared with those of mothers living in the same area who didn't eat lake fish. After socioeconomic factors, maternal age, drinking, smoking, breastfeeding, and number of other children were all corrected for, the investigators found that PCB levels in the babies increased with the amount of fish consumed by the mothers. Moreover, children most highly exposed as fetuses showed delayed development and cognitive deficits that persisted well beyond toddlerhood (in contrast to the findings of the North Carolina study). Even at eleven years old, the children most highly exposed to PCBs during their prenatal lives were three times more likely to have below-average IQ scores and twice as likely to be two years behind in reading comprehension. Clearly, as the study concluded, "*[I]n utero* exposure to PCBs in concentrations slightly higher than those in the general public can have long-term impact on intellectual function."

Two lakes east from Lake Michigan is Lake Ontario, on whose south bank is the city of Oswego, New York. This is the location for the most recent PCB study, which is still ongoing. Using a study design similar to that used in Michigan, researchers are finding similar results. Oswego mothers who eat fish from Lake Ontario have higher PCB levels, and these are associated with poorer neurological functioning in their babies. More specifically, newborns at the high end of exposure have poorer autonomic regulation, decreased responsiveness, and more abnormal reflexes. This group of children is still being followed to determine if these deficits persist (as in Michigan) or eventually resolve themselves (as in North Carolina).

Meanwhile, in the Netherlands, a number of carefully constructed long-term studies have been completed on Dutch mothers and their children. I became particularly interested in these because I know that one of the principal investigators is not only a topflight researcher but a new mother herself. By the time I read the conclusions she drew from her study, I wonder why the issue of POPs is not discussed in every prenatal clinic on earth:

> Among 18-month-old children, we found a negative effect of prenatal PCB exposure on neurological development. . . . Prenatal exposure to PCBs was found to have an adverse impact on general cognitive development and play behavior. . . . PCB body burden at 42 months negatively influenced attentional processes in preschool

children. . . . Thus, early exposure to PCBs has long-term negative effects on most aspects of child development.

Under the large, blocky body of mainland Alaska, the Kenai Peninsula hangs like a stretched-out mitten. On the west side is Cook Inlet, named for none other than Captain James Cook, who sailed through it in 1776 looking for the elusive Northwest Passage. This wasn't it. In fact, the voyage was Cook's last; he would soon be slain on a beach in Hawaii. On the east side of the peninsula lies Prince William Sound, the site of an even more star-crossed voyage. In 1989, the tanker *Exxon Valdez* spilled 38 million liters of crude oil into the sound in an accident whose ecological effects are still felt on the Kenai.

In a one-day journey that we hope will prove luckier than either of those, we are traveling down the Cook Inlet side of the peninsula, heading for the town of Homer. The first thing we notice is that the highway has no exits. It's the only road there is. The next thing we notice is how thin this thoroughfare seems—not because its lanes are unusually narrow or few in number but because the world crowds up against it. Just to our left, Dall sheep pose along the exposed cliffs. On the other side, moose swim through thickets of willow and birch, antlers just visible above the branches. The streams and rivers we cross over are crowded with fishermen and running salmon. Fishing buoys hang from fences. Fireweed blooms in every open patch of ground.

There is no other world than this one. It's a notion that first occurs to me while I'm scanning a menu in a roadside restaurant in Soldotna, a coastal town that was once a Russian fur-trading outpost. The choices basically boil down to delicious just-caught salmon or mushy spaghetti with canned tomato sauce. When we finally arrive in Homer and stop for supplies, we are faced with similar options. The imported produce in the grocery store is expensive and shriveled. By contrast, the charter boats docked at the spit are unloading fresh halibut the size of garage doors. I realize how unaccustomed I am to the stark contrast between local and long-distance food items.

I have lived in plenty of places where the locally produced food is too contaminated to eat—catfish from the Illinois River, flounder from Boston Harbor—but there was always an infinite number of other choices. How easy it is to dismiss the loss of garden-grown carrots in Somerville when local supermarkets offer plenty of cheap, good-looking vegetables trucked in from elsewhere. How easy it is to sit on the banks of the unfishable, undrinkable rivers of Illinois while munching a McDonald's Filet-O-Fish and sipping bottled water. But in rural Alaska "elsewhere" is so remote from life here as to be irrelevant. The food from this place has to feed me and my baby for another week. The food from this place will become the body of my baby. It is irreplaceable.

There is no other world than this one.

In Homer, we are guests of Ed Bailey and Nina Faust, biologist and mathematician, respectively, who have spent years studying birds on the Aleutian Islands. Their house is located high on the promontory overlooking Kachemak Bay, an inlet within the inlet. Out their back window is a postcard view of ocean and forested mountains. Nina points out the glacier in between two of the highest peaks. Glaciers, of course, are the immediate reason for Illinois's wide-open landscape, and I've learned about them since grade school. Whenever annual snowfall exceeds annual snowmelt, a glacier starts forming. As the snow piles up and turns to ice, internal pressures begin to move it in whatever direction downhill happens to be. I've always imagined glaciers as icy bulldozers, scouring and churning the earth as they advance. But this one looks more like a deep, slow river.

The night before my lecture, I can't sleep, and so I come out to the picture window. In the indistinguishable glow that is either twilight or dawn, the glacier is a translucent lavender bowl. Just seeing it fills me with such peace that I wrap a quilt around me and perch on the back of the couch to look at it for a while. Within me, the baby remains quiet. I remember that Yolanda encouraged me to keep a count of fetal movements. In any given twenty-minute interval, she said, the baby should move at least twice. I don't have a watch on, but I decide I can probably estimate pretty accurately. Twenty minutes is about half a lecture.

Most women experience weeks twenty-nine through thirty-eight of pregnancy as the period of maximum fetal activity. The baby's nervous system is well developed, and yet it still has room enough to move freely. Just before we left Boston, I noticed that my baby was developing a rhythm to her day that was different from mine. She slept later than I did, waking only after I had finished breakfast. Her biggest movements—turns and twists and repositionings—came late in the afternoon. Then she sprang into motion again just as I was lying down to sleep.

Childbirth anthropologists call this growing awareness of a two-in-one-self "motherselfhood." It's the sensation that one is now inhabited by another conscious being whose moods, needs, and habits are not identical to one's own. What I am experiencing in Alaska during my seventh month of pregnancy is another kind of identity shift. Call it mother-earth-hood: an awareness of how my own doubled self is contained within the body of the world. The same snow that falls on the glacier across the bay also fills Ed and Nina's well, from which I drink, and in my so doing it becomes the well from which the baby drinks, too. The glacier's meltwater fills the inlet that feeds the fish on which we two both feed. Prenatal care means taking care of water, fish, and glaciers. *There is no other world than this one.*

There! I feel a shimmy! Another shimmy! And two kicks in quick succession! I laugh out loud. Across the bay, the glacier pours itself slowly into the sea.

Of the many dangers that PCBs pose for human health perhaps the most insidious is their ability to lead astray thyroid hormones.

Thyroid hormone is essential during fetal brain development. We know this because infants born with thyroid deficiencies are at risk for mental retardation, as are children born to mothers with lower than normal levels of thyroid hormone. The evidence for a brain-thyroid connection goes back a long way. Members of the Clinical Society of London alerted the British medical community to the relationship between thyroid disease and congenital feeble-mindedness as long ago as 1888. They called it cretinism.

At first glance, brains and thyroids seem unlikely conspirators. Located just below the voice box, the thyroid gland secretes iodine-laden molecules of thyroxine, which are then ferried through the bloodstream by special carrier proteins. Like bicycle messengers, these proteins deliver thyroxine to cells throughout the body, where, among other tasks, it quickens the pace at which oxygen is burned. Stimulating oxygen consumption raises metabolic rate, which in turn helps maintain a high body temperature. In an adult, none of these activities has directly to do with the electrical firing of the brain. However, in a fetus, the story is much different. Here, the carrier proteins speed thyroxine directly into the tissues of the developing brain, where the hormone spurs all kinds of projects: the migration of neurons, the spidery growth of axons and dendrites, the wrapping of myelin insulation around these webs of electrical connections, and the creation of synaptic junctions. A grown person who is short on thyroxine will experience slow heart rate, sensitivity to cold, fatigue, and puffy cheeks, but a fetus in the same situation will lose brain functioning. Adult symptoms are reversible; fetal damage is not.

The exact source of fetal thyroxine is still a mystery. The brain appears to require it as early as the first trimester, but the fetus's own thyroid gland is not up and running until mid-gestation. Presumably, the fetus obtains thyroxine from its mother until it is able to make its own. In other words, a few short months ago, hormones produced by a gland in my own throat were carried across my placenta and into the body of my daughter, where they helped direct the creation of her mind. A more noble assignment my seldom-regarded thyroid has never had.

PCBs prevent thyroid hormones from attaching to their carrier proteins. Unattached molecules of thyroxine are not deliverable: they are flushed from the body and never reach the fetal brain. This appears to be the means by which prenatal PCB exposure extinguishes human intelligence, the capacity for language, and the ability to pay attention.

The sign over the front door to the Homer hospital reads PLEASE REMOVE ICE CLEATS BEFORE ENTERING. I've decided to come in for a nonstress test, despite my feeling that everything is probably okay. The baby has quieted down again. Also, I now feel a strange twitching—like a spastic eyelid—deep inside my uterus. It's come and gone since yesterday, and it doesn't feel like fetal movement. The nursing staff is more than happy to accommodate me. It's not a busy shift. No one's having a baby in Homer today.

I'm led into a labor and delivery room. Although the obstetrical unit is a small one, I am nevertheless back in the land of tubes and curtains and pieces of large machinery parked in corners. And although the nurses are nice enough, none of them touches me the way Yolanda did. The difference becomes immediately apparent during the search for the fetal heartbeat. Yolanda has been the only one of my many caregivers who could locate it immediately. The staff today spend considerable time gliding the black transducer back and forth, up and down, heads cocked to one side. I feel all the old anxiety rush back in the long seconds before rapid, unmistakable thumping pours out of the amplifier. By trial and error, they eventually stumble on it in the exact same spot—down and to the right—where Yolanda somehow knew to find it right off.

The mystery of the episodic twitching is solved immediately: fetal hiccups. Very normal, I'm assured.

A nonstress test is a twenty-minute procedure that uses ultrasound not to create a visual image of the fetus but to monitor the activity of the fetal heart. "Stress," in this case, refers to the pressure of uterine contractions during labor. A nonstress test, therefore, is one that takes place in the weeks before labor's onset. The premise behind the test is that changes in heart rate are an indirect measure of fetal activity. Because the fetal nervous system is immature, the heart beats faster in response to physical exertion. As adults, we are pleased when our hearts are not reactive to exercise. A slow, steady heart rate is a sign of physical fitness; a racing pulse after mounting the stairs is not. But with fetuses, fast and erratic is good. Lots of sudden accelerations mean both that the placenta has adequate oxygen reserves and that the fetus is active. At 120 to 160 beats per minute, a baseline fetal heart rate is double that of an adult. What we want to see in this little birthing room is a minimum of one acceleration that exceeds the baseline by 15 beats and lasts at least fifteen seconds.

The nurse attaches two stretchy bands over my exposed belly. The first is down low and holds a transducer tight against the place where the fetal heartbeat was located a few minutes earlier. This sends out a beam of ultrasonic energy and records the returning echo. The echo is then converted into an audio signal as well as a mechanical one that moves an ink-filled nib across a moving scroll of paper. The resulting trace is a diagram of fetal cardiac activity. The second band is attached up high. It also presses a black disc tight against my abdomen, but this is a passive receiver. It records uterine activity—the weak contractions that periodically sweep across the surface and that are too faint for me to feel—and likewise leaves a wavering line along the turning drum of paper. Were I in labor, the two parallel traces could tell us how strong the contractions are and how well the baby is tolerating them.

The only other marks recorded on the graph are the ones I leave myself. The nurse gives me a hand-held gadget with a red button to push, as though I were a contestant on a game show. If I feel the baby move, I am to depress the button, which will leave a mark on the cardiac trace. In this way, we can judge how the baby's heart responds to exertion.

After reassuring me that there is still plenty of time to airlift me to Anchorage "if we have to take the baby," the nurse leaves the room. Alone, I instantly hate this procedure in which I am both subject and scribe. I try to concentrate on fetal movement but get distracted by the sound of the baby's heart as it pours out of the enormous machine, which has been wheeled from its corner and into the center of the room expressly for this purpose. A baby in a machine. It is an eerie displacement. The whole experience transports me back to the day of my cancer diagnosis when I lay in a hospital bed just like this one, strung up with cords and cables, burning with fury.

Why did I sign up for this?

Nonstress tests are good early warning systems, I remind myself. However disconnected they make me feel from my own baby and my own body, they can serve to enhance human perception. Ultrasound can detect fetal movement during the second month of pregnancy, even though the quickening does not occur until months four or five. The first movement is the pulse of the cardiac muscle. Thereafter, fetal movement starts at the top of the body and moves progressively downward over time: first the head bobs, then the trunk wiggles, then the legs kick. Thus, the heartbeat is detectable at six weeks, head rotations at about seven weeks, and the rising and falling motions of breathing at ten weeks. When the fetus is in trouble, movements are lost in the same order that they first developed: accelerations in heart rate are the first to go, then breathing motions, then limb movements. This is why nonstress tests can identify problems early.

Finally, the test is over, and my scroll of paper shows plenty of fetal activity and lots of squiggly leaps and stutter steps in the graph's cardiac trace. On the uterine front, all is quiet, with no signs of premature labor. Perhaps, the obstetrical team suggests, the baby has simply rolled over so that her kicks and pokes are directed back instead of out and are therefore less noticeable. Or perhaps the four-hour time change between Boston and Alaska has thrown our sleep-wake cycles out of sync with each other. Or perhaps, speculates another, the endless daylight here has somehow quieted her down. In any case, all agree, according to the data the baby looks fine.

That's all I need to hear. Within minutes I am back outside, walking among black spruce trees where everything is growing and growing in unceasing light.

8

Green Corn Moon

*B*oston. August. The air blurs and thickens. Trees drone with cicadas. Our third-floor apartment fills up with fans and extension cords and lots of discussion as to exactly how and where they should be placed and which windows should be opened or closed at which times of day or night in an elaborate and mostly futile campaign to draw a cooling breeze through our three small rooms. Real relief comes only when the westerly winds turn around, and a steady sea breeze blows through the east windows, levitating the gauze curtains. On those nights, we sit out late on the balcony, eating ice cream straight from the box. We are invariably joined by my dog and Jeff's two elderly cat sisters, who now leave the cool tiled bathroom floor only after the sun goes down.

As my thirty-ninth birthday approaches, all physical evidence of my own birth vanishes. I no longer have a navel. The space it once occupied is now a flat, purply, translucent disk the size of a silver dollar. A porthole made of skin. It is so thin, I feel I should be able to peer through it and see what is going on in there. It looks like the round window on a front-loading washing machine, Jeff teases. If I tap on it, the baby kicks back, but doing so makes me queasy.

Other parts of my body are also becoming unrecognizable. My fingers and ankles are puffed into sausagelike shapes that no longer resemble the originals. When I wake up, the hand lying on the pillow looks like a stranger's. So do the feet that walk me to the bathroom. Before my very eyes, I am turning into someone else.

In the middle of the month, we start childbirth education classes. Led by an obstetrical nurse who works in Beth Israel's maternity ward, they're taught right at the hospital. On the first day, I'm way too excited. At the corner store, I buy a new notebook just for the occasion and two new pens. I'm eager to meet other pregnant women whose birthing calendars roughly approximate mine. I imagine us comparing notes, cheering each other on, and performing silly exercises intended to get us in touch with our inner warriors. Boston, after all, is the city that produced the women's health manifesto, *Our Bodies, Ourselves*. I start brushing up on the birth chapters in the old edition I've saved since college.

"Do you think our instructor will make us roar like lions?" I ask Jeff on the car ride to the hospital. "Do you think I should start practicing now?"

My insufferable enthusiasm requires that Jeff take on an air of skepticism and reserve.

"Let's just take things one step at a time."

I'm quickly divested of my expectations. We're a large group—there are twelve other couples—and a diverse one. Black, white, Latino, the age range is about twenty to forty. What unites the class—and separates Jeff and me from the rest—is fear. During the introductions, nearly every woman expresses how afraid she is of labor. One proclaims that all she wants to know is when she can get anesthesia. This brings nervous laughter all around. Another says, "I'm just really scared," and bursts into tears. This elicits sympathetic nods. The fathers-to-be don't have much to say for themselves, except that they are here to support their wives. They project a kind of blank awkwardness. Jeff and I exchange looks. Have we missed something? When it is my turn, I say as calmly as I can that I hope to have a natural childbirth. There is a moment of silence—no nodding of heads—and then the mother next to me clears her throat, states her first name, and says she has a really low tolerance for pain.

Now it's the teacher's turn to speak. Her name is Michelle. She is young, blond, and deeply tanned. Like a popular gym teacher or aerobics instructor, she has a confident, jocky manner about her.

She refers to us collectively as moms and dads. Michelle immediately puts the men at ease with sports jokes and stories about dads so engrossed with the NBA finals they fail to notice their wives panting away in active labor. The husbands in the room visibly relax. However hapless they feel, they are quite sure they won't be that oblivious. Michelle quickly wins over the dads.

As for us moms, Michelle outlines the curriculum for the next six weeks of classes. First we'll learn the basic stages of labor and birth. Then we'll become familiar with the medical procedures that often accompany them: epidurals, episiotomies, external monitoring, internal monitoring, stress tests, forceps deliveries, pitocin drips, amniotomies, and cesarean sections. These discussions will fill most of our class time together. Along the way we'll visit the labor and delivery unit, learn breathing exercises to help us stay focused, and see some videotapes of actual births. She issues a couple of warnings, too. One: We should all pay close attention to the information on cesarean sections. Even though no one ever *wants* a c-section, the fact is that 20 percent of laboring women receive them, which means at least two moms in this room are likely to have their babies this way. Two: As valuable as the breathing techniques are, they don't take the pain away. "Labor hurts," she finishes simply.

Back at home, I repair to the balcony. The master of cross-ventilation, Jeff opens the door to the fire escape, adjusts the transom, turns on the fans, and then follows me outside, carrying two quart-sized drums of ice cream and two spoons. He hands me one of each and settles into a lawn chair with the other set. The breeze is delicious. I turn so it blows against the back of my neck. Inside the apartment, white curtains float sideways, like a magician's trick. The bay window in the bedroom is missing a gauze panel. Its absence is deliberate, intended to remind me of the night Jeff and I fell in love.

It was midsummer. After a long date at a jazz club, we walked back to my apartment. There was a moon, an ocean breeze, a box of ice cream, wine. We undressed each other slowly. There was Billie Holiday, candlelight, the scent of roses. The wind blew through the open windows. And then, just as we were standing skin to skin for the first time, one of the curtains fluttered over one of the candles. There was a soft *poof*, like the sound of a cork being pulled from a bottle. Suddenly, the window was a sheet of fire. In the slow-motion seconds that followed, I watched my new lover vault across the bed and tear the burning cloth from the rod. And this is my first memory of Jeff without clothes on: a naked juggler rolling an enormous ball of light in his hands. The flaming sphere grew smaller, smaller, darker, darker, until it disappeared altogether. The fire was out. Jeff was unhurt. For one long moment, we stared at each other from across the width of the mattress, the only sound the matched inhaling and exhaling of our breath. And then the dog jumped up on the bed and peed on it. With that, Jeff flipped on the overhead lights, blew out the remaining candles, threw the remains of the burned-up curtain into the bathtub, and changed the sheets—all the while reassuring both me and the dog that everything was okay. Looking him over, I thought to myself, *Here is a man good in a crisis.*

"Hey, remember the night I set the curtain on fire?"

Deep into his cylinder of strawberry mango swirl, Jeff laughs. "What made you think of that right now?"

"Oh, I don't know. I was thinking about our class. And then I was thinking about our first night together. We were brave then. We took care of things ourselves—or at least you did. We weren't scared."

"Are you scared now?"

"I wasn't until tonight."

Jeff looks up at me. "We're still just as brave, Sandra. I think we both just got caught up in all the collective anxiety in that room tonight."

"I think I hate our class."

In spring 1971, when I was in sixth grade, my mother took me to the local YWCA to watch a Very Special Filmstrip with a group of other preteen girls and their moms. After the film there was to be a discussion, led by a health teacher with experience in sex education. All the way there, I huffed and whined. "Why do we have to go? I know all this stuff already."

Part of my complaint was actually a compliment to my mother, who had always been so forthright about bodily functions. When I began to ask where babies come from—a question made complicated by the fact of my own adoption—I was given a clear description and presented with an oversized gold-edged tome called *The Human Body*. The illustrations were fabulous, and I went to work reproducing in crayon the development of the human fetus from fertilized egg through full-term neonate. Thus, since at least the first grade, I've been happily setting my friends straight on the origins of babies. What was missing from the text of my first anatomy book, however, was an explanation for how the sperm reached the egg. Initially, I presumed they swam across the mattress at night while husbands and wives slept together. Which is how I explained it to my younger sister. At some point, my mother recognized the missing element in my rendition of human creation, and filled me in on coitus. By age eleven, I had long since recovered from the shock of this revelation and was convinced nothing more remained for me to learn—and certainly not from the place where I took swimming lessons.

Au contraire. What I hadn't anticipated was the scene in the movie where the labeled diagram of the male penis suddenly stood up in the air! The concept of male erection shed a whole new light on the mechanics of sex. When the lights came back on, I glanced sideways at my mother. Why had she neglected this critical detail?

On the car ride home, Mom inquired casually if I had learned anything. "No," I said, sighing deeply. "I told you I knew everything."

Now, a year shy of forty, I settle down with the thick gray booklet entitled *The Gift of Motherhood: Your Personal Journey Through Prepared Childbirth*, handed to us by Michelle on the first night of childbirth class. Perhaps there is something else about human reproduction I've overlooked. In any case, my previous aversion to descriptions and pictures of childbirth have yielded to curiosity and wonder.

What I learn is that giving birth is essentially a three-stage process and that these three stages are exactly the same ones that organize a good novel. Stage one is otherwise known as labor. During this time, the cervix—that narrow entryway between uterus and vagina—gradually opens its round doorway, which is called the os. This period is characterized by increasingly frequent and powerful uterine contractions—or, to speak narratively, by a buildup of tension, suspense, and conflict. The second stage, otherwise known as delivery, is the climax of the story: it starts with the urge to push and ends when the baby comes out. During the denouement, stage three, the placenta is expelled and all is resolved. The events of childbirth pick up speed as they progress because they operate on what's known as a positive feedback loop, meaning that each hormonally mediated response triggers a bigger response, which in turn triggers yet an even bigger response. Momentum builds, and so each stage is shorter than the one before it.

Because the first stage is the longest, it is traditionally divided into three phases, which are defined mostly by how far the cervical os has opened. If the laboring woman has never before become intimate with the metric system, she will now. In the first phase of stage one, also called early labor, the os opens two to three centimeters (about an inch or so). The next phase, called active labor, widens the cervical opening to about seven centimeters (a little more than two inches). Finally, during the last phase, called the transition, the os expands to a full ten centimeters (or about four inches) in diameter. Which is about as big as the human doorway gets.

Each of the phases of stage one labor demands increasing attention from the mother. At first, contractions feel like menstrual cramps and they are several minutes apart. Women in early labor are typically talkative and highly social and often go about their normal activities. In active labor, which is shorter in duration, contractions come frequently, last longer, and intensify in strength. Women stop talking and turn their thoughts inward. The transition is the shortest but most intense phase. It is the eye of the needle. Contractions come one on top of the other with little rest in between. The list of possible physical sensations during transition includes trembling, nausea, hot and cold flashes, rectal pressure, and back pain. Cognitive reasoning decreases while sensitivity to sensory input—voices, smells, images, touch—increases. And then, what remains of the cervix slips over the baby's head, and labor becomes delivery.

The breaching of the cervix in stage one is actually accomplished in two different ways. One is by dilation. The other is by effacement. Imagine a house with a front vestibule. Over a period of hours or days, the front door slowly opens. This is dilation. At the same time, the vestibule itself is retracted into the house and disappears almost entirely. This is effacement. Normally, the cervix is one to two inches in length, an inch or so across, and tough as a tendon. But in the month before birth, the cervix begins to soften. Its fibrous strands relax and stick to each other less tightly. This allows for both dilation and effacement. As the contractions of early labor massage the baby further and further down into the pelvis, the growing pressure of its head on the cervix begins to force the os to dilate. These same contractions draw the now soft and pliable cervical fibers up into the uterus itself. The cervix gets shorter and shorter and thinner and thinner until it is just a circle of gauzy tissue.

On to stage two. Once the cervix is out of the way, the baby can be propelled into the world. This requires an effort not unlike rocking a car out of a snow drift. You can't just gun the engine once. Instead, you have to push and let go, push and let go, the baby moving forward and backward, forward and backward, the top of its head appearing briefly between the vulval lips and then disappearing again into the mother's body. When the head no longer slips back inside between contractions, the baby is said to be crowning. It is at this moment that the obstetrician is usually summoned to the scene.

The moment of crowning is also the point of maximum tension on the perineum, that trampoline of flesh between the vaginal opening and the anus. At every other time in a woman's life, her perineum is less than an inch wide. But in the final, dramatic moments of pregnancy, it stretches to many times its resting width and balloons out like a sail in a windstorm. An essential component of the pelvic floor, the perineum is made of several criss-crossed layers of muscle, nerves, and erectile tissue, and it is the main reason the baby doesn't just shoot out once stage one is over. Indeed, helping the perineum stretch around the crowning head is one of the main skills of delivering babies, at least according to the traditions of midwifery. Obstetricians are more likely to cut the perineum with scissors to speed up delivery (and then sew it back up again once the baby is born). This procedure is called an episiotomy, and it is the most common surgery performed on women in the United States. At the Beth Israel hospital in Boston, 90 percent of first-time mothers receive one. With or without an episiotomy, rips of the perineum are not uncommon in stage 2, and a whole classification system exists to describe their severity.

Studying the labor and delivery timeline in *The Gift of Motherhood*, I suddenly have an epiphany. Births are really not about vaginas. In fact, the journey down the vaginal tunnel is actually the briefest part of the passage. Consider that for a first-time mother, an average labor from start to finish is thirteen hours. This is about the length of time it takes to drive from Boston to Cleveland. It's a good day's work. Of those many hours, the baby spends only a few minutes in the highly mythologized, deeply symbolic vagina. The real work of birthing a baby comes at either end of the tube and involves two obscure parts of one's anatomy that a woman almost never thinks about under any other circumstance: the little keyhole called the cervical os and the rubbery band of skin and muscle called the perineum. The great effort that goes into opening up the first and the trickiness of getting the baby past the second are the two big reasons why birth is painful and women require assistance during childbirth. Passing a baby through a six-inch-long vagina is, by contrast, no big deal.

I begin to dread the weekly trips to the heavily paneled, deeply carpeted hospital conference room where portraits of the grand old fathers of Harvard Medical School gaze beneficently upon us as Michelle leads us in breathing exercises. The more she tries to put us at ease with c-sections and episiotomies, the more tightly I fold my arms across the shelf of my belly and fight the urge to flee. I had arrived the first night with valedictorian aspirations. By the third week, I was the sullen one with the attitude problem in the back row, notebook kicked under my chair. I spend a lot of time gazing up at the row of silver-haired dons in their gold frames. What did any of them know about childbirth? I glance around at the other mothers. They all treat Michelle like she is captain of the cheerleading squad. On the other hand, she is the only one who knows how they do things upstairs. I wonder whether she's ever had a baby. Doesn't look like it.

Pay attention, I scold myself. But instead of following the details of her upbeat presentation on the use of the synthetic hormone pitocin to augment a stalled labor, I draw up a list of my childbirth education grievances. First of all, there is not enough time for discussion. For all my fantasies of joining a supportive union of pregnant mothers who would embolden and encourage each other, none of us ever speaks except to murmur a few hellos as we scramble to take our chairs at the beginning of class. Between the breathing drills and the lectures on various kinds of obstetrical procedures, no time remains for talking among ourselves.

Second, there is way too much emphasis on medical intervention. Getting chummy with all the latest drugs, technologies, and surgical techniques has the effect of making them seem harmless, normal, and expected. This is no more true than for the epidural, an injection of anesthesia into a space near the spinal cord that numbs the lower body during active labor. At Beth Israel, epidural rates are twice what they were in the 1980s and now stand at 80 percent. In our class, narcotics and epidurals ("the good stuff") are presented as rewards for endurance and progress. To wit: "Once you're four centimeters dilated, you can get your drugs. But not before." The breathing exercises themselves seem intended to keep laboring women behaving calmly until the time when they can receive epidurals. To her credit, Michelle does acknowledge that the surrender to drugs is not compulsory ("And if you don't want an epidural, then we just keep rolling right along"), but she offers no alternative methods of pain relief other than just toughing it out.

Finally, the relentless attention to what can go amiss at every phase and stage—the Murphy's Law approach to childbirth preparation—seems potentially self-fulfilling. At the very least, all the lectures on aging placentas, prolapsed cords, malpresentations, failure to progress, premature rupture of membranes, and fetal distress seem doomed to undermine a woman's trust in her own body and her own abilities. It occurs to me that reviewing all injuries that could possibly occur is probably *not* the tack that coaches take with their star athletes right before the big game. And it is definitely not how cancer survivors face the future. As my own mother might say, it's all enough to make you lose your nerve.

I look up in time to hear Michelle say we should assume our labor will be overdue, long, and difficult. Then, if it is not, we will be pleasantly surprised.

The weather stays hot and muggy. Each morning, we shut all the windows and blinds to hold in the bubble of cool night air as long as possible. By 11 A.M. it's gone, and I lumber on my great puffy feet to the air-conditioned chill of the Somerville Public Library. Upstairs, in adult nonfiction, someone has thoughtfully positioned an easy chair right next to the large shelf of books on childbirth. Each morning I set up camp there and move through the volumes in call number order, picking up where I left off the day before.

When one of the authors recommends a title not found on the shelf, I send away for it via an interlibrary loan request and thus quickly find myself surrounded by stacks and stacks of books and journal articles on human birth. I'm trying to figure out a couple of things. One: Whatever happened to natural childbirth? Two: What is my emerging desire for it all about?

Many of the books I find on natural childbirth date back to the 1970s and '80s, the heyday of the movement, but a few are recently published, too. They describe a variety of methods for managing the pain of labor and for bringing forth babies from women's bodies, and they put forth divergent goals. For example, some advocate midwifery and home births, whereas others seek a change in the way obstetricians are educated. All decry the growing medicalization of birth and advocate a return to fewer intrusions during labor and delivery.

The central complaint leveled by critics of current obstetrical practice is that it too often sets in motion a "cascade of intervention," a running sequence of medical procedures, each of which necessitates the introduction of the next. For example, anesthesia and narcotics can slow down contractions so much that labor grinds to a halt. To speed things back up, uterine-stimulating pitocin is dripped into the mother's veins. This procedure requires fetal monitoring to ensure the baby is not overly stressed. Tethered to IV poles and ultrasound equipment, the now actively laboring woman is unable to change her position to alleviate pain. She therefore calls for more drugs. Lying on her back also places the perineum at risk for tearing during delivery and leaves her without the assistance of gravity to help ease the baby out, so she soon receives an episiotomy to widen her vaginal opening and hasten delivery. Thus, anesthesia requires pitocin requires monitoring requires anesthesia requires genital surgery. Considerable data in the medical literature support these allegations.

There are other problems, too. Because anesthetics can diminish the urge and ability to push, epidurals also raise the risk of forceps delivery and cesarean section. They can also prolong labor. They can also interfere with the ability to urinate and thereby necessitate catheterization. As for ultrasound, there is no evidence to suggest that continuous monitoring improves outcome in either high-risk or low-risk pregnancies, in spite of deeply cherished beliefs to the contrary. Furthermore, several large, well-designed studies show that episiotomies do not prevent perineal tearing and may indeed contribute to it. They also contribute to urinary incontinence, weakening of the pelvic floor musculature, and sexual discomfort.

Most attention-getting of all, midwives, who rely less on medical technologies and interventions, have a better safety record than obstetricians. One recent study examined all vaginal births at 35 to 43 weeks gestation that did not involve twins or other multiples and that were delivered either by physicians or nurse-midwives in the United States in 1991. After correcting for social and medical risk factors, the researchers compared midwife and obstetrical deliveries. Much to their own surprise, they found that risk of fetal death was actually 19 percent *lower* when midwives attended the births, and risk of newborn mortality was 33 percent lower with midwives. The authors conclude that "certified nurse midwives provide a safe and viable alternative to maternity care in the United States, particularly for low to moderate risk women."

In spite of evidence like this, natural birth has fallen out of popularity during the 1990s. Defenders of mainstream approaches claim it's because natural childbirth proved punishing and inhumane. They also point out that obstetrical drugs—particularly epidurals—have been perfected over the years. "Having a child in great pain when pain relief is available is no more a great transforming experience than having a tooth extracted without anesthesia," posits one obstetrical anesthesiologist in a letter to the *New York Times*. Another notes, "There is no other condition in medicine where we allow patients to have severe pain and not treat them."

But from my reading of the literature, these kinds of statements misrepresent natural childbirth. The choice is not between anesthesia and unremitting agony. One is not asked to lie in a hospital bed and, like the recipient of a battlefield amputation, bite a bullet and suffer. Rather, natural childbirth seeks to substitute nonpharmaceutical methods of alleviating pain. These include continuous emotional support, relaxation techniques, meditative breathing, warm baths, changing positions, acupuncture, music, walking, and massage. Natural childbirth advocates would also say that the perception of the laboring woman as a patient with a medical problem on par with an impacted molar is exactly what has always been wrong with medicine's view of childbirth.

Especially interesting to me in this regard is a 1996 investigation of labor pain published in a medical periodical with the curious title *Journal of Psychosomatic Obstetrics and Gynecology*. The central question of this study is one of my own: What determines how severe the pain of childbirth will be? The authors of this article first review previously published reports on the experience of labor pain. They find the literature shot full of contradictions. For example, in controlled questionnaires labor pain is often ranked the most intense of all human pains—receiving higher scores than the pain of cancer or phantom limbs—and yet some women claim they enjoy almost pain-free labors. No single explanation for this variability exists. Education, social class, wealth, and maternal age have little influence on the severity of pain in labor. Neither is there a clear association between length of labor and amount of pain. Nor is the weight of the infant predictive of pain level. Nor is a history of severe menstrual cramping. Nor, for that matter, is enrollment in a childbirth preparation class.

Nevertheless, the authors did unearth a few intriguing patterns. One is that anxiety consistently correlates with high pain scores, while self-confidence is faithfully associated with lower scores. Most revealing, "Women who expected labor to be very painful were more likely to find it was." These women were also more likely to use drugs.

The authors also conducted their own interviews among several hundred women who delivered their babies in three large urban hospitals in Sweden. As in previous studies, the range of women's reported experience with pain was huge, some new mothers describing their labor pain as the worst possible imaginable and others dismissing it as easily bearable. As before, expectation of pain was associated with more painful labors, whereas continuous support during labor correlated with lesser pain. And yet, all these variables together still could not predict an individual woman's experience. The authors thus began to suspect that *attitude* toward pain may influence the perception of it. So they also interviewed women about this. Much to their own amazement, the researchers found that a full 28 percent of the women they questioned—almost a third of the total—recalled their labor pain as a positive experience. The authors, sounding baffled by their own findings, concluded that for these women, "labor pain has another meaning than pain related to disease."

I feel I have stumbled onto the missing piece of the jigsaw puzzle. Trained to treat trauma and disease, physicians tend to see pain as a problem to be fixed and the refusal to accept analgesics as an exercise in masochism. But in the human experience there are many kinds of pain besides the pathological. There are the searing lungs of the mountain climber who nears the summit. There are the burning quadriceps of the ballet dancer who has just executed a triple *tour en l'air*. There is even the victorious ache between the shoulder blades of the writer who finishes the final paragraph as the first rays of sunrise fill the window. As more than one advocate of natural childbirth has pointed out, if labor and delivery were viewed less as medical events and more as Olympic ones, this distinction would be obvious. Who, after all, would rush up to a marathon runner in the final stretch with a needleful of narcotics?

The claim that undrugged childbirth can be a euphoric, life-transforming experience attracts no small amount of ridicule. Reporting on the threefold rise in U.S. epidural rates between 1981 and 1997, magazine and newspaper writers could not resist such sarcasm. One elated columnist announced that the "reigning cult of birth as an athletic event" had been overthrown at long last. The real orgiastic moments of childbirth, she declared, are those "simultaneous with that first welcome sensation of anesthetic coursing through one's veins." And yet, among the natural childbirth books of the 1980s are many photographs of undrugged, laboring women who appear truly caught in the throes of ecstasy—or at very least, who look powerful, wild, and unafraid, including one in the midst of a breech delivery. Why are we so eager to sneer at these images? I don't remember anyone ever laughing at our high school football team—true believers all in the cartharsis of physical pain—when they chanted "Blood makes the grass grow!" as they ran onto the field before cheering throngs.

I start to wonder if there are reasons other than improvements in the formulation of anesthetics to explain natural childbirth's current unfashionable status. A lot of thinkers and critics have weighed in on this question. Some believe that the culture of the hospital itself works against nonintervention in childbirth. For example, seldom are there enough nurses working on any given shift to provide the kind of steadfast emotional support that is known to shorten labor and reduce the need for drugs. This problem has intensified in recent years under managed health care systems. One former obstetrical nurse—now a practicing midwife—recalls that, in the hospital where she worked, electronic monitoring allowed her and her overworked colleagues to attend several labors simultaneously while also providing precious time to complete paperwork. Thus, data sent from bedside to nursing station sometimes substitutes for one-on-one care. Epidurals serve much the same purpose. Laboring women hooked up to monitors, numbed from the waist down, and confined to bed are easier for nurses to handle when they are overseeing multiple patients.

What's more, nurses and obstetricians are not routinely trained in alternative methods of pain control. If a woman desires to forego drugs and other interventions, she's on her own; all the knowledge in the world about how to manage pain using other techniques won't help if no one in the know is there to deliver it, and her choice truly does become anesthesia or agony. Alone, frightened, and soon overwhelmed by the intensity of labor, even a woman absolutely resolved to avoid drugs will call for an epidural, a change of heart that further convinces obstetricians and anesthesiologists that the pain of normal childbirth must be extreme and unbearable.

At the same time, those few physicians who do hold noninterventionist philosophies say they find it almost impossible to practice natural birthing in "hospital settings brimming with technocrats." As places of crisis and emergency, hospitals induce both stress (a physiological state that inhibits the progression of labor) and anxiety (an emotional state that magnifies its pain). As for that all-important element, self-confidence, it is undermined, say the critics, as soon as a woman assumes the identity of a patient. Dressed in a hospital gown, arm ringed with hospital bracelets, laid out in a hospital bed, she soon becomes passive and deferential. According to Barbara Katz Rothman, one of the most outspoken writers on this issue, "A woman cannot view herself as healthy while all the external cues proclaim illness."

This is not to say that the natural childbirth movement has left no lasting impressions on hospital childbirth practices. Not so long ago, laboring women were routinely shaved of pubic hair, purged with enemas, isolated from family members, and forbidden food or drink. And after delivery, they were immediately separated from their newborns. All these rituals were once justified with medical reasons. Thanks to women's health activists and certain forward-thinking obstetricians, these practices have largely been retired. Women can choose to have whomever they want in the birthing room with them. They can drink and eat when they need nourishment. They can take showers, soak in hot tubs, and assume whatever position feels most comfortable. And for all these hard-won privileges, I am grateful.

In the afternoons, I leave my library chair and walk, blinking, into the smudgy sunlight to find a bench to eat my lunch. Tomatoes, green peppers, and peaches from the farmer's market. Slabs of dark bread. An icy thermos of lemonade. Sometimes a slice of cheese pizza from the corner store.

Watching the neighborhood kids wheel around on their skateboards, I start to wonder whether planning for a natural birth in one of Harvard Medical School's flagship teaching hospitals isn't like trying to organize a peace rally in the Pentagon. Wrong venue. I've also discovered that I don't want to become a mother surrounded by the same instruments and clothed in the same blue, backless cotton gown that I wore when I became a cancer patient. I want new symbols. New ceremonial garments. I want a birthplace far away from latex gloves, surgical masks, IV drips, heparin locks, catheter tubes, gurneys, and heart monitors.

And yet I also feel reluctant to make enormous changes at this point. The alternatives seem out of reach. Though the data on home births show that they are just as safe as—if not safer than—hospital births for women at low risk for complications, they do require one key prerequisite: that one be in possession of a home. Our tiny, steamy flat hardly seems to qualify. One has to inch sideways just to get to the bed. If walking and changing positions frequently are good tools for managing pain in labor, I'd have better luck in a hospital. As for other hospital-independent places to have a baby, such as free-standing midwife-supervised birthing centers, the sheer number of calls I'd have to place to make such arrangements defeats me. The last thing I feel like doing right now is sitting in front of a fan arguing on the telephone with my HMO.

I also have something else at stake here. Beth Israel may indeed brim with medical technology, but it's also my lucky mitt. During the four years I've lived in Boston, it's provided my follow-up cancer care. Until I enrolled in childbirth classes there, I'd come to see it as a place of security and vigilance where I speak the same language as my caregivers. My physicians there are thoughtful, cautious, and knowledgeable people. Some are world-renowned.

For that matter, most of my friends from high school and college are practicing physicians. Right or wrong, I tend to sympathize with doctors. I've sat with these friends at 10 P.M. while they field emergencies over the phone. I've talked with them about the financial debts they shoulder, about split-second decisions made after going twenty-four hours without sleep, about litigious patients, about the immorality of profit-driven health care. I also tend to rely on medical thinking rather than intuition when making decisions about my health. Before Jeff and I nearly burned the house down, we had HIV tests conducted. When a routine blood test once showed I was mildly anemic, I insisted on testing for the presence of blood in my stool. When this test turned up "slightly" positive, I insisted on a colonoscopy. When the colonoscopy uncovered a precancerous growth, I felt grateful to this invasive intervention for possibly saving my life.

At the same time, a wealth of data clearly show that conventional obstetrics suffers from some glaring blind spots. One of them is an inability to see how the immediate, external physical environment profoundly affects the physiological course of internal events. Another is an interventionist ideology that fosters submission on the part of laboring women and that keeps alive certain antiquated habits, such as routine episiotomies, even when very good evidence shows they do more harm than good.

Tucked in a corner of Boston's Public Garden stands an obscure sculpture that may be my favorite public statue of all time. Erected in 1867, it is a monument to ether. More specifically, it is dedicated to THE DISCOVERY THAT THE INHALING OF ETHER CAUSES INSENSIBILITY TO PAIN, FIRST PROVED TO THE WORLD AT THE MASS. GENERAL HOSPITAL IN BOSTON.

It can't be easy to fulfill a commission for a statue commemorating a volatile organic chemical, but the sculptor carries it off magnificently, employing the best traditions of Victorian excess. Atop enormous pillars, wrapped with oak leaves and acorns, sits a bearded gentleman in robes and turban. He looks wise. Caught in his embrace is a beautiful, naked youth whose muscular limbs hang limply down, as if in blissful slumber. The bearded man presses a cloth to the sleeper's chest, as though stanching a wound. God and Christ come to mind. The pillars themselves rest on a marble pedestal carved with lotus blossoms and chiseled in bas-relief. One scene depicts an angel appearing to an injured man. Another shows the attending of the war-wounded. Another features a mother with a babe in her arms, sitting atop medical instruments.

I've come here in the hope that a historical perspective will help me figure out what to do. To that end, I've brought two sets of research notes with me. One outlines the history of obstetrics as told by obstetricians and their sympathizers. The other is the history of obstetrics as told by midwives and their supporters. I settle into a bench facing the side of the pedestal that is inscribed with a verse from Isaiah. Its implied message is that anesthesia is a gift from the Almighty himself: THIS ALSO COMETH FORTH FROM THE LORD OF HOSTS WHICH IS WONDERFUL IN COUNSEL AND EXCELLENT IN WORKING.

I start with the obstetricians' version of history. It is a story of enlightenment triumphing over superstition and helplessness. In their own telling, obstetricians are venerated as heroic, sensible, and scientific—but above all, humanitarian. One obstetrical anesthesiologist, also the author of a recent history of his profession, describes labor pain as a social ill that ranks alongside "poverty, torture, mental illness, imprisonment, and slavery." All these torments, he points out rightly enough, were once considered inevitable components of life. Gradually, social reformers began campaigns to abolish these afflictions from the human experience; relief from the pain of childbirth was an essential part of this honorable crusade. It was an effort that pitted physicians against fundamentalist clergy who argued that travail in bringing forth children was retribution for Eve's sin and therefore part of the natural order.

In addition to fighting the Church for the right to lessen women's suffering, obstetricians also credit themselves with saving their lives. Before the dawn of modern obstetrics, they say, pregnancy almost always carried with it the risk of death. Indeed, diaries from previous centuries show that women routinely prepared to die before every childbirth. Women with difficult labors were sometimes abandoned by unscrupulous midwives. The most wretched complication was probably the transverse fetal lie, when the baby was positioned sideways in the womb. This condition was usually fatal for both baby and mother. Today, however, babies positioned sideways, or any other direction, can be delivered surgically with ease.

The first important development in the field of modern obstetrics was the invention of forceps. First put to the test by a British surgeon in 1598, these instruments became commonplace tools of the trade by the eighteenth century. What eventually necessitated their routine use, say obstetrical historians, was European industrialization. With poor nutrition and inadequate exposure to sunlight in urban areas, girls grew up so deficient in vitamin D that their pelvises became constricted with rickets. These kinds of childhood deformities guaranteed painful, protracted labors years later. With forceps, male obstetricians could, under such adverse conditions, extract living infants from living mothers. With this demonstration, midwifery began to wane.

The nineteenth century ushered in the use of anesthesia. Which brings us to the turbaned fellow on his marble throne. On October 16, 1846, a Boston dentist proved to an audience of onlookers that ether could relieve surgical pain. Three months later it was being used on laboring women in Scotland. Three months after that, none other than Fanny Longfellow—proper Bostonian wife of Henry Wadsworth Longfellow—became the first woman in America to be etherized for childbirth. Afterward she became a major advocate for the provision of anesthesia during labor, helping to popularize the practice. Meanwhile, in England, Queen Victoria was given chloroform for the birth of her eighth child, Leopold. Her attending physician was none other than Dr. John Snow, one of my true heroes in this world. Snow, a champion of public health, once halted a cholera epidemic by determining the outbreak was due to contaminated wells and initiating preventive measures to ensure the purity of drinking water. Interestingly, it was Snow who, having smelled ether on the breath of newborn babies, first became concerned that anesthetics might cross the placenta.

The nineteenth century also brought important advances in obstetrical surgery. Most notably, the American gynecologist James Marion Sims learned to repair vaginal tears that extend into the bladder. These birth injuries, called fistulas, were a terrible scourge, and those with rickets-deformed pelvises were at special risk. To suture these tears, Sims had to see what he was sewing and so invented the speculum. He eventually trained legions of doctors in his techniques, but first had to overcome the medical taboo of exposing women's vaginas to examination.

The twentieth century brought hospitalization. According to two obstetricians writing in 1970, moving births out of bedrooms and into hospitals was a stunning achievement. Early in the twentieth century, "Only the derelicts of womankind and the destitute sought hospitalization [for childbirth]. The present popularity of the hospital, then, has been achieved against great odds, and can only mean that hospital care has proved its values to millions of satisfied mothers."

To be sure, the introduction of the drug scopolamine in 1914 also played a direct role in bringing laboring women into hospitals. Inducing a semiconscious state known as twilight sleep, this drug, mixed with morphine, blocked not only the sensation of giving birth but all memory of the experience. Because women in twilight sleep often hallucinated, they had to be restrained and watched closely. A hospital setting was required. It should be said that early feminists, including many women doctors, campaigned hard and long for the right to receive scopolamine during labor. By the 1950s, spinal anesthesia began to replace twilight sleep as the pain relief method of choice. The spinal was gradually refined and perfected into today's epidural. Those who now advocate for drug-free childbirth, say the defenders of modern obstetrical practice, romanticize women's suffering in the name of "naturalness." The fact that women come to childbirth classes asking for epidurals by name is, they say, testament to their effectiveness.

I walk around the statue. The Bible verse on the opposite side is from the book of Revelations: NEITHER SHALL THERE BE ANY MORE PAIN. Then I turn to the history of obstetrics in the Western world as told by midwives and their tribe of sympathizers. Their story is an accusatory one: For centuries, medicine considered childbirth beneath its purview and was more than happy to cede the whole business to midwives. Birth was a woman-controlled event that took place at home. Then came the Inquisition. Half of the women burned at the stake as witches between the fifteenth and eighteenth centuries were midwives, and much of their collective knowledge was incinerated with them. Midwives were especially vulnerable to accusations of witchcraft because they traded herbs and potions and had access to human body parts, such as umbilical cords and placentas. By the middle of the sixteenth century, English midwives were tightly regulated—not as a means of quality control but as a way of monitoring their possible involvement in the black arts.

During the 1700s and 1800s, surgeons began developing formal training programs in the nascent field of obstetrics, from which women midwives were excluded. Forceps were kept from midwives as well, so that when faced with an arrested labor which their hands alone could not put right, women midwives were forced to turn to male physicians for help. Midwives were also barred from training in anatomy and surgery, allowing physicians to then turn around and challenge their lack of credentials. Physicians eventually seized legal power over midwifery licensing requirements (which they still control today). In the United States, doctors waged deliberate campaigns to put midwives out of business. By the early twentieth century female midwives had lost control of birth, both in Europe and in the United States.

This obstetrical takeover might be less tragic, say these authors, if physicians truly provided safer deliveries than midwives. No evidence suggests they ever did. Throughout the nineteenth century, midwives had lower rates of childbed fever than medical students. Two famous frontier midwives, Martha Ballard in Maine and Patty Sessions in Utah, each attended thousands of births, many under extreme conditions, and lost very few mothers. As for the heroic application of obstetrical forceps, their use probably caused as much suffering as it eased. For example, forceps contributed greatly to the risk of death by childbed fever and to vaginal tearing into the bladder. As for the lionhearted Dr. James Marion Sims, who overcame violent prejudice in order to win the right to fix these injuries, a recent historical account reveals that, in fact, he perfected his techniques on slaves, whom he kept for a period of several years and on whom he experimented repeatedly and without anesthesia.

And as for the transformation of maternity hospitals from filthy death traps to safe, sanitary facilities, this change occurred, say the obstetrical critics, only after women reformers in the 1870s threatened to go to the press with stories of physicians spreading disease from patient to patient. The rate of hospital births accelerated during World War II in no small part because the shortage of civilian doctors necessitated centralizing the process and few midwives remained in practice to oversee births at home. Far from "proving their value to women," hospital maternity wards were pressed upon mothers as the only possible setting for birth. Like it or not, they were admitted, drugged into a stupor, and tied into beds with restraints, their babies pulled out of them with forceps. Mothers were often so undone by the whole experience—as were their intoxicated newborns—that their ability to breastfeed was compromised.

Midwives and natural childbirth advocates reserve special ire for a gynecologist named Joseph DeLee. More than any other individual, DeLee was responsible for introducing aggressive intervention into obstetrical practices. DeLee published a famous, influential paper in 1920, which outlines his ideas. I find the original article, "The Prophylactic Forceps Operation" in a yellowed, moldering volume of *American Journal of Obstetrics and Gynecology*. It is everything the critics claim—and more. DeLee describes labor as a violent event, comparing the perineum to a door that slowly crushes the baby's head and likening the baby's head to a pitchfork driven through the pelvic floor, causing trauma and permanent disfigurement to the mother. He minces no words: "Labor is a decidedly pathological process." The answer is episiotomy and forceps. He promotes a militaristic approach. Women's pelvic floors are the battlefield. The obstetrician is the general. His weapons are surgery, drugs, and medical instruments.

Thanks greatly to DeLee's influential paper, episiotomy was recast as a routine procedure rather than one to be used only in emergencies. In addition to DeLee's original argument that it spared injury to the neonatal brain, all kinds of other claims were made for it as well. That episiotomies could restore the vagina to its "virginal condition" is the most eye-opening. Noting that medical students were once taught to call the final suture "the husband's stitch," some critics are quick to claim that the real purpose was to sew women up tight for the pleasure of men. Fueling the practice of episiotomy today, say other observers, is probably the more mundane factor of physician exhaustion. Wakened in the middle of the night to attend births, with a full day of surgery and office visits ahead of them, obstetricians rely on episiotomies to speed up delivery and save time otherwise spent suturing the perineum afterward. Straight cuts are easier to repair than jagged tears, as Michelle has emphasized to us in childbirth class more than once.

But easier to repair does not mean easier to heal, as midwives point out. The outcry over episiotomies from activists has launched several investigations into their alleged benefits. None has ever been found. Episiotomies do not prevent birth injuries to the baby nor trauma to the perineum. Unlike spontaneous tears, episiotomy incisions extend deeper and damage more, rather than less, tissue. This is probably why women with episiotomies report more sexual pain and more problems with bowel and urinary functions—even many months after birth—than women with spontaneous lacerations. Moreover, episiotomies actually make such lacerations more, rather than less, likely to occur—in the same way that a cloth nicked with scissors is more prone to rip than uncut fabric. (A typical episiotomy is one to one and a half inches long and extends a bit less than halfway to the anus when the perineum is stretched taut during stage two labor. It is usually done in between contractions, right before the baby's head comes out.) Episiotomies and spontaneous tears can both be avoided, say midwives, if the attendant takes a more patient approach—allowing the baby's head to descend slowly and then delivering it in between contractions. Squatting during delivery also minimizes the risk of tearing.

In short, the ongoing claim that routine episiotomies prevent trauma appears to be a medical myth. Ian Graham, a medical sociologist, in his book on the history of the episiotomy, reaches a similar conclusion: "None of the benefits claimed for episiotomy were evidence-based. Therefore, the subsequent adoption of routine episiotomy by American physicians suggests the greater influence of the claims-makers . . . rather than scientific research." Graham believes that episiotomies appealed to obstetrician's surgical aspirations at a time when the field was seeking prestige and attempting to distinguish itself from old-fashioned midwifery.

In the 1940s and '50s, a backlash against obstetrical interventions of all kinds was brewing as those receiving them began to suspect their real purpose was for the convenience of the doctor, not the well-being of the mother. Ironically, it was a maverick English obstetrician, Grantly Dick-Read, who first coined the term "natural childbirth." He advocated pain relief through relaxation. At about the same time, an American obstetrician, Robert Bradley, brought husbands into the delivery room and gave them an active role to play in bolstering women's sense of confidence and security. Shortly after, the French obstetrician Ferdinand Lamaze demonstrated how controlled breathing and attention to focal points could obviate the need for anesthesia. All these physicians borrowed ideas and techniques from midwives, who had been quietly using them many long years. The collective efforts of these doctors challenged the old obstetrical notion that birth is a pathological event. Their highly publicized successes made many women wonder why their own obstetricians had so much trouble keeping their hands in their pockets.

I close my notebook. High above, in the arms of an old man, a swooning youth dreams on.

In the end, I make just two phone calls. One is to Janet Collins, a long-retired nurse midwife in Canada whom I befriended at an international cancer conference a year earlier. Janet once delivered babies up and down the Labrador coast of Newfoundland. Would she be willing to come to Boston for the birth of my daughter? Not as a midwife but simply as a kind of . . . courageous presence? She says yes. And then I call Sheila Bogan, an obstetrical nurse at Beth Israel who is said to be skilled in natural childbirth methods and midwifery techniques and likes working with women who want drug-free childbirths. She is also rumored to send Harvard medical residents trembling away in fear. Would she be willing to attend my birth as my private nurse? She says, "Let's talk about it. Why don't you come into the hospital tomorrow at two? I'll be on the floor." I say yes.

The next day, Jeff and I take the elevator up to labor and delivery. It feels like a dress rehearsal for the real thing. We're ushered into a waiting room. Moments later, the most powerful-looking woman I've ever laid eyes on opens the door and walks in. I have a hard time not staring at her forearms and biceps, which seem to burst out of her green surgical scrubs. The first thing she does is stride over to the thermostat and fiddle with it.

"It's too hot in here for pregnant women and menopausal nurses. Now what can I do for you?"

For the better part of an hour we chat about the history of obstetrical practice and growing medicalization of birth. Sheila is happy to hear that I'd like to try for a drug-free childbirth. While she won't make any promises, she does say she has a bag of tricks—including perineal massage—that can improve my chances of avoiding various interventions. Everything else is unpredictable. I like her self-confidence and honesty.

After listening patiently to my descriptions of the various medical procedures I've undergone without narcotic pain relief, she nods.

"Okay, then. I'll keep the anesthesiologist from sneaking in the door." She escorts us to the elevator and shakes our hands. And then she walks down the hospital corridor, as if on her way to roof a house or butcher a hog.

"Are you scared now?" Jeff asks on the ride down.

"Nope. I feel pretty brave."

9

Harvest Moon

*T*he heat lifts. The days turn blue. The world comes back into focus.

I reoccupy my writing desk but spend a lot of time just looking out the window at the massive tree across the street. *Ailanthus altissima*. It's an exotic species whose vernacular name, tree-of-heaven, can only be understood as ironic. Its members are most commonly found in railroad yards and abandoned city lots, pushing their orange, foul-smelling stems through razor wire, trash, broken glass, and gravel. They are nevertheless welcomed as shade trees in city neighborhoods where pollution, disease, and poor soil would defeat more discerning species. This one, a female, provides shade for our entire block. Buckling the sidewalk, she rises from a three-foot-diameter trunk and dwarfs our neighbor's two-story house. I'm keeping a close eye on her. Day by day, her clusters of winged, red seeds droop heavier on the branch. Her leaves are already beginning to pale and curl upward.

Soon after Labor Day I begin to experience what midwives call "the lightening." Although my maternity dresses grow tighter and tighter, I feel more and more buoyant. The baby has begun its descent into the bone funnel of the pelvis. Paradoxically, the further the baby drops, the lighter the mother feels. Pressure on ribs and diaphragm lifts so that breath can again flow easily into the lungs.

177

It's as though time is moving backward. Not only do I feel airier, I sense the two of us are fusing together again. We are now so pressed against each other that when she moves, I move too, my belly lurching from side to side. "You're all baby," the obstetrical nurse said with a laugh during my latest checkup, as she moved her hands up and down my torso. Since January I've gained forty-two pounds. "Is she going to be . . . big?" I asked, not sure what answer I wanted to hear. "Well, this isn't some scrappy six-pounder," was all she would say.

We are as physically close as we will ever be, she and I. And yet I am increasingly aware of our imminent separation. All that is joined together must be torn asunder. This prospect doesn't frighten as much as fill me with a kind of wondrous disbelief—as when one discovers, on a late-summer afternoon, the first yellow leaves of the next season.

From field mice to elephants, almost all mammals are born in the spring, despite gestations that vary from three weeks to two years. Some species rely on tightly prescribed mating seasons to help synchronize birth with the return of warm weather and abundant resources. Others make use of delayed implantation. This means the fertilized egg floats around for a while—sometimes for months—until the calendar is right for a pregnancy to begin. There are a couple of exceptions to the springtime birth rule. One is humans. The other is bears. Polar bears are all born around Christmas. On the other hand, these births happen while the mother is hibernating, and she and her cubs don't tunnel out from their den until spring arrives; so, in a practical sense, humans really are the odd species out.

It wasn't always this way. Up until a few centuries ago, most humans were also born as the days grew longer (save for northern Europeans, who have long had an excess of September births, likely owing to the return of fishermen from the sea each December). With industrialization, however, the spring birth peak shifted. In the United States, most birthdays are now clustered in the fall. There is no good explanation for this.

There is also no good explanation for what causes human labor to begin—regardless of the season in which it occurs. Or, as a recent study states, "Despite the vast array of biochemical data, the final word on human parturition remains elusive." In other words, we know labor represents an avalanche of biochemical changes—one initiating another initiating another—but no one knows what sits at the top of the mountain and pushes that first stone over the edge. Even though the choices of initiator really come down to only three—baby, mother, or placenta—no one knows who or what ultimately controls the timing of birth.

Until the 1960s, the initiating agent was thought to be the maternal hormone oxytocin. This is the naturally occurring version of the synthetic hormone pitocin, which has long been used to induce labor in women and with reasonable success. If oxytocin were the initiator, then the mother would be the prime mover of the birth process. But an observation in the barnyard made researchers begin to suspect the story was more complex: mothers of lambs with brain defects involving the hypothalamus never go into labor at all. This odd fact made some wonder whether the fetus might actually stand upstream from its mother in determining the timing of birth. Perhaps the baby is the prime mover after all. Various experiments have confirmed that in sheep, the fetus indeed holds the switch that sets the whole drama in motion. The sequence of signaling events is roughly this: When a lamb is ready to be born, its hypothalamus sends a message to the fetal pituitary, which sends a message to the fetal adrenal glands sitting atop the fetal kidneys. Once stimulated, the adrenals produce a hormone that directs the fetal lungs to pump water out of the air sacs and prepare them for inflation. This same hormone, cortisol, also passes through the placenta and begins converting the mother sheep's progesterone to estrogen, a hormonal shift that allows uterine contractions to proceed.

Naturally, everyone was eager to believe the same story applied to us. A number of mysterious phenomena would be explained if it did. For example, the births of human infants suffering from anencephaly are usually overdue. This would make sense if the master controller were located in the absent part of the fetal brain. But—it's not. In humans, cortisol doesn't initiate labor. Instead, another chemical is used to rev up placental estrogen production. And though this chemical does originate from the fetal adrenal gland, its production is not governed solely by the fetal brain but instead is controlled by a conspiracy between the fetal pituitary *and* the placenta. This complicated operating schema was finally decoded by Roger Smith and his graduate student Mark McClean in Australia. In doing so, they demonstrated that the human placenta acts as a kind of clock that controls when labor will begin. But, like the kid who asks, "Yeah, but who made God?" we can inquire what causes the placenta to manufacture its all-important hormonal timer in the first place and what controls how much of it is made. "These fascinating questions remain unanswered," admits Smith.

Here are some things we know for sure. Throughout most of a pregnancy, the onset of labor is prevented by the placental hormone progesterone. Its purpose is to keep the muscular layer of the uterus quiet and relaxed, like the surface of a pond on a calm day. Estrogen, also made by the placenta, seeks to trouble these waters, but its actions are deftly thwarted by progesterone. As in the sheep, human labor begins once progesterone loses its grip, and the balance of power shifts toward estrogen. But even when it finally gains the upper hand, placental estrogen alone cannot bring on the tempest of full-blown labor. It requires the assistance of oxytocin, which is manufactured by the mother's pituitary gland. The mother and the placenta thus work in tandem to initiate the birth process. The uterus, however, will not respond to oxytocin until its muscle fibers are stretched taut, which only occurs when the baby's body grows to a certain size. Moreover, uterine contractions can accomplish little until enzymatic proteins finish dissolving the cervical collagen fibers. The production of these cervix-tenderizing enzymes is directed by chemicals called prostaglandins, which are produced by the placenta (among other sources). And what triggers the release of prostaglandins? The baby. Or to be more specific, the growing pressure of the baby's head on the cervix. Thus, human labor does not, after all, follow a one-way chain of command. Determining what ultimately sets childbirth in motion is less like tracing a path up to the top of an avalanche-prone mountain than like searching for the headwaters of a swiftly flowing river. What one finds at the source is a nexus of interconnecting creeks and springs, each feeding the other.

At the beginning of the second week of September, I wake up feeling absolutely full of energy, the best I have felt in nine months, if not nine years. Coincidentally, I have a new realization: "I am having a baby!" It's the same new realization I've been having every day since January, but the emphasis is different. For the first seven months of pregnancy, the accent fell on the subject of the sentence: *I* am having a baby! Then with the advent of childbirth education classes, my attention shifted toward the verb: I am *having* a baby! Now, two weeks before my due date, the sentence's direct object suddenly dawns on me: I am having a *baby*! The apartment I deemed unfit for a home birth is nevertheless soon to become home to an infant. And don't infants require a certain amount of . . . stuff?

I dedicate myself to organizing the household. I scrub baseboards and clean out closets. I send out kitchen knives to be resharpened and shoes for resoling. I inventory closets, alphabetize spice bottles, replace missing curtains, rearrange furniture, and banish beloved objects to the storage space in the basement. I balance the checkbook, return library books, and drop the dog off at the veterinary dentist for a long-overdue appointment. I draw up a to-do list for Jeff that is three pages long. It begins with changing the oil in the car. It ends with finding a diaper-changing table.

With Jeff out of the house, I begin washing loads of baby clothes bequeathed to me months ago by mother friends more foresightful than I. Pinning them in the sunlight to dry, I am suddenly scared. They all look impossibly tiny and full of complicated snaps, and I don't even know what some of them are. Pajamas? Undershirts? Bath wear? I try to read the faded tags. Their mysterious sizes—6M, 2T, NB–3M—confuse me.

I read up on baby care. I look up the word "layette" in the dictionary. Outside the window, a fall wind blows through the tree-of-heaven, and a few small leaves float away over the rooftops.

The timing of human birth—both its seasonal patterns and its biochemical origins—is an unsolved mystery. It would be a more enjoyable mystery if premature births were not such a stubbornly persistent problem. Because no one fully understands what initiates normal labor, no one fully understands either what initiates spontaneous preterm labor—or how to prevent it. Although advances in neonatal medicine have made it possible to keep many such babies alive— even a few born as early as at twenty-four weeks—prematurity is still the number one killer of babies after birth defects. Preterm birth is also a leading cause of disability, some forms so severe that many have questioned whether saving younger and younger babies at all costs is a worthwhile goal. About 10 percent of babies born in the United States arrive more than two weeks before their due dates—that is the official definition of prematurity—and the rate has been steadily increasing. Those who have studied the data carefully say this rise in incidence cannot be attributed to changes in medical practice, nor to variables such as maternal age or prenatal care. A third of preterm births are thought to be due to infections; the remaining two thirds of cases remain unexplained.

Because the uterus and placenta are known to be highly susceptible to interference by hormone-disrupting chemicals, recent attention has shifted to looking at the role environmental exposures might play in triggering labor before its time. The pregnant uterus, for example, appears to be a special target for PCBs. Experiments conducted in the 1970s found that lipids extracted from the uterine muscles of women in labor contained impressively high levels of PCBs, higher than concentrations found in either fetal or maternal blood. This discovery spurred further investigations into PCBs' possible effects on the timing of birth. These showed that PCBs can trigger contractions in strips of uterine muscle isolated from rats. Also, women exposed to PCBs on the job have higher rates of preterm births. Reviewing the human evidence, the authors of a recent report by the National Academy of Science concluded that, "collectively, these studies indicate that prenatal exposures to PCBs can cause . . . shorter gestation."

A series of experiments conducted at the University of Michigan has unveiled the apparent mechanism behind this effect. When applied to uterine tissue, PCBs increase the production of a chemical messenger that directs the flow of calcium ions into special channels within its muscle cells. The resulting influx of calcium in turn stimulates contractions. In addition, PCBs provoke the release of a chemical called arachidonic acid. This substance can generate uterine contractions in its own right. It's also the stuff of which prostaglandins are made.

Closely related to the question of when a baby will be born is the question of how big it will be. It is pounds rather than inches that is the critical variable here. This is because the growth spurt in length occurs much earlier (during the fifth month of pregnancy) than the growth spurt in weight (not until the end of the eighth month). Thus, at seven months' gestation, a human fetus has already reached most of its full-term length but only a fraction of its final weight. Obviously, then, premature babies are much lighter than babies born near their due dates.

But even independent of prematurity the incidence of low birth weight is rising in the United States. In other words, more and more full-term babies are being born unusually small. Low birth weight in this context means weighing less than 2,500 grams (about 5.5 pounds). Or, to describe the problem in another way, more babies are being born small for date, which is defined as falling below the tenth percentile in size—whether by weight, length, or head circumference—for a particular week of gestation. Such babies are said to suffer from delayed growth, or, more officially, from intrauterine growth retardation. This condition is a very different problem from being born too soon and carries its own special dangers. A risk factor for infant mortality and illness, low birth weight also raises the risk for adult problems such as diabetes, high blood pressure, and heart disease; reduced head size correlates with poor cognitive functioning and school performance.

As with prematurity, the recent rise in low-birth-weight full-term babies is an unsolved mystery. Some, but not all, of the increase is due to the rise in multiple births. However, even among singleton births the rates are rising. Incidence is also up among mothers who have the lowest risk of having a small-for-date baby, those twenty to thirty-four years old. Since it is well known that alcohol consumption, cigarette smoking, and drug abuse are all associated with low birth weight, researchers began suspecting that other environmental factors might play a role as well.

The mechanism for such an effect has not yet been uncovered, but the evidence for its existence is growing. In Germany, for example, occupational exposures to wood preservatives among pregnant daycare workers was linked to lower birth weight in ways not explained by gestational age. Several studies have found a relationship between drinking-water contamination and low birth weight. In North Carolina, mothers whose drinking-water sources were contaminated with dry-cleaning fluids were significantly more likely to have infants small for gestational age. Similar patterns were seen in Iowa in communities where water supplies were tainted with herbicides. They were also found in New Jersey and

Colorado in places where tap water contained high levels of trihalomethanes, the chemical by-products of water disinfection.

Still other investigations have found associations between living near toxic waste sites and having low-birth-weight infants. The best of these studies have been able to document a depression among birth weights during the time of dumping and a subsequent rebound to normal birth weights after the problem was remedied and exposures presumably mitigated. There are at least three such reports. One comes from Love Canal, the famous neighborhood in Niagara Falls, New York, that was built on top of a noxious chemical dump. Significantly more low-birth-weight babies were born to Love Canal mothers during the years of maximum contamination. This change could not be explained by various confounding factors (smoking, education, length of gestation, or birth order). When exposures declined, birth weights recovered.

Researchers uncovered a similar pattern among families living near the Tinker Air Force Base in Oklahoma. From 1956 to 1967, airplane maintenance and paint-stripping activities made exposure to airborne solvents very probable. During these years, mothers who lived in the neighborhood near the base were three times more likely to give birth to small-for-date infants than mothers living in other areas of Oklahoma City. When operations were later modified to reduce emissions, birth weights rebounded. In fact, families living in the same housing development began having babies with above-average birth weights.

The third and most comprehensive study comes out of New Jersey and focuses on babies born near the most highly-ranked toxic waste site in the nation, the Lipari landfill. Originally a gravel pit, Lipari started out as a fifteen-acre hole in the ground. Then, beginning in 1958, it was slowly filled up with liquid chemical wastes. Its contents—which include heavy metals, cleaning solvents, and paint—eventually seeped into a neighborhood lake and evaporated into the ambient air. During the years of greatest chemical leakage, 1971 to 1975, infants born to parents living in this area had twice the risk of low birth weight than infants born to families living farther away. This difference is especially significant because, both before and after this period, families living near Lipari tended to have bigger babies than those in comparison areas. Furthermore, after the landfill was closed, birth weights near

Lipari rebounded dramatically. By contrast, birth weights in communities farther from the contaminated zone held steady, showing neither slumps nor recoveries. As in other studies, differences in maternal age, prenatal care, education level, and other personal risk factors were all taken into account and corrected for.

In all three of the studies described above, air rather than water is thought to be the medium by which pregnant mothers were exposed to toxic chemicals. A large group of other studies shows that ambient air pollution can indeed affect fetal growth—quite apart from living near a dump site.

Beijing and Los Angeles are the respective study sites of two such investigations. In the former, researchers looked at the birth records of all pregnant women in four city districts between 1988 and 1991 and compared them to daily air pollution data collected from these same areas over the same time period. They found that the most highly exposed mothers had the highest risk of bearing full-term infants who weighed less than 5.5 pounds. Air pollution during the third trimester was the best predictor of low birth weights. Cigarettes were presumed not to play a role because so few Chinese women smoke. Similarly, in Los Angeles, researchers analyzed records for 125,000 babies, all born full term between 1989 and 1993, whose mothers happened to live near a carbon monoxide–monitoring station. They found that exposures to high levels of ambient carbon monoxide during the final months of pregnancy significantly increased the risk for low birth weight—even after adjusting for confounding factors, such as prenatal care, age, ethnicity, and education.

Several corroborating studies come from that heavily industrialized zone of eastern Europe known to public health researchers as the Black Triangle. This area includes the Czech Republic, Poland, and the former East Germany. In the Czech Republic, researchers analyzed all singleton births in 1991 within sixty-seven different districts where air-pollution monitoring is carried out. They discovered that low birth weight, as well as prematurity, was associated with air pollution indices. However, in contrast to the findings from California and China, the relationship was strongest for exposures occurring in the first, rather than the third, trimester. Similarly, within the district of northern Bohemia, risk of intrauterine growth retardation rose when air pollution levels were high in early pregnancy.

What is it about air pollution that shrinks babies? And why do some studies show that air quality is critical in the early months whereas others find it more important nearer to birth? As yet there are no answers to these questions. Air pollution is not a single class of chemicals. It is a soup of sulfates, suspended particles, carbon monoxide, heavy metals, nitric oxides, ozone, and volatile organic compounds. Depending on whether the main source of the pollution is car exhaust (as in Los Angeles) or coal-burning industrial operations (as in eastern Europe), the relative mix of contaminants is different. Some ingredients may poison fetal hemoglobin, while others may disrupt placental functioning.

In spite of this uncertainty, we do know of at least one ingredient in polluted air that plays, all by itself, a villainous role in fetal development. It is not a single compound but a family of chemicals called PAHs, polycyclic aromatic hydrocarbons. Their quaint middle name reflects the history of their discovery: the first PAHs were isolated from scented plants such as anise and vanilla. Not all PAHs are fragrant, but by definition they all consist of long carbon chains looped around to form a series of hexagonal rings. Naphthalene, the active ingredient in mothballs, is a PAH. Some occur naturally, others are synthesized in the laboratory, and still others are created inadvertently when organic substances burn; the members of the last subfamily are uniformly toxic to human health. When formed as by-products of combustion, PAHs can disrupt the endocrine system, alter liver enzymes, and cause cancer. They are the reason why tobacco smoke is carcinogenic and why charbroiled meat, smoked fish, and backyard barbecue are not recommended as dietary staples. Because they are formed when gasoline, wood, diesel fuel, coal, and fuel oil are burned, PAHs are ubiquitous in urban air.

In documenting how PAHs undermine fetal growth, the work of Frederica Perera, a molecular epidemiologist, is the standard-bearer. A professor at the Columbia University School of Public Health, Perera measures fetal exposures directly and then documents how this exposure correlates to injury. Making the case against this class of chemicals is a bit easier than trying to catch other air pollutants in the act of harming fetuses because PAHs actually glue themselves to human chromosomes. Perera can therefore quantify exposure by counting the number of such adhesions, called DNA adducts, in white blood cells. Working in Poland, Perera and her team of researchers showed that high ambient air pollution is associated with high numbers of adducts in both mothers and their infants. Moreover, newborns with high levels of adducts have decreased birth weight, body length, and head circumference. She also found that newborn babies consistently had higher levels of adducts than did their mothers, implying that fetuses are missing some defense mechanism that adults use to ward off damage from air pollution.

This is the first molecular evidence that a common airborne contaminant crosses the placenta and compromises fetal development.

The third week of September is hot and summery. I turn on the fans and keep scrubbing. Never has housework seemed so pleasurable. By now, word of my nesting frenzy has leaked out. My childhood friend, Gail Williamson—internist, pediatrician, and mother—checks in by phone.

"How long has this been going on?"

"Oh, about a week."

"A burst of energy at the end of pregnancy usually means that labor will start within a week."

"But my due date is still twelve days away. I thought first babies were usually late."

"I've never heard of anyone cleaning longer than a week."

The next morning I'm washing dishes in my nightgown when I feel something strange working its way down through some deep, hidden part of me. Before I can turn off the water, a mass resembling an egg white splats on the floor between my feet. I blink at it for a few seconds until I realize what it is.

"Jeff!"

"What's wrong? What is it?" He trips over the vacuum cleaner as he dashes into the kitchen.

I point to the floor.

"What is it?" he asks again.

"I'm not sure, but I think it's the mucus plug."

"The what?"

"Oh my God, it's happening. It's really happening. Gail was right! I can't believe it." Now I'm crying, mostly from sheer astonishment.

"Sandra, please explain to me what this is. Do I need to call the hospital?"

I finally look up, take a deep breath, and burst out laughing.

"It's the plug, a mucus plug. It's what seals up the opening of the cervix. It stays in there for nine months, and when it falls out that means labor will start."

"Always? Or sometimes?"

"Sometimes. I think. I don't know."

I call Sheila, who is on vacation this week. Fortunately, she's using the time off to refinish her bathroom. I imagine her with sleeves rolled up, ripping out tile and spreading spackle. She listens closely to my description, asks a few questions, and then encourages me to go about my business, stay calm, and stay in touch. Loss of the mucus plug may or may not signal the onset of labor.

The next morning, I wake up at 5 A.M. It's barely light. My back aches. When I sit up, a vague, crampy pain radiates around to the front. I feel my way to the bathroom. When I turn to flush, something catches my eye, and I flip on the light. The toilet water swirls with red—not the heavy velvet of menstrual blood but something lighter, more akin to grenadine. The weave of tissues holding the baby in place has begun its unraveling. This is the so-called bloody show, another sign of imminent childbirth. But rather than allowing me a glimpse of the future, the image pulls me into the past. I see myself at age thirteen, staring into a toilet, realizing I just got my first period and life would never be the same. It happened on an early morning much like this one, with the world bathed in peaceful gray air.

I call Janet in Canada first, then the on-call obstetrician at Beth Israel, and finally Sheila. Janet advises me to spread a piece of plastic under the sheets. If my water breaks while I'm in bed, the high protein content of amniotic fluid can ruin the mattress. In the meantime, she'll catch the next bus to Boston. The obstetrician says the cramping may progress into regular contractions or it may stop, in which case real labor may not set in for several more days. Or for another week. Or two. Sheila says, "I think you're going to have a baby within forty-eight hours."

But by the time we pick Janet up at Harvard Square later that night, eat rye bread and borscht soup together at the neighborhood deli, and deliver her to a friend's house up the street, the contractions have stopped. Back at home, I dig out the ground cloth we use on camping trips and smooth it over the mattress, per her suggestion. A few pine needles flutter out from the folds. I've spent a lot of nights sleeping on top of this piece of nylon. Sometimes on the tops of mountains. Sometimes near streams. Sometimes during storms. At least once in the company of bears. But never in my own bedroom. Tucking the sheets over it, I tell myself to cultivate the same attitude of wonder I adopt when hiking in the backcountry. Be receptive but without expectations. Watch for blazes along the trail. Keep an eye on the clouds.

In the past two days, I've been given two signs. Whenever the next one comes I'll need to recognize and welcome it. Sometimes the weather changes slowly. And sometimes it changes all at once.

Compared to human birth, labor and delivery among other mammals is a day in the park. A mother rat pulls her babies out with her own mouth after contractions lasting a few seconds. Kittens are born after two contractions; elephant seals require three whole minutes of pushing. Other primates have a more difficult time of it, but not when compared to what human women must endure. Gorillas, who have been heard to scream while giving birth, have labors lasting eighteen to thirty minutes. Squirrel monkeys labor for up to two hours. But, as many primatologists point out, estimating length of the birthing process in other species—especially among animals in the wild—is really sheer guesswork as no one knows when it starts. Much of human labor is also relatively painless in the early stages, requiring little change in behavior. We are able to record its onset only because women can verbally indicate when they feel contractions begin. Nevertheless, most researchers agree that human labor is probably three to four times longer than that in other primates.

Many people assume that our babies' big heads are what makes human births so arduous. This is part of the story. All primates have heads large for their body size. In most, however, the skull is deeper than it is wide, and the forehead therefore leads the way down the birth canal. The result is that monkeys are born face-up. This arrangement allows a mother monkey to pull her baby up to her chest as it emerges. But human babies are born face-down because the crowns of their heads serve as the leading wedge. For a human mother, pulling the emerging baby up to her chest would force the newborn to execute a backbend. Furthermore, with the baby's face turned away from her, she cannot easily clear its airways. These are but two reasons why the midwife and evolutionary anthropologist Wenda Trevathan believes that attendance during childbirth has been part of human heritage for at least a million years, making midwifery the world's oldest profession.

But the prolonged nature of human birth has as much to do with hips as heads. Among four-legged mammals, and even among knuckle-walking primates, the sacrum—that flat, bony triangle at the end of the spine—is located high above the pubic bone, allowing the fetus to pass under one limbo bar before encountering another. By contrast, an upright, two-legged posture requires a narrow pelvis with the sacrum positioned directly opposite the pubis. A birthing infant is thus forced to contend with two closely opposed unyielding surfaces simultaneously. Thus, from a Darwinian point of view, the travail of childbirth is the price women pay not for Eve's sin but for bipedalism, a novel means of locomotion that has freed our hands for tool-making, fire-making, art-making, the playing of musical instruments, and manifold other clever activities. It should all be enough to make us fall upon our knees and thank our ancestral mothers for all they have endured over the millennia just so we can type and wave hello.

Bipedalism has another consequence relevant to birth. It requires that the entire weight of the pregnant uterus be held up by the very structures that must later open and let the baby out, to wit: the cervix and the perineum. Compare this situation to that of our barnyard friends. In a pregnant sheep or cow, the unborn baby hangs within a bowl of abdominal muscle, and the birth canal is located safely uphill, like the spout of a teapot. Pushing a fetus through tissues that do not also have load-bearing requirements is a much easier task.

Happily, evolution has not left us defenseless in the face of some stiff engineering challenges. We members of *Homo sapiens* are equipped with two remarkable adaptations that allow contradictory demands to coexist. First, our babies come with semicollapsible heads. During the process of birth, the plates of the skull slide over each other as the head passes through the pelvic outlet. This process is called molding. Second, human women are outfitted with the most powerful uterine muscle of any mammal. Within its fibers lies the strength to push a baby through a narrow pelvis wrapped with materials designed to bear the weight of the prenatal world.

I do not have to wait long before the next sign arrives. A few hours after falling asleep on my nylon-covered bed, I wake up wet. Not floating in a puddle but definitely wet. When I stand up, the trickle stops. It starts up again when I lie down. For this reason, I guess it is not urine, which I've also been leaking lately but only when upright. It also doesn't feel like urine. It's slippery—like contact lens wetting solution—and smells like semen or the ocean. I rub it between my fingers. Is this the texture of amniotic fluid? Craving sleep, I decide not to ring all the alarm bells this time. Let the night be unbroken by analysis and surmisings. Let morning come when it will.

I sleep late. The next day, the autumnal equinox, is sunny and mild. Other than damp sheets, there is no evidence of further change. I feel equally poised between pregnancy and birth.

Except in Hollywood movies, most births do not begin with bags of water bursting open. This notable event usually occurs well into active labor. In about one in every ten pregnancies, however, the amniotic sac breaks, or is otherwise breached, before the onset of uterine contractions. Most women who experience what is officially called premature rupture of membranes go into spontaneous labor within twenty-four hours. The tiny minority who do not start laboring make their obstetricians very nervous because the chance of infection mounts with every hour that goes by. It's not a great risk, but it's a real one. During the phase of my pregnancy in which I interviewed almost every mother I encountered about her experience with labor, I heard two stories involving early ruptures. Both involved planned home births. In one, a forty-year-old giving birth to her fourth child walked around for two weeks leaking amniotic fluid and then went on to have a healthy baby girl at home with the assistance of her midwife. In the other, a forty-year-old giving birth to her first child walked around for three days with ruptured membranes, spiked a fever, and was driven to the hospital by her midwife where she received a cesarean section at the hands of doctors furious that labor had not been induced right after her water broke. In the end, her baby was also fine, but only thanks to medical heroics.

I call Sheila. She prohibits baths and sexual intercourse; she endorses long walks and nipple stimulation, both of which are known to promote uterine contractions. It's time for this baby to be born. And so we walk, Jeff and I, stopping every now and again to make out like a couple of teenagers. We walk up and down the hills of Somerville. We walk past soccer fields and churches, past bakeries, video stores, retirement homes, fruit stands, consignment shops, tobacco shops, pasta shops, bridal shops, used-car lots, and at least one nunnery. Behold, my little one, the city waits to welcome you. It is full of things both wondrous and absurd. Come out. Come out.

Nothing happens.

I spend the night much like the previous one, wakening periodically to the sensation of warm dripping. The next morning we set out for the Middlesex Fells, a forest preserve about ten miles from Somerville. We scramble up rocks, watch a heron skim the surface of the reservoir, look for signs of color among oaks and maples. Behold, the wind and trees and water call you forth. Come out, come out, wherever you are.

Still nothing.

That night I dream the baby and I have become separated. She is alone in a forest, and I am miles away in a city. I commandeer a car but it crashes en route. I climb onto a picnic table, which turns into a soapbox derby racer, but I don't know how to steer it. There is a snowstorm. Finally, on foot, I find her. She is cold but alive. Together, we run to the hospital.

The next morning I call my obstetrician, who wants to see me right away. I go to Beth Israel. She is cheerful and encouraging. A nonstress test shows the baby is fine. My cervix is one centimeter dilated. There are still no signs of uterine contractions. But because I've been leaking fluid for more than twenty-four hours, she wants labor induced by this afternoon if it doesn't start spontaneously before then. Unfortunately, my obstetrician is not the one on call tonight. However, she assures me I am in good hands with Sheila, who knows her way around a pitocin drip. She wishes us both good luck and hugs me on her way out the door. The exam room is suddenly very quiet. Jeff and I look at each other. I'm about to become a hospital patient. Our baby will be delivered sometime tonight by a physician we have never met, and we're stepping on the train of medicalized childbirth not knowing when we can get off.

Back at home, I get very determined. Let's walk, I say. And we climb the tower at the summit of the hill where General Washington once monitored the movement of British troops. Not stopping to admire the view, we walk back home again. Fast. Let's dance, Jeff suggests and turns on the stereo. Patti Smith. The Rolling Stones. Loud.

Finally, at 4 P.M., I give up. Pack a suitcase, I tell Jeff. I'll make some last calls. And then, as I stand by the phone flipping through the day's mail, a gush of slippery fluid soaks the floorboards. Within fifteen minutes, I feel a contraction. Which is to say, I feel something like a sharp menstrual cramp. It lasts about a minute. And then it's gone. Ten minutes later it comes back. And then comes back again.

It's 10 P.M. by the time Jeff and I leave for the hospital. Janet, who is still housed up the street with a friend, will get some sleep and join us later. The streets of Boston are uncharacteristically empty of traffic, the cause of which we can't identify until we whiz by floodlit Fenway Park. The Red Sox, World Series contenders, have gone into extra innings. In a reversal of a lifelong opinion, I decide professional sports are a boon to womankind. We find a place for the car (freshly tuned, new oil, infant seat correctly installed) in Beth Israel's parking garage. I choose to walk outside to the front door rather than enter the hospital through the connecting leeway. It's a clear, warm night, and the moon is already up—a bright, left-pointing crescent. Babies born under waxing moons are said by the old farmers' almanacs to be strong and grow quickly. I decide to believe this.

Sheila meets us at the triage station, smiling. She doesn't seem fazed by the prospect of spending a vacation night at the side of a laboring woman. "Just get me home in time for breakfast," she requests, jokingly. Earlier in the day she had encouraged me to bargain with the obstetricians for more time. Even arriving at the hospital at 6 A.M. would allow me one last blessed night of sleep. But my appeal had been denied. Regular contractions or not, my leaking fluids have apparently moved me into another medical category. The decision as to when I should be admitted seemed to be based solely on the number of hours since onset of rupture, not on how my labor was progressing since then. No one but Sheila seems impressed by my successful efforts to get labor started on my own. This includes the on-call obstetrician, a small, quiet man who seems nice enough but thoroughly uninterested in my hike up Prospect Hill and the labor-inducing properties of Patti Smith. He is on his way to bed and will see me again when the baby is ready to emerge.

Then the anesthesiologist drops by for a visit, peddling his wares with all the soft-spoken earnestness of a Mormon missionary. Sheila stands by silently, arms crossed. Her presence clearly makes him nervous, and with every sentence his eyes dart over in her direction. After asking me to summarize my entire medical history, he inquires about my teeth. Any bridgework? Dentures? Could I please open my mouth so he can count my fillings? It's an Alice in Wonderland moment. I'm guessing he needs this information in case unforeseen complications lead to surgery, but the incongruity between his questions and my state of mind is disorienting. He wants to know about my past; I am immersed in the sensations of the present. He wants to hear about my physical fallibilities; I want to speak about courage and stamina. He invokes hypothetical emergencies; I am trying for grace and repose. In the exhausting push and pull of our conversation, it becomes clear why home birth advocates claim that the act of entering a hospital is hostile to the birthing process.

Satisfied with my dental history, the anesthesiologist launches into a presentation of various narcotic and anesthetic options. At some point, Sheila decides our guest has crossed a line between describing epidurals and promoting them. The latter is apparently against hospital policy. She lets him have it.

"You can't say that," she asserts, cutting short his pitch. "You are NOT allowed to say that."

He objects but is quickly reduced to sputtering.

"And we won't be needing your services," she concludes firmly and steers him by the elbow to the door.

Thanks to Sheila, bouncer as well as bodyguard, the atmosphere in the room relaxes considerably.

But I don't escape the pitocin drip.

"I don't think we can get away with that," she says.

Still so proud of my labor-initiating achievement, I am surprised, but I don't think to refuse or even question why. The showdown with the anesthesiologist was my last act of resistance. I now feel aware of a growing need to conserve strength, turn aside from conflict, be open to direction, trust what I hear. And so, shortly after midnight, the intravenous line goes in. I am sitting in a rocking chair near the window, four centimeters dilated with contractions coming every 5.5 minutes. Sheila assures me this is a good place to start from.

And here is what labor contractions feel like to me. They come in from the sides, like bands of tightness. They progressively increase in strength and intensity—which I do not mean as euphemisms for pain—until they are literally breathtaking. Except that it helps to keep breathing anyway. The childbirth books all describe contractions as oceanlike waves, with lulls between the peaks. To me, they feel more like the periodic tightening and loosening of a corset. The moments of looseness give me a chance to regroup. I tell Sheila and Jeff that I had expected contractions would exert a downward pressure, not this lateral squeezing. I had also assumed I would want to walk around during this stage—which I am free to do—but in fact I am content just to sit and rock. Jeff suggests that perhaps I've filled my quota of walking for the day.

Sheila encourages me to look out the window at the city lights. Find one, she says, that attracts me. I do—and cast my attention out the window toward my chosen dot of light as the contractions intensify further. Now my pelvis feels as though it is caught in an ever-tightening vice. This is when I recall the unequaled strength of the human uterus. The power of my own body becomes amazing to me, thrilling. The force in whose grip I am held is generated by my own muscle. I am both the squeezer and the squeezed. Both the boa constrictor and the mouse caught in its coils. The sensation of being squeezed verges on the overwhelming, but the real labor of labor is the involuntary work of doing all the squeezing.

As the contractions clamp down with even more force, the skyline of Boston seems to rush toward me and then swing away again as the pressure subsides. And then I am the one who rhythmically flies out into the night sky and back. I try to describe my perceptions to Sheila and Jeff but discover I can no longer speak in full sentences. My legs begin to tremble. I ask to lie down. Instead, Sheila suggests I kneel in the middle of the mattress and hold on to the head of the bed, which she elevates to vertical.

Next, she stations Jeff behind the bed so that our eyes are level. She gives us a mantra: the word OUT. As I feel a contraction coming on, we are to hold hands, lock eyes, and chant OUT until the pressure subsides. Right away, the word pleases me. OUT OUT OUT. I say it fast; I say it slow. The more I utter it, the more it comforts me. OUT. What a perfect syllable. I explore each of its sounds—the long moaning vowel and the finality of the consonant. I notice how my lips first dilate then contract, how the tongue slowly rises up to the palate as the jaw closes. OUT OUT OUT. I listen to the shape of the sound as it uncurls from the back of my throat to the back of my teeth. I see the architecture of each letter—the endless cycling *O*, the hairpin turn of the *U*, the intersecting timbers of the *T*. OUT is the sheltering tree in a storm. OUT is a bubble of air under the ice. OUT is the train pulling away from the station. OUT is the bed at the top of the stairs. OUT OUT OUT OUT.

And now there is pain. I am still being squeezed, but something is pushing against my back from the inside, and it hurts. And now Sheila is up on the bed, holding me in a kind of football tackle, applying counterpressure. The pain subsides. I cast around for the word OUT and I find it in Jeff's eyes. OUT is the color blue. OUT is the bottom of a lake. Fish swim through the word OUT. It is peaceful inside the word OUT. OUT is deliverance. OUT is love. OUT is God.

And it goes on like this, the three of us shouting OUT OUT into the hours of the night.

Until a deep shuddering pain descends through my bones, and I lose my way. Do not misunderstand me. On the scale of sheer physical torment, I have experienced pain more acute than this pain. A finger smashed by a hammer hurts worse. Back spasms hurt worse. So do certain orthodontic procedures. But I have never felt a more *profound* pain. It is like the chords of a pipe organ filling a cathedral. It is like an earthquake.

San Francisco. 1989. I am standing in the doorway of my office, the floor rocking like the deck of ship. I look into the eyes of a coworker across the hall, who is also standing in his doorway as it lurches back and forth. His name is Federico. We hardly know each other. File cabinets fly open absurdly and slide down the hallway. It occurs to me he is the last person I will see before I die. I know he is thinking the same thing. And then it stops.

It doesn't stop.

Utah. 1995. Two friends and I hike up a mountain. Near the top, between two peaks, we discover a blue lake full of clouds. Only they are not clouds at all. They are pillows of snow rising and sinking, sinking and rising. Transfixed by this loveliness, we stay too long. When we finally begin the hike down, we hear a roaring sound beneath our feet. The sun has melted the snow above us and sent it rushing under the snow pack we are walking on, which begins to collapse and give way. We lie down and separate, crawling like spiders along the slope. Below, trembling aspens beckon to us from solid ground. When we finally reach them, we stand up, laughing and weeping.

There is no tree line here.

Somewhere in the distance, I hear Jeff's voice and navigate toward it. Now, I hear other voices. Sheila, urging me to keep it together. A kind of bellowing that seems to be coming from my own throat. And then my lips round up, my tongue finds the roof of my mouth, and the bellow becomes a word. OUT OUT OUT. I emerge from Jeff's eyes and reinhabit my body. OUT OUT OUT OUT. And the word becomes flesh.

Slowly, I become aware that the room is filling up. In a corner, the obstetrician is washing his hands. A Harvard medical student chats about a paper she once wrote on midwifery. Janet arrives, summoned by telephone. The lights are dimmed. A spotlight goes on above the bed. Sheila tells me I am fully dilated. The transition phase is over. I'm done with stage one.

If you have ever studied the anatomical charts that hang in gynecologists' offices, or inspected the plastic three-dimensional models that sometimes adorn their desks, you may have noticed that the uterus and vagina actually lie at right angles to each other. The uterus slants down and back, toward the rectum, and the vagina slants down and forward, toward the pubic bone. Between them is a neat, 90-degree turn. This arrangement requires a birthing baby to negotiate a serious curve, which some have likened to putting one's foot into a cowboy boot. The head-down, side-lying baby usually manages this task by rotating its body a quarter turn so that it faces backward, toward the mother's rectum. It then tucks its chin to its chest so that the crown of the head—the narrowest part—leads the way around the bend. When the head finally emerges from the vaginal opening, it turns to the side again as the entire body rotates internally. This second rotation allows the upper shoulder to slide out from under the pubic bone and the lower shoulder to pass in front of the rectum. Thus, human birth is rather like getting a large piece of furniture through a doorway: first you pivot it one way and then you swivel it around the other way to allow the various parts to pass through.

I'm thinking about all this as Sheila begins the perineal massage, which includes the application of hot compresses and warm oil. "We don't want any episiotomies here," she exclaims loudly, to no one in particular, but I am hoping the obstetrician catches the drift. At this point, I am uncomfortable and tired but not in any particular pain. The hot compresses are wonderfully soothing. As she works the oil in, she tells me the grunting sound in my voice indicates to her that I am ready to push.

Push? Now? I don't think so. I'm enjoying the intermission too much to return to my seat. Just let me stay out here in the lobby a little while longer. As a matter of fact, I'd like to go home. Or, at least, let's go back to the part where we were all shouting OUT together; that was okay. Sheila lowers the head of the bed to semireclining and adjusts pillows behind my back. She instructs me to grab hold of my thighs and pull them toward my chest. Now, take a deep breath, hold it, and bear down.

It is the most ridiculous suggestion I have ever heard.

Sheila and Jeff confer.

Jeff leans down and explains the concept to me in Zen-like terms. Before, I needed to let pain pass through me, like wind through a tunnel. Now, I need to push into it, not cast my consciousness away. There is no way out but through.

Shifting from passivity to action is going to require some kind of internal rotation of my own. I need to turn a psychic corner, reconnect with the stubborn, damn-the-torpedoes part of me that, earlier today, marched up the steps of a Revolutionary War tower in a defiant attempt to get labor underway. After meditating on this image for a few minutes, I recognize a need to push. With surprise, I realize this sensation has been coming and going for a while, but I hadn't acknowledged it.

I push, and everyone takes their places. Janet stands near my head and reminds me to keep my chin tucked. Jeff is at my right side. Sheila moves between the foot of the bed and my other side, and the doctor and his assistant stand quietly in the background like a Greek chorus.

The idea that there comes a point in labor where the need to bear down becomes an overpowering desire is not, in my experience, correct. For me, this urge is more reflex than desire. It's like the need to throw up. You can resist it. You can let it happen. Or you can encourage it. But you wouldn't exactly call it a desire. And, as in vomiting, I prefer to let the urge build a bit before throwing my weight behind it.

Pushing quickly takes on a rhythm and momentum of its own. I stop taking direction and start narrating the show. "Wait, let me rest a minute. All right, here it comes. Okay . . . NOW!" Once I discover that pushing doesn't hurt as much as I imagined, I let go of all remaining tentativeness and am once again amazed at the power streaming through me. At some point, the stretching tissues around the mouth of my vagina begin to tingle and burn. Soon they become numb, like a foot that has gone to sleep. This is useful. I go on, letting my body swing between resting and pushing, resting and pushing. Then I hear the two doctors exclaim in unison, "Wow! *Look* at all that hair!" A voice asks me to reach down and touch the baby's head as it crowns. I obey but am not in the mood. I also wave away the mirror that someone offers. Too many distractions. Can't you see I'm trying to work here?

And then, without warning, I am ordered to stop pushing. At the foot of the bed, a big conversation ensues as to whether or not I should receive an episiotomy. I am listening to this discussion as though from the bottom of a well, as though to a radio show that keeps cutting in and cutting out. I catch about every third word.

Finally, I hear myself say, "I would rather. Have a first-degree tear. Than an episiotomy."

I watch the obstetrician shake his head. "I'm afraid . . . not going to be . . . degree tear." He is a minor character in a scene from a foreign film.

Now there is more discussion. I am reading badly translated subtitles. I am getting bored and annoyed.

I hear myself say, "Okay. Then do it."

It is a decision I will curse for months to come, and as soon as I feel the scissors sliding into my vagina I know it.

But there is no time for regrets now. I am carried off by an enormous, pent-up desire—yes, now it is a deep, deep desire—to push. And then again. And someone is saying the head is out. And then again. And then something is rushing through me like a waterfall of snowmelt down a mountain and suddenly there is space inside me and tremendous sense of relief and a voice saying, "Sandra, reach down and grab your baby," and a tiny, perfect body appears in my hands.

Spiky feathers of wild, luxuriant black hair.

Dusky skin, greased with vernix that is smooth as the finest lotion.

Lips I recognize from a school picture of myself in the first grade.

Oh, who are you?

Two eyes open, black as mystery. They ask, *And who are you?*

It is 2:56 A.M., September 25, 1998.

PART TWO

There was a child went forth.
The early lilacs became part of this child,
And grass and white and red morning-glories,
and white and red clover, and the song of
the phoebe-bird. . . .
Winter-grain sprouts and those of the light-
yellow corn, and the esculent roots of the
garden,
And the apple-trees cover'd with blossoms and
the fruit afterward, and wood-berries, and
the commonest weeds by the road. . . .
The horizon's edge, the flying sea-crow, the
fragrance of salt marsh and shore mud,
These became part of that child who went forth
every day, and who now goes, and will
always go forth every day.

—Walt Whitman

10

Mamma

The nicest mammary glands I ever saw belonged to an American Alpine goat at a county fair in upstate New York. Talk about your velvet orbs! Your snowy white hemispheres, gently trembling! Down to their two erect and perky nipples, these were show-stoppers—the kind of bosoms dissatisfied women empty their bank accounts to have surgically recreated on their own chests.

These are not my breasts. To say I have small breasts is even an exaggeration. My chest most closely resembles that of a sixth-grader whose nipples have just begun to show through her T-shirt. What I have are not so much breasts as breast *buds*, a physician once informed me. That he happened also to be my lover endeared the term to me at the time, but when his ongoing fascination with both me and my breast buds proved tiresome, I left both him and the phrase behind. I began to think of myself, once again, as simply a woman without breasts. *La Femme sans mammae.* By and large, this has been a liberating identity, although breastlessness did not seem liberating in adolescence. At fourteen, it was a condition of sufficient cruelty to make me declare myself an atheist. By the end of my twenties, however, I had made two discoveries. The first: There exists a large subset of interesting men for whom breast size is utterly inconsequential. The second: According to several men within this subset, my nipples are notably . . . enthusiastic. And as someone French once said, when it comes to sex, there are no tricks; there is only enthusiasm. With these revelations, all remaining doubts about my minimalist, unadorned torso evaporated, and by the time I met Jeff, a man more captivated by shoulder blades than mounds of quivering flesh, the whole issue of breasts had become deeply irrelevant to me, and so it remained.

Until now.

Inside the human breast is a tree. Its branches increase in number as you move back toward the chest wall. At the tips of the branches hang fruitlike structures called lobules. Milk is made inside these lobules and then flows down through the branches, called ducts, and into the nipple. You are forgiven if you think the human nipple is like a faucet or a garden hose. This is indeed how the mammary gland of a cow is designed, with a single large canal draining milk from all the various ducts and conveying it through the teat to the outside world. This is also how the breasts of rats and goats are set up. But the human nipple is more like the head of a sprinkling can, with ten to fifteen ducts emerging at various points on and around it.

You will also be pardoned if you have assumed that breastfeeding is, like the urge to push during labor, an instinctual act. For most mammals, it is. But for humans, nursing is an activity that both mothers and infants must learn. And, like the tango, it can only be mastered with a partner. You can study up on it all you want—I myself enrolled in a breastfeeding class during my last month of pregnancy—but ultimately, you just have to get out there on the dance floor and do the best you can. Plenty of women have failed at nursing—and not just since the invention of bottles and formula. Medieval French poets wrote about new mothers who did not know how to breastfeed. So did Sigmund Freud. Wealthy white women of the antebellum South apparently had a particularly difficult time of it and relied heavily on wet nurses—sometimes enslaved ones.

We humans are not completely alone in our unknowing. Certain other apes are also unable to nurse their own young if they have never seen breastfeeding carried out by others. Nursing women and their human babies are sometimes invited to zoos to demonstrate the basics to captive chimpanzees and gorillas in need of instruction. It works.

Quite possibly the greatest achievement of breastfeeding advocates is their challenge to old, widely held beliefs that some women are simply incapable of nursing. La Leche League, the oldest and most venerable of these groups, contends that virtually all mothers possess both the anatomical equipment necessary to feed their babies and the ability to learn how to use it. From the League's point of view, any obstacle in the way of successful breastfeeding is a surmountable obstacle. Breastfeeding problems are not caused by inherent flaws within the mother's body, its leaders insist, but by external conditions that can be changed. An inadequate milk supply is not caused by inadequate breasts but by exhaustion, anxiety, and infrequent suckling. Colic and rash are not caused by allergies to mother's milk—which is hypoallergenic—but, very often, by reactions to specific food items within the mother's diet that can be eliminated (dairy products, broccoli, beans, etc.).

Most reassuring to me in the breastfeeding literature is the oft-repeated statement that milk production has absolutely no relationship to the size of the breast. This disconnect makes sense because something as crucial to reproductive success as the ability to nurse an offspring should not be yoked to a trait as whimsical as breast size. Evolution is too conservative a force to permit such dependencies. Thus, the milk-producing glands—the lobules and their latticework of ducts—are doled out in equal portions. Whatever her bra size, each woman possesses about the same amount of glandular tissue per breast. As the writer Natalie Angier has observed, this simple fact renders the grand assortment of breast sizes and shapes an utter, baffling mystery. The volume of a woman's breast is a function of how much fat and connective tissue it contains. And yet, these tissues apparently play little direct role in its ability to make milk. Breast fat is normally not metabolized during lactation.

The young, handsome pediatrician is worried. Not very worried, just a little worried. Forty-eight hours after birth, Faith has lost 10 percent of her body weight. Born at eight pounds, four ounces, she is now seven pounds, seven ounces. A drop like this is not unusual, but 10 percent is the maximum weight loss pediatricians like to see in newborns. In accordance with HMO regulations, Faith and I are about to be discharged from the hospital, so he suggests we stop by the office tomorrow and have her weighed again. He is a kind man, and when he's done with his exam, he shows Jeff and me how to swaddle.

"Everyone has their own method, but this is how I do it," he says, with obvious pleasure, spreading out the regulation blue-and-white flannel blanket on the bed next to me and placing Faith on it. "First you fold down this corner, and *then* you bring the far corner up like this . . ." His slight clumsiness makes the demonstration all the more enjoyable. ". . . and now, you fold this up, and go around this way, and you tuck it in over here." Voilà! A baby burrito. He smiles down at her adoringly. His eyes are red, and he needs a shave. He's probably been on call all night. He's only a little worried, not very worried.

"How do your breasts feel?" he asks on his way out. "Are they warm to the touch? Any sense of fullness yet?"

"No."

"Hmm. Well, don't worry. Milk usually comes in by the third day postpartum." After the door swings shut, I unbutton my nightgown. I don't see or feel any difference. When I press on the nipples, nothing comes out. Several mothers had told me to prepare for a huge growth spurt, first during pregnancy, and then again after the birth. I would almost certainly, they warned, need to wear a bra for the first time in my life.

It didn't happened. Tricked again.

I forget all my biology and burst into tears. I am failing, failing, failing motherhood.

Helpless in the face of my grief, Jeff rings for a nurse. Every few hours, day and night, the neonatal nurses have instructed me in the art of breastfeeding, demonstrating how to position the baby correctly, induce her to open her mouth, help her create a seal between lips and nipple, and then break the vacuum and switch sides. They have been wonderful teachers all, but Faith is losing weight, and I don't have any milk. And I don't have any breasts. And there is no God. Failing. Failing. I am failing.

A nurse sweeps in—one of the helpful ones from yesterday's early-morning shift—and in a flash has Faith latched on and suckling.

"What's the matter?" she finally asks.

"How can I breastfeed when I don't have any breasts?" I'm still sobbing.

"Honey, everybody's got glands. I've never met a woman yet who didn't have glands."

The breast is one of only a few human organs not fully developed at birth. Certainly, no other structure undergoes such dramatic changes in size, shape, and function. It all starts in the female embryo in the seventh week of pregnancy, when the embryo is the size of a rice grain, and a mammary ridge rises up from its ectodermal layer. By the sixth month of fetal life, most of the building blocks of the future mammary gland are in place: nipples, lobules, fat pad, ducts, and even the sheath of muscle around the ducts that is designed to help propel milk out of the lactating breast.

The breast stays like this until puberty, when the ducts begin to divide and grow under the influence of ovarian estrogen. With a girl's first ovulation, progesterone kicks in, too, and lobules begin to bud. None of this activity is visible from the outside, however. When we say that a girl's breasts have begun to develop, what we are noticing is a growing accumulation of fat under the nipples. Fat deposition is also under the direction of estrogen.

Long after puberty, many women recognize that their breasts change in size throughout the yin and yang of their menstrual cycles. Breasts are at their largest about eleven days after ovulation. This proliferative peak is then followed by a period of cell deletion once menstruation begins. Although these seasons of growing and shrinking mostly balance each other, the breast never fully returns to the starting point of the preceding cycle. With each round, new structures bud, and the mammary gland becomes incrementally more elaborate, like a house onto which additions are constantly added but only worked on one weekend a month. In this way, the breast continues its leisurely development until the women reaches the age of thirty-five or so.

During pregnancy, the pace picks up. Assisted by the placental hormone lactogen, progesterone encourages further development of the ducts, while estrogen stimulates them to elongate. Estrogen also causes the breasts to enlarge by increasing their fat content, but if this happened to me, it was scarcely noticeable. By mid-gestation, the lobules have begun to differentiate into actual milk-secreting units, called acini. Meanwhile, concentrations of a hormone from the pituitary gland, prolactin, rise. It carries instructions to begin milk production. But as long as the placenta rules the kingdom, prolactin's chemical signal is intercepted by progesterone before it can activate the acini. No milk is made.

Once the baby is delivered and the placenta evicted, prolactin can finally deliver its message to the mammary glands. It takes anywhere from twelve hours to a few days after a birth for progesterone levels to fall far enough to dismantle the prolactin blockade. During that time, blood flow from the uterus is redirected into the breasts as part of a massive demolition and reconstruction project. Meanwhile, the baby waits patiently. Full-term infants are born with enough fluid to last for five days, with or without milk.

The lactation consultant is not worried. Not a bit. Even though four days have gone by, I still have no milk, and Faith still weighs 10 percent less than she did at birth.

Lisa McSherry welcomes us into her tiny Beth Israel office and sits me down in a rocking chair to observe how I feed Faith. She leans her head close to my chest to listen for the soft click that means the baby is swallowing. As is the usual pattern, Faith falls asleep after a few short sips. She's not interested. She is a good baby. Perhaps too good for her own good.

None of this is unusual, Lisa reassures me. Nevertheless, intervention is required. And here's what we're going to do. She begins to write instructions on a pad of paper. First, I'll rent a top-of-the-line breast pump to simulate nursing until Faith finally rouses herself from her dreamy slumber and decides she is hungry. Then, whatever drops of milk I manage to collect will be mixed with a few ounces of infant formula and poured into a breastfeeding supplementer. She shows me the required equipment, which resembles a doll-sized IV bag. The milk is poured into the top and drips through a soft plastic tube thinner than a strand of spaghetti. The open end of the tube will be taped against my nipple, like an extra mammary duct, so that when Faith nurses she gets a bigger reward for the effort. This should keep her suckling longer. The more she suckles, the more milk I will make. Eventually, the supplementer will be entirely filled by my own milk, and I can dispense with the formula and, within a few weeks, the supplementer. At that point, we'll be a blissful, breastfeeding couple. In the meantime, I'll nurse Faith every three hours and pump in between feedings. If she doesn't wake up at night to eat, I'll set an alarm clock. It's also important to offer no bottles and no pacifiers until breastfeeding is established. These will confuse her and sabotage the process. Also, we must count the number of wet diapers. As long as she has eight to ten within a twenty-four-hour period, we'll know she's not becoming dehydrated.

Jeff and I look at each other. It all sounds bizarre but manageable. After two days at home with the bizarre and unmanageable, it is nice to have a plan.

Lisa holds Faith as we fumble with the diaper bag, the water bottle, the baby carrier, and the buttons on my blouse. She smiles broadly as she hands her back to me.

"I think she looks like you," she says with a wink.

"I'm adopted," I say blankly. It's a telling response. I'm so accustomed to discounting the physical resemblance people claim they see between me and my own mother that I forget that Faith and I are related. Even though I have the episiotomy stitches to prove it. Which, right now, are hurting me a lot.

Lisa studies me for a while.

"So am I," she replies slowly. Then she shows me a picture of her own (breastfed) daughter, now eight years old. Bright eyes, mile-wide grin, she looks like a miniature version of her mother.

And that's when I know it is no accident that Lisa has devoted her career to helping mothers forge abiding, biological bonds with their babies. Nor is it any accident that I desire this relationship so deeply. Your body out of mine. From my body into yours. First blood. Then milk. These are the living threads that weave mother and child together. As much as I love my adoptive mom, this bond is a connection we never had. And as for the unknown woman who gave birth to me, we were lost to each other before I was even as old as Faith is now. And for about the twelfth time today, I begin to cry.

Just as the breast has a life history, so does its milk. From midpregnancy on, the mammary glands produce a thick, yellow fluid that breastfeeding advocates like to extol as "liquid gold." This is colostrum, and perhaps no other human bodily fluid is as highly revered. Rich in proteins and fat-soluble vitamins, it swarms with antibodies, growth-promoting substances, and living immune cells. It also contains a laxative that helps flush meconium out of the gut. (So startling in appearance to new parents, meconium is the black, tarry material that forms the newborn's first stool. Hoarded in the intestine for nine long months, it contains dead skin cells, amniotic fluid, body hair, bile, blood, and mucus.) Sometimes drops of colostrum begin to ooze spontaneously from the breasts during the last few weeks of pregnancy. But plenty of mothers never see their colostrum even after they give birth—except perhaps as sticky, glistening strands suspended between their nipples and their babies' mouths at the conclusion of an early breastfeeding. Colostrum is produced in only tablespoons per day.

Once progesterone is cleared from the bloodstream and prolactin can take charge, a massive increase in synthesis and secretion gets underway, and milk volume increases tenfold. This jump in production usually occurs suddenly and is perceived by the mother as the coming in of her milk. The breasts often become engorged during this time, undergoing yet another astonishing increase in size. This transformation is not caused by overfilling but by a kind of edema. Milk leaks from the ducts and accumulates in the spaces between cells. The surrounding breast tissue becomes temporarily turgid. After a few days, engorgement subsides and the breasts soften again.

Over the next week or so, the milk becomes paler and thinner as it evolves from colostrum to transitional milk—which is the color of melted butter—and finally to mature milk. As the volume increases, sugar and fat content are stepped up and protein levels drop, along with the concentration of antibodies. Eventually, the volume of milk produced levels off at just under one quart per day. This figure is remarkably consistent among exclusively breastfeeding mothers around the world, although there are important exceptions. Among very lean women, milk volume is increased 5 to 15 percent to compensate for the milk's lower fat content. The daily milk volume in mothers of twins and triplets plateaus at two to three quarts per day. Most impressive, some wet nurses in the 1930s were found to be capable of producing nearly a gallon of milk every twenty-four hours.

Even after its daily volume stabilizes, mother's milk remains dynamic. It has its own seasons and biorhythms. Morning milk has the lowest fat content, noon milk the highest, with evening milk somewhere in between. The composition of human milk changes even within a single feeding. The milk stored at the front of the breast—the foremilk—is high in water and sugar but low in fat. It quenches thirst and provides quick calories during the first few minutes of nursing. As the baby drains the milk stored in the ducts, another pulse of milk rushes forward from the back of the chest wall. This second wave—the hindmilk—is 30 percent creamier, stays in the stomach longer, and, many mothers believe, helps to promote sleep.

The fifth day after Faith's birth is golden and summery. Through a fog of exhaustion, I notice that the thorny tangle of roses in the perpetually unkempt yard next door is blooming one last time. I am so tired I am starting to twitch. After a night of alarm clocks and flashlights, of syringes and pumps and frantic conversations about how best to tape a tube to my nipple, I am not sure what to do with myself. Jeff and Faith are napping together in the living room. I shuffle out to the kitchen, where Janet is sterilizing tubes and milk-collecting bottles on the stove. The breast pump sits on the counter, and I momentarily mistake it for a car transmission. It occurs to me that I should ask why there is a transmission next to the coffee grinder, but by the time I formulate the question, the answer doesn't seem to matter. Between my perceptions and responses is a strange time delay, which, if I thought about it further, would unnerve me. I sit down on a chair and then stand up again. The episiotomy. It hurts. I should probably take a sitz bath. I should probably pump again. I should probably eat something.

Janet, who has been a workhorse since we arrived back home—doing laundry, washing dishes, overseeing the wet diaper count—turns and looks at me.

"Take a nap, sweetheart. Everything's fine out here." I turn and shuffle back into the bedroom. It feels strange to lie down without Faith next to me. She has been such a constant presence, her peaceful, black-haired spirit breathing next to me through all this chaos. How is it that I've known her for only five days? And then I am asleep.

I dream my breasts turn into two bottles of Coca-Cola. Someone is trying to shake them up. When I open my eyes, I am in my own bed, but I am still caught in the dream. My chest is fizzing. I sit up, trying to escape. The front of my nightgown is soaked. Bewildered, I walk to the bathroom and undress. In the mirror is my own face, pale and confused. Beneath it are a pair of enormous breasts. They begin at my collar bone and extend under my armpits. They are hot, lumpy, and hard. I am awake. My milk is here.

Prolactin is only one of two crucial pituitary hormones that make breastfeeding possible. The other one is oxytocin, the hormone that plays a leading role in labor. (Oxytocin also plays a role in female orgasm. It's a versatile actor.) Where prolactin causes the milk to be made, oxytocin causes it to flow.

Since the pituitary gland is located underneath the brain, far from the breast, it needs to receive a quick message about when to release milk. The communications device it uses is the fourth intercostal nerve, whose starting point is the areola, that pigmented halo that surrounds the nipple. When the baby begins to suckle, the muscles beneath the areola contract and cause the nipple to become erect, the better for the baby to latch on to. The areola also releases from its own bumpy glands an oily lubrication that both protects the nipple from the friction of suckling and serves as a natural antiseptic to keep yeast and bacteria from infecting either the mammary glands or the baby. But most critically, the areola lets the brain know that milk is needed. Now.

About thirty seconds after suckling commences, oxytocin, which is released into the general circulation, reaches the mammary ducts and causes the muscular layer that surrounds them, the myoepithelium, to contract. A surge of milk moves out of the lobules, down the ducts, and sprays out of the nipple's showerhead and into the mouth of the baby. Meanwhile, the oxytocin molecules still coursing through the mother's bloodstream trigger physiological changes that bring on a sense of calmness and well-being. Just as it does after orgasm.

Stress, fatigue, and anxiety can inhibit this cascade of events. Just as it can inhibit the momentum during sex.

The plan is working. The refrigerator fills up with bottles of breast milk. The baby grows. The mother rejoices. Or, at least, she would, if she were not so tired.

My physical connection with Faith is reestablished and reconfigured. Ten to twelve times a day—and into the night—we two become one again. As with a lover, the world contracts when we are together. She and I enter a little bubble of our own making. The larger, outer world we leave behind seems ridiculous, overstimulating, vulgar, unmiraculous. Let's just stay here in this rocking chair, this bed, this couch, and drown in milky abundance. I think I will burst with pride. We figured it out, you and I. First we came through the birth, and now we've learned the tango.

At the start of a feeding, Faith sips, like a gourmet cook tasting the broth. Then she closes her eyes, latches her suction cup of a mouth around the entire pinky-brown circle, and begins in earnest. I wait for the oxytocin to hit, which feels like a velvet curtain falling inside my breasts. Tingly, warm, sumptuous. Lactation specialists call this the milk ejection reflex, but I prefer the old-timey term: the let-down. The old dairy farmers were on to something when they remarked of a milk cow, "If you don't gentle her she won't let down." Milk blooms around the edges of Faith's lips, and she presses in harder, gulping, gulping. She stops periodically and looks up into my eyes as if she had just remembered something she wanted to say. But then again, never mind, and she goes back to work. If her hand should fall against my other nipple, she grabs hold of it, as if to anchor it in place until she is ready for it. When she is finished, she pops off the nipple with the sound of a cork flying from a champagne bottle, rounds her mouth up into a little O, and then throws her head down onto my chest, arms splayed, like a drunken sailor slumped to the decks. Sometimes she lies for hours with my nipple in her ear, as though listening for the milky tide to come rushing back in. No one has ever enjoyed my breasts more. Faith is the consumer. I am the consommée.

Suckling is not the same as sucking, which is simply the creation of negative pressure. Sucking is what draws water up a straw when we pull our cheeks together. Suckling, on the other hand, is complex activity that can only be done by infants. It involves three simultaneous actions. First, the tongue strokes the nipple and the lower part of the areola. At the same time, the ridges of the baby's gums compress the milk sinuses, the flared-out portion of the milk ducts located just under the areola. This double motion pulls the foremilk out of the sinuses and sends a message to the pituitary gland, which both stimulates the let-down reflex (via oxytocin) and speeds up milk production in the acini (via prolactin). In the meantime, the baby's lips and cheek muscles create the suction that draws the nipple up against the baby's upper palate and into the back of its throat. In the vacuum created by this motion, the mother's nipple thins out to half its normal width and elongates to double or triple its normal length.

Mathematicians have looked closely at this arrangement. ("We describe a mathematical model of the flow and deformation in a human teat. . . . Our model is based on quasi-linear poroelasticity whereby the teat is modeled as a cylindrical porous elastic material saturated with fluid. We impose a cyclic axial suction pressure difference which mimics infant suckling.") They have filled many pages with calculations—"With these assumptions, equation 4 becomes____where Newton's third law implies_____ Substituting the interaction term of equation 7 into equation 5 and using____leads to_____ Taking Darcy's law and expressing it relative to the movement of the solid it is easy to obtain____." Finally, they reached their conclusion: "During suckling, both the suction pressure and compressive force applied by the infant are equally important." What this means in practical terms is that no machine can precisely mimic suckling. Breast pumps recreate only the rhythmical sucking, not the attendant peristaltic stroking and compression. Not surprisingly, then, pumps can only extract a fraction of the milk that a month-old newborn can. This is why a new mother is instructed not to despair when, after twenty minutes of motorized tugging by a $500 machine, the collecting bottles contain only a measly ounce or two of milk. As long the baby produces ten wet diapers a day, she's getting a lot more than that.

Faith is the consumer, and I am the consumed. We sit down to breastfeed, and the world disappears, just out of reach. The newspaper sits unread, inches away, but I cannot quite reach it. As soon as the let-down hits, my mouth turns to ashes. The glass of water, too, is just out of reach. I call for Jeff, but he is down in the basement doing laundry. I now have tendinitis in my wrist from holding the baby to my breast four hours a day, five hours a day, six hours a day. I leak urine every time I cough. There are supposed to be solutions for these kinds of problems, but the books that provide them are over there on the shelf. Just out of reach. The tea kettle starts its insane whistling, and there is nothing I can do about it. The phone rings and there is nothing I can do about it. I haven't taken a shower in two days, and there is nothing I can do about it.

According to evolutionary biologists, breastfeeding is a form of matrotropy: eating one's mother. To this end, all mammary glands share fundamental aspects of structure and function. Their number and placement, however, are highly variable. The current record holder, with twenty-four mammae, is an insect-eating, hedgehog-like mammal that lives in Madagascar. In general, the number of mammae is roughly twice the litter size, making two the minimal number. Pigs and rats have twelve. Opossums, for some reason, have thirteen. In many mammals, the mammae are located in two lines along the underbelly, but the glands can be confined either to the groin or to the chest. At least one aquatic rodent, the nutria, has breasts on its back.

As a general rule, mammals that hold their young with their upper limbs—bats and primates—wear their mammae on their chests, whereas animals that stand up to nurse—cows, horses, sheep, goats—have them tucked into their groins. Inexplicably, elephant mothers nurse from their chests. So do manatees, those gentle, floating sea cows, although in their case, it's an arrangement that allows for simultaneous nursing and breathing. Other marine mammals have breasts capable of shooting jets of milk into the mouths of their submerged young. These include whales, dolphins, and hippopotamus, whose babies also feed while underwater.

According to historians, the Latin word *mamma*, meaning "breast," the singular form of "mammae," makes its first appearance in the English language in 1579. It probably derives originally from the syllables "ma-ma" uttered spontaneously by babies, who are encouraged in many different cultures to use it as their name for mother.

I am milk. My milk is me. When Faith cries for me, she cries for milk, for the breast stuffed into the mouth. It is all the same thing. I am eaten. I have never felt more alive. I am eaten. I have never felt more abolished. The oneness of breastfeeding is totalizing. We even sleep and wake in tandem, my eyes opening just before she begins to stir in the bed next to me. I pull her down to my breast, check for a wet diaper. I'm getting good at this. We drift back into sleep, conjoined.

In the meantime, I bleed for six long weeks. Except it is not really blood but lochia, the digested matter of the postpartum uterus. The human womb has the power of autolysis, the breaking down of tissue by self-produced enzymes. The excess uterine muscle once used to push the baby into the world must be consumed. So, too, the blood pooled in the holes left behind by the placenta's deep roots.

The baby eats the mother. The mother eats herself. Everyone comes to feast upon the body of the mother.

It was the Swedish botanist and taxonomist Carolus Linnaeus who, in 1758, named the warm-blooded, hairy branch of the animal kingdom Mammalia. It was an attention-grabbing choice and certainly parted company with the previous name, Quadrapedia, which had been in place since Aristotle first tried classifying creation some 2,200 years earlier. In fact, Linnaeus's decision brought immediate hoots of derision from rivals and colleagues, who were swift to point out that the possession of mammae was a feature of only *half* of the members of the group. Many were outright offended that Linnaeus would heap honor upon a female organ by naming a whole class of animals after it. But the title stuck anyway.

Despite the fact that an entire taxonomic category is named for the mammary gland, very little is known about its origin. Breasts do not fossilize, and unlike the situation with, say, the bones of the inner ear, no homologue can be found among living reptiles. The mammary gland is believed to have evolved from an ectodermal structure, but the commonly held notion that breasts are modified sweat glands is an oversimplification. In their cell structure, they have as much in common with oil glands as with sweat glands.

Equally mysterious is why, in males of all species, mammary glands are present but never become functional. (Well, almost never. Male fruit bats in Malaysia have been captured with milk-filled mammary glands, but no one knows whether they are actually used to nurse offspring.) Curiously, the degree to which the male breast remains undeveloped is highly variable. Human males, possessing well-formed nipples and ducts, occupy the far end of the male mammary continuum. Our males even respond to nipple stimulation with a pituitary surge of prolactin. Men are also susceptible to breast cancer, albeit to a much lesser degree than women. At the opposite pole are rodents, whose males typically possess neither ducts nor nipples.

What we do know is that lactation apparently made it possible for mammals to inherit the earth from dinosaurs. At least two leading evolutionary biologists, Daniel G. Blackburn and Caroline

Pond, believe breasts are responsible for the phenomenal success of the whole class, for they permitted its penetration into harsh ecosystems, including the ones where reptiles fear to tread, such as the Arctic. In addition, as Caroline Pond has pointed out, breast-feeding allows mothers to dispense with foraging expeditions in search of suitable food for their newborns, and the babies themselves can grow faster because they are not expending energy looking for food. Furthermore, calories and key minerals such as calcium can be stored up in the mother's body over a long period of time and then transferred via breast milk to the offspring, even when these materials are not immediately available in the surrounding environment. Compare this situation to that of reptiles. Even within the same species, individuals of different sizes and ages require very different diets. Babies may dine on one set of foods and juveniles another, while the adults choose something else altogether. All the items on the grocery list may or may not be consistently available. Breasts are thus a hedge against food shortages.

Biologists think that mammary glands arose very early in the Darwinian game, almost surely predating the advent of live birth. The strongest evidence for this suspicion is the existence of a queer little group of mammals called monotremes, which includes the platypus and spiny anteater. Monotremes lay eggs and yet also lactate, indicating that breasts are older on the evolutionary timeline than placentas.

When Faith turns three weeks old, she wakes up. Her quiet serenity gives way to keen insistence—but for what? I guess she might be going through a growth spurt, so I leave my shirt open for easy access. But even after feeding off and on all day, she still longs for something she cannot express except through an unceasing cry that cuts through me like a police siren. Janet has gone back home, leaving Jeff and me to sort this one out by ourselves. We try to have a calm, thoughtful discussion about what to do but are reduced to hand-waving, charades, and attempts at lip-reading, as the baby is crying so loudly we cannot hear each other. I look up "crying" in the index of every baby-care manual I own and run through their checklists of possible reasons, all to no avail. Finally, at 4 A.M., Jeff stumbles upon one last untried recommendation: take the baby for a walk. He holds up a hand-lettered sign that reads GOING OUT

FOR COFFEE. Then he plops Faith into the baby sling and heads out the door. The last thing I hear before drifting off to sleep is the Doppler sound of a baby's cry disappearing into the distance like a train whistle.

For the first time since I went into labor, I am alone.

An unshaven, unwashed man with a sleeping infant slung around his neck walks into a twenty-four-hour doughnut shop in Union Square, Somerville. It is 4:20 A.M. Except for two cab drivers, the place is empty. Ragged with exhaustion, the man steps up to the counter and orders a large coffee and a jelly doughnut. The cashier narrows her heavily mascara'd eyes. "Where," she demands to know, "is that baby's mama?"

Humans stand out among mammals for the runny quality of our milk. In fact, ours is the most dilute of any mammalian milk, and it also has the lowest protein content. This thin gruel apparently suits us, however. Though human babies are the fattest of all the mammals at birth, we are among the slowest-growing. The idea is to provide us a long childhood for ample learning and lots of water so that we can sweat to regulate body temperature.

The nutritional content of mammalian milk is also a function of nursing style. Animals that are infrequent nursers, leaving their babies in nests while they graze or hunt, have the richest milk. Because the mothers return at widely spaced intervals, they must provide their young with a concentrated energy source. Rabbits nurse every four hours. Rabbit milk is 10 percent fat. Lions nurse every eight hours. Lion milk is 19 percent fat. Constant nursers are those whose young remain close to the mother. Because feedings are frequent, their milk is lower in nutrients. Members of this category include grazing animals as well as primates. Thus, cow's milk and human milk are both about 4 percent butterfat.

It's ugly. Let's be honest. Compared to the crisp purity of cow's milk, mother's milk looks dim, blurry, and out of focus when poured into a bottle. It's not even white. Breast milk is the yellow-gray color of an old undershirt. And after the milk sits in a bottle for an hour, a thin scum of cream forms across the top, leaving underneath a liquid of pale green. Perhaps this is why breastfeeding mothers who return to work complain about the lack of privacy not only for the act of expressing their milk but also for its storage. Working mothers say they feel uneasy about parking bottles of breast milk in the employee refrigerator where all can see. Before I became a breastfeeder myself, I didn't understand this. You wouldn't feel strange about putting a bottle of cow's milk on a shared shelf; why would you feel shy about your own? Now I find myself hiding the bottles of pumped milk behind the mustard and the olives in the back of my own refrigerator, just because it's so . . . homely.

Perhaps our collective squeamishness about breast milk goes deeper than misgivings over its appearance. Infant formula wouldn't win any beauty contests either, and it smells a hundred times worse. And yet, in one recent book on breastfeeding, a new mother tells of her mother-in-law's refusal even to touch a bottle of breast milk, announcing firmly that she isn't going to feed that stuff to her grandson. Whatever this aversion is about, it's relatively new on the cultural scene. Museums are full of paintings of the lactating Virgin Mary, her milk a symbol of mercy and holiness. Indeed, as Natalie Angier points out, vials of fluid alleged to be the milk of Mary filled Catholic reliquaries throughout the Middle Ages. Throughout antiquity, mother's milk was believed to possess all-purpose powers of healing and was variously prescribed to adults as a cure for deafness, consumption, constipation, and fever.

Even our own galaxy was named because it resembled a wash of breast milk across the night sky. *The Origin of the Milky Way*, Jacopo Tintoretto's famous Mannerist painting, celebrates the story. In it, Jupiter's wife, Juno, releases the suckling infant Hercules from her breast in mid-let-down and instead lactates out into the cosmos. The jets of milk that spurt upward become stars. Those falling to earth give rise to lilies. I myself stood in front of this painting in the National Gallery of London when I was four months pregnant and still waiting for the results of my amniocentesis. Looking at the white arcs shooting, fountainlike, in all directions from Juno's two nipples, I laughed, thinking, "how exaggerated and improbable." But it's not. Tintoretto was the devoted father of seven children. He probably knew a thing or two about the milk ejection reflex.

Lilies and stars. I pull a bottle of breast milk out of the back of the refrigerator, pour it into a wine glass, stir it up with a spoon, and take a big swallow. The first thing I notice is how surprisingly sweet it is, like sweetened condensed milk that's been diluted several times. (Which is not so surprising, really, since condensed milk was first marketed as a breast milk substitute.) As the initial sugariness wears off, a series of musky, earthy notes linger on the tongue. Finally, one is left with a faint, mysterious flavor that tastes like how the breath of a baby smells.

Although containing an identical percentage of fat, human breast milk has nearly twice the sugar (lactose) of cow's milk. It also has more vitamin A, C, E, and K. However, cow's milk contains more than triple the protein of human milk and a lot more salt. Calves need more protein than human babies because they double their birth weight in less than two months. Humans take a full half year to do this.

Also, the type of protein is different. Or, more specifically, the ratio of curds to whey is different. Curds are casein, the chunks in the cottage cheese; whey is lactalbumin, the fluid that floats on top of the yogurt. Cow's milk has twice the curds and one third the whey of breast milk. This is why feeding unmodified cow's milk to newborns is not recommended. The high level of protein and salt is a burden to the kidneys, and the large, solid blobs it forms in the stomach cause colic and cramping. On the other hand, breast milk would make lousy cottage cheese.

Early motherhood is an extreme sport.

Sleep deprivation is part of the problem. This will not come as news to anyone who has ever had a baby, but before I gave birth, I had naively assumed that some mystical, mother-love hormone would kick in and make it possible for me to endure sleeplessness in ways that non-mothers cannot. I am somehow astonished to discover that being awakened at 2 A.M. feels just as awful as it ever did. For me, the accumulating sleep deficit manifests itself as a growing inability to find things—even when they are in plain view and directly in front of me. Thus, making dinner takes two or three times longer than it would if I could just see the salt shaker on the counter, the paring knife in the sink, the salad bowl in the dish drainer. Jeff, on the other hand, loses vocabulary words. So our conversations now go something like this:

"Honey, have you seen the paper towels?"

"They're on top of the . . . thing."

The direct consequence of sleep deprivation is a gradual slowing down of routine activities at precisely the time when they need to be sped up. The disparity between what needs to be done and what actually gets done leads to chronic frustration, which, if unchecked, leads to despair.

But sleeplessness is really only part of it. More profound is having to pay attention all of the time. One is not merely awakened at 2 A.M. One must solve complicated and alarming problems at 2 A.M. (Example: Why is the baby's poop green?) The need always to pay attention leads to another kind of dispossession that I can only call thought deprivation. In my life as non-mother, I had moments even during very busy days in which I was free to entertain an old memory, replay a conversation, form a political opinion, or just daydream. Such opportunities might come while walking to the bathroom, getting dressed, opening the mail, feeding the dog. One does not even notice these moments until they are confiscated, stripped of conscious thought, and filled with listening for the baby, wondering if the baby is still breathing, trying to distinguish between the sound of a hunger cry and a pain cry, and imagining the various ways the baby could die. At some point, when one is offered a short reprieve from new-mother-ness—as when the new father says, "Why don't you take a walk?"—all the suppressed and unthought thoughts come rushing up at once. This can feel like a form of insanity.

Finally, there is the inability to have expectations. For example, the baby falls asleep, and peace descends upon the household. But one does not know if the baby will stay asleep for two hours or two minutes. Therefore, one does not know whether it is more appropriate to write a quick thank-you note, take a nap, too, or finally deal with the insurance claim mess. Every time I guess wrong I feel defeated, and a string of defeats gradually leads to a kind of helpless confusion. When the baby is not sleeping, the ability to accomplish tasks goes completely out the window. Breastfeeding happens every two to three hours, an interval that extends from the start of one feeding until the start of the next one. If Faith feeds for an hour, then I might have only one hour before the next round. During this hour, the baby needs to burp, and I need to pee. The pitcher of water needs refilling. The baby needs a diaper change. The baby needs a bath. Suddenly it's time again.

The home front looks like . . . a front. One load of laundry is washed but not dried; two loads are ready to go into the washer; and one load is washed and dried but needs folding. Half of the mail has been opened. Three out of nine bills have been paid. Two others are ready to go, but we need more stamps. The other four bills are still unopened, at least one of which fell behind the radiator and needs to be retrieved with a broom handle, which I can't do while holding the baby. Three out of seventeen phone messages have been returned. The cat has been fed but not the dog. Six out of eight house plants have been watered. A few dishes have been done, but the rest are marooned in the sink. The mental list of half-finished tasks splinters and grows exponentially, and the mental inventory I carry around in my head threatens to undo me.

Other mothers are my lifeline. The antidote to the despair factor, they all agree, is to get out of the house every day. With or without the baby. No matter what. No matter how briefly. One says, "There is a fine line between saying 'I spent the whole day picking Cheerios up off the floor' and saying 'The only thing I'm good for is picking Cheerios up off the floor.' Getting out every day keeps you on the right side of that line."

So why *did* Linnaeus name the mammals mammals? It's tempting to imagine him as a kind of prescient proto-feminist who understood before his time the power of the female breast in shaping evolutionary history. Alas, this does not seem to be case. As is convincingly argued by Londa Schiebinger, a historian of science, Linnaeus's peculiar and radical decision seems to have been deeply influenced by his strong opinions on breastfeeding. And these opinions were part of a larger political agenda that was anything but progressive.

At the time Linnaeus was compiling his magnum opus, *Systema Naturae*, in which he names all the animals of the world, Europe was caught in the throes of a debate over wet-nursing. This was a common practice in the eighteenth century, especially in Paris, where most infants were farmed out to professional lactators during their first year of life. Linnaeus was actively involved in a campaign that sought to outlaw wet nursing and require women to breastfeed their own babies. Like Tintoretto, he was the father of seven children—all of whom were nursed by his wife. Linnaeus was also a practicing physician, and shortly before coining the term "Mammalia" he authored a treatise that thundered against the abuses and evils of wet-nursing. One of his arguments was that it deprived a baby of colostrum, which he (correctly) claimed helped purge meconium from the gut. In the United States, wet-nursing also contributed to the deaths of the nurses' own biological offspring, who were often abruptly weaned and delivered into the care of others when their lactating mothers turned professional.

But Linnaeus's objections were more than biological. He warned that the character of upper-class children was being corrupted by the milk of lower-class nurses. In ordering high-born women to return to their rightful places as loving, lactating mothers in the home, he appealed to them on the basis of natural law. Be like the beasts of the field, he urged them—which is always frightening advice when directed by men at women. Indeed, as Schiebinger goes on to explicate, the anti-wet-nurse campaign was but one part of a larger social crusade to rein in women's growing political power and curtail their opportunities outside the home.

Linnaeus was coming fresh from this political battlefield when he christened the human race *Homo sapiens*—wise man—and embedded us firmly within a class of animals he called mammals.

11

Loaves and Fishes

As a young bride, my mother underwent emergency surgery when an ectopic pregnancy ruptured one of her fallopian tubes. When her doctor told her she could never become pregnant again, she and my father turned to their Methodist minister for help. He led them to a Methodist adoption agency in neighboring McLean County, whose social workers led them to me, a three-month-old infant who had been surrendered at birth at a hospital in Champaign, one more county farther east. I was fed 5.5 ounces of infant formula every four hours; my diaper was folded into thirds with a twist in the middle and pinned on both sides; and I took three scheduled naps per day. Already sleeping through the night, I was considered by all to be a very cooperative baby. Or so goes the family story.

My parents named me after a teenage girl in their church, Sandra Miller, who, it seemed to them, was particularly bright, outgoing, and happy. And with this new identity, I was baptized a Methodist. For most of my childhood I went to Sunday school every week and Bible school in the summer. As a teenager I took confirmation classes, competed in New Testament trivia contests, and played the part of Mary in the annual Christmas play. When it was time to go to college, it seemed natural for me to consider the Methodist-affiliated university forty-five miles away, which is how I ended up at Illinois Wesleyan.

It is also where I left Methodism behind. This was not a big decision, or even a conscious one. Years passed before I realized, with some relief, that I could no longer remember the last time I had been inside a church. Nevertheless, in a recent conversation with a lapsed Baptist and stay-at-home-father, I discovered that I do carry a genuine appreciation for all those Bible verses we were made to memorize. So, my friend admits, does he.

They come back to me while I am breastfeeding. Take the fourteenth chapter of Matthew. This is the one where Jesus sails off to "a desert place apart." But solitude is not his for long, for he is joined by a multitude of 5,000 followers. He spends all day healing their sick. When night falls, his disciples urge him to disband the crowd and send them home because everyone is hungry. Instead, Jesus orders the throngs to be fed from five loaves and two fishes, which he personally blesses. Miraculously, after all eat their fill, twelve baskets of leftovers remain.

It's those overflowing baskets I most often think about while I nurse. At six weeks old, Faith has resumed her old identity as a peaceful, self-assured baby. Only now she eats and sleeps according to almost-predictable patterns. Now she smiles. Life gets easier. I take daily showers again. Letters are written. Dishes washed. Laundry folded. Best of all, Faith weighs nine pounds, ten ounces. "Growing like a weed," according to the pediatrician, a phrase to gladden the heart of any breastfeeding mother. I feel my milk supply expanding along with the baby and no longer have to pump on the side.

This, then, is the daily miracle of breastfeeding: the more milk the baby drinks, the more milk the mother makes. There is no need for rationing and measuring. Instead, hunger itself produces a surfeit of food. There is no end to it. By giving all I have, I have more to give. The breast is a self-replenishing vessel, not a pantry that can be depleted. The breastfeeding handbooks call this phenomenon the principle of supply and demand. I prefer to think of it as the principle of loaves and fishes. Wherefore didst thou doubt?

The ability to heal the sick is another miraculous property of breast milk not shared by its inferior pretender, infant formula. Breastfed infants have lower rates of hospitalization and death. They develop fewer respiratory infections, gastrointestinal infections, urinary tract infections, middle ear infections, and bacterial meningitis. They succumb much less often to that most dreaded of all maladies, Sudden Infant Death Syndrome. They also produce more antibodies in response to routine immunizations. These patterns hold for infants living in wealthy, industrialized nations as well as in poor, rural ones.

Breastfed babies even breathe differently than bottle-fed babies. Babies who drink from a bottle have longer exhalations and a reduction in breathing frequency while they are feeding. These changes contribute to a decrease in oxygen intake during bottle-feeding that is not seen in breastfeeding. A difference in the mechanics of extracting milk from a breast and an artificial nipple is probably the reason. This difference also helps explain why ear infections are so much higher in bottle babies: the Eustachian tube—that narrow tunnel linking the ear to the sinuses—does not close properly during bottle-feeding, allowing nasal secretions and formula to back up into the tubes. By contrast, the faster and more vigorous suckling required by breastfeeding seals off the Eustachian tubes.

Studies documenting the benefits of breastfeeding on infant health are not as easy to undertake as they might at first seem. Breastfed and formula-fed babies differ in ways other than their methods of nutritional delivery. Breastfeeding mothers in the United States tend to have more money and education than mothers who bottle-feed. They also smoke less. The best studies take these social factors into account and correct for them. One of the most convincing studies, published in 1998, investigated 2,000 Navajo infants in New Mexico before and after a breastfeeding promotion program. Before the program, only 16 percent of infants were breastfed. After, 55 percent were. After the program, infant pneumonia fell by a third and gastrointestinal infection by 15 percent. The authors conclude, "Increased incidence of illness among minimally breastfed infants is causally related to lack of breast milk."

The fortifying effect of mother's milk on health endures long after weaning. For example, the ability of breastfeeding to protect against respiratory illness extends for at least seven years, according to a Scottish study that followed a cohort of 600 breast- and bottle-fed babies into their school years. Seven-year-olds who were breastfed as babies also had significantly lower blood pressure.

These differences remained even after correcting for factors such as weight, maternal blood pressure, and economic class.

Thus, breastfeeding offers benefits beyond simple protection from infectious diseases. Studies consistently show that children and young adults who were breastfed as infants suffer less from allergies, asthma, type I (juvenile) diabetes, Crohn's disease, ulcerative colitis, and juvenile rheumatoid arthritis. All these various disorders share in common a misdirected immune reaction. In Crohn's disease, antibodies attack milk proteins and bacterial flora in the colon, resulting in inflammation and ulcers. In ulcerative colitis, the immune system attacks the intestinal lining itself, resulting in damage that raises the risk for colon cancer and, in severe cases, necessitates surgical removal of the entire colon. (Interestingly, when human milk is fed to rats with chemically induced colitis, they are cured.) In rheumatoid arthritis, the target is the connective tissues of the joints, which are erroneously identified as foreign proteins. In type I diabetes, the wrongfully attacked body part is the pancreas or, more specifically, the cells of the pancreas that produce insulin.

How exactly breastfeeding safeguards against the onset of these diseases is not clear. However, some light is now being shed on the link between formula feeding and diabetes. Bovine insulin, which is present in milk-based formulas, is very similar in structure but not identical to human insulin. The infant's immune system sometimes begins to manufacture antibodies in response to the foreign insulin protein in formula. Later on—sometimes many years after the fact—these antibodies begin to attack the pancreatic cells that make human insulin. In one study, 10 percent of children drinking cow's milk formula had formed the kind of antibodies that are known to be associated with diabetes, which means they are at increased risk of contracting the disease. Another recent study compares diabetes rates in Cuba, where breastfeeding is universal, with those in Puerto Rico, where less than 5 percent of mothers breastfeed. Type I diabetes is ten times more prevalent in Puerto Rico.

Breast milk may also safeguard against obesity and cancer. At twelve months, breastfed babies are leaner than formula-fed babies. This difference is due partly to the higher caloric content of formula. However, breastfed babies continue to regulate their own calorie intake at lower levels even after they start on solid foods. Again, these benefits linger. A recent study in Germany found that babies breastfed for a year were one fourth as likely to be obese as schoolchildren as those breastfed for less than two months. Whether these differences persist into adult life is not clear.

Several carefully designed studies have found that artificially fed infants, as well as those who are breastfed only briefly, go on to suffer significantly higher rates of Hodgkin's lymphoma than babies breastfed for six months or more. A rare cancer that is most prevalent in adolescents and young adults, Hodgkin's lymphoma is a cancer that originates in the lymph system, that far-flung network of canals and nodes that is a leading player in providing immunity. According to the leading hypothesis, breastfed infants are made more resistant to this cancer by their receipt of some as-yet-unidentified component in human milk that bestows an ability to ward off carcinogenic threats to the immune system.

What's good for the gosling is good for the goose, too. Breastfeeding also protects the health of mothers. The consistently high levels of oxytocin maintained by suckling more quickly returns the uterus to its prebirth size, which is approximately that of a plum. Because breastfeeding women don't resume menstruation immediately, they lose less blood during the sleepless, stressful days of early motherhood. High prolactin levels suppress ovulation, providing a natural form of birth control for at least three months— and often longer (though not foolproof) if mothers continue to nurse at night, when prolactin levels are highest. Nursing mothers also have lower rates of ovarian and premenopausal breast cancer, two big killers of younger women. A recent study conducted in Iceland found that breastfeeding significantly reduced the chance of contracting breast cancer before age 40. The longer the duration of nursing, the greater the protection afforded. The relationship between breastfeeding and postmenopausal breast cancer is, however, unclear. Some research shows a modest reduction in postmenopausal breast cancer among women who practice prolonged breastfeeding. A recent study of Chinese mothers found that women who breastfed for more than twenty-four months per child cut their risk of breast cancer by half.

Several investigators have tried to express the health-promoting aspects of breast milk in economic terms. According to one, in the first year of life alone breastfeeding saves between $331 to $475 per infant in medical treatment, owing solely to decreased incidence of lower respiratory illness, ear infections, and gastrointestinal illnesses. (This is on top of the average $1,000 per year saved by not feeding a baby formula instead of breast milk; breast milk may be the only free lunch in the economic world.) These calculations, of course, do not include the savings—in dollars and in lives—from decreased rates of diabetes, allergies, asthma, obesity, rheumatoid arthritis, lymphoma, leukemia, colitis, Crohn's disease, breast cancer, and ovarian cancer.

By the time Faith is seven weeks old, I've figured out how to breast-feed while lying down, breastfeed while walking, breastfeed while talking on the phone, breastfeed while reading the paper, breastfeed while taking a bath, and breastfeed while typing at the computer (one-handed). How is it that only a month ago I couldn't even fig-ure out how to make a cup of tea? I'm ready to accept social invita-tions again, but the phone—which for so long has gone unanswered and its dutifully recorded magnetic messages unreturned—has stopped ringing. I stare at it from across the room. "Ring," I order it. When suddenly it does, I nearly jump out of my skin.

It is the secretary of the president of Illinois Wesleyan Univer-sity. The president, who is traveling along the East Coast, has in-vited a few New England–area alumni to a dinner tomorrow night at Boston's Harvard Club. Would Jeff and I like to join them?

Yes, oh yes, oh yes. "Well, that depends," I say slowly. "I have a new baby I would need to bring along. Would she be welcome, too?"

Of course, is the breezy answer.

"Umm. I also breastfeed. Is that a problem?"

"Let me get back to you."

"Okay, thanks."

"Okay, bye."

I pace around, waiting for the phone to ring again. Why did I say that? Why ask permission to nurse a baby? On the other hand, what if we went, I did, and everyone was mortified? For all my bravado, I haven't attempted public breastfeeding yet, unless you count the waiting room of the pediatrician's office.

The phone rings. Yes, of course it would fine. The president explicitly says that it is fine. Terrific. Thanks. Bye.

I don't lose my nerve until we walk into the private room filled with bejeweled women and pinstriped men holding martini glasses. I quickly surmise this is a fundraising party, but why I—who just applied for a deferment on my student loan—am on this guest list escapes me. Happily, Faith is the picture of slumbering tranquillity. Our silver-haired president makes his way over to pump Jeff's hand and admire the baby.

"Right out of central casting!" he enthuses. I look toward the dining room, where waiters are preparing the tables. There are ten pieces of silverware at each plate.

Everything goes swimmingly until the soup course, when Faith wakes up and decides she wants to eat as well. The president has just begun his pitch for the new library. Having read up on how to breastfeed a baby in fine dining situations, I slip off my jacket and deftly take the baby from Jeff with one hand. With the other, I draw my linen napkin up over her head and my shoulder to create a little tent. Then I reach under it and unfasten the top two buttons of my blouse. She latches on and begins to suckle. Perfect.

A second later I learn something new about my daughter which will hold true for her entire life as a nursling: she does not abide covers over her head while she is eating. With some kind of flailing martial arts move, she knocks the napkin off my shoulder and into the soup bowl, which catapults my soup spoon out of the bowl and onto the other row of spoons lined up next to it and sends soup flying into the centerpiece. Faith continues to wave and kick wildly, managing to wedge a foot in between two buttonholes and thereby causing two more buttons to pop open. Caught under her heel, the front edge of my blouse is pushed all the way over to my arm so that both breasts are now completely exposed and I am essentially sitting naked at the table. Meanwhile, the clanging of silver has caused all eyes to turn away from the president and in my direction, where Jeff is now attempting to throw his own napkin over both wife and child. All eyes instantly revert back to the president, who doesn't miss a beat of his speech, and no one looks in our direction again.

The rest of the dinner goes by uneventfully. As the secretary said, of course it would be fine.

Outside the sterile environment of the womb, a human infant immediately encounters roving gangs of bacteria, viruses, and fungi, many of which cause disease. But a newborn is armed with only a rudimentary immune system that won't completely mature for at least two more years. At first glance, this situation seems like a terrible evolutionary oversight. Since immunity is so important to early survival, why wouldn't it be robustly developed by birth? It turns out that all mammals are immunologically incompetent as neonates, which means not only that we humans are in fine company but that there is probably a good explanation besides.

The best hypothesis put forth so far is, basically, you can't do everything. If an infant can defer one big project—like setting up a workable immune system—then it can throw its resources into another one, like brain or lung maturation. This is an especially good idea if the deferred project can be compensated for by agents transferable from the mother into the infant via the milk. If you can get it from Mom, you don't have to invest energy into making it yourself.

For all its reputation as a benevolent nurturer, human breast milk is also a very effective assassin. It kills on contact giardia and trichomonad protozoans, dysentery amoebas, and *E. coli* bacteria. Its ability to do so derives from an arsenal of weapons, both living and nonliving. The living elements within breast milk are leukocytes, white blood cells. These were not even discovered until 1966, when two researchers examined the debris obtained from spinning a tube of colostrum around in a centrifuge for a while. They found it teeming with leukocytes. In other words, they discovered that breast milk is alive. (To be fair, these living cells were first observed by a photographer in 1844—he happened also to be a microscopist—but no one was interested in his findings.)

Now we know that the white blood cells in breast milk actually consist of three different types: macrophages, lymphocytes, and neutrophils. They work both collaboratively and independently. Macrophages are scavengers that engulf and destroy microorganisms that don't belong inside the human body. Macrophages also process foreign substances so that they can be recognized by the lymphocytes, which then escort them away. Lymphocytes hold down two other jobs as well: they manufacture antibodies, and they destroy cells infected by viruses. Neutrophils mediate inflammatory responses, as when tissue is injured or infected. They surround and kill invading bacteria in a bath of enzymes and hydrogen peroxide.

The nonliving immune elements in human milk include interferon, lysozymes, antibodies, and anti-inflammatory agents. Interferon disables viruses by preventing them from reproducing.

Lysozymes slice bacteria into little bits. Antibodies prevent pathogens from sticking to the intestinal-tract lining and also bind to the toxins the pathogens produce. Some milk-borne antibodies can also pass through the intestinal tract through special passageways and circulate within the baby's bloodstream.

How antibodies find their way into breast milk is a fascinating story. It all begins in the gut, which is where our immunological memory is stored. More specifically, the tale begins within special patches of lymphatic tissue associated with the small intestine. These patches are filled with B-cell lymphocytes, more commonly called memory cells. B-cells hold grudges. Each remembers a past encounter with a particular pathogen and holds instructions for how to make antibodies against it, should it ever show its face in these parts again.

As soon as a woman begins lactating, B-cell lymphocytes migrate from her intestines into her breasts, where they secrete large volumes of antibodies. In this way, a mother transfers to her child temporary immunity to the various diseases that she herself has overcome during her lifetime (including some she was vaccinated against as a child). These relocated memory cells will also suffuse breast milk with antibodies for new pathogens to which the mother is exposed during the course of lactation. If a nursing mother gets the flu, her milk may protect her infant from the same fate.

When Faith is eight weeks old, Jeff notices that her right eye seems to be tearing excessively. We mention this to the pediatrician, who guesses the problem is due to a blocked tear duct, a common problem among infants that usually fixes itself by six months. In the meantime, we are instructed in the art of tear duct massage, the purpose of which is to stretch open the membrane obstructing the duct. Faith gladly puts up with this, but the problem persists, and soon her eye is red and inflamed. I wake up one morning to discover, to my horror, that both her eyes are sealed shut with gooey yellow pus. Conjunctivitis.

The pediatrician prescribes an antibiotic cream, which quickly clears up the yellow discharge, but the rims of her eyes remain an angry pink. Every time I administer a dose of cream, she cries out in pain. The pediatrician reassures us that the continued inflammation is probably due to the ointment itself, which is chemically irritating to the eye. It's all enough to break a mother's heart. Finally, the antibiotic regimen is completed. And within three days the gooey discharge comes back. We're in a vicious cycle.

The pediatrician offers another suggestion. Try a topical application of breast milk. Really? I do a little research. It turns out that treating eye infections with human milk dates back to 1500 B.C., when it was prescribed by Egyptian physicians. Ancient Sumerians and eleventh-century residents of Baghdad also advocated the practice. I try it first in my own eyes. The milk feels soothing enough, and, because it's body temperature, I hardly notice it going in. I try it on Faith. She doesn't mind it either. So before each breastfeeding session, I squirt a few drops of my milk into her eyes. Within two days all her symptoms disappear. Her eyes become clear and sparkly again. I continue to give her a daily dose until her tear duct finally opens two months later.

I did it. I healed you.

Breast milk does more than just provide temporary immunity through the baby's vulnerable early months. It also helps set up the infant's own permanent immune system. One of the most important pieces of evidence for this phenomenon comes from the thymus gland, which in infants and children is a large spongy mass that fills much of the chest cavity, lying over the lungs and heart and extending into the neck, almost reaching the thyroid gland. The thymus is a kind of finishing school for white blood cells. Immature lymphocytes in the bloodstream migrate into the gland and emerge as fully functional killers called T-cells. In contrast to B-cells, T-cells dispense with the complications of making antibodies and, instead, just slay all cells displaying foreign proteins. Some studies show that breastfed babies have larger thymus glands and better T-cell responses than their formula-fed counterparts.

The ways by which breast milk programs the infant immune system are just beginning to be understood. We know, for example, that cells in the infant immune system have receptors on their outer membranes for substances called neuropeptides found in breast milk. However, we don't yet know the implications of this finding. It's like discovering locked doors inside a baby that open with specific keys found within its mother's milk—but why and for what purpose? We do know that milk-borne immune cells themselves play a role in jump-starting immunity in infants. Maternal phago-cytes, for example, release chemicals that cause infant B-cells to make antibodies. Still other chemicals in breast milk work to *suppress* certain aspects of immune response, which is probably why children breastfed as infants have fewer allergies.

Essentially, then, an infant is born with most, but not all, of its essential life-support systems up and running. Within a few minutes after birth, it can breathe on its own. Within a few days, it learns to eat on its own. It takes a year or more to fight off infections on its own and learn to distinguish between truly harmful invaders and benign ones, between self and non-self. During this time of transition, the breast is perfectly prepared to take over from the placenta the role of nurturer and teacher. Like the placenta before it, the breast sends into the bloodstream of the baby a steady stream of chemical signals that guide and direct development.

In some ways, breastfeeding is a relationship more intimate than pregnancy. Whereas the placenta disallows direct transfer of maternal blood into the infant, breast milk carries white blood cells from the mother directly into the baby. Every time I breastfeed Faith, antibodies and living cells from my blood are sent coursing through her blood, physically enacting the hopes of every mother for her child—that I can keep you from harm, that you can learn from my past sufferings.

When Faith is two months old, I pack our suitcases and bring her home to Illinois for Thanksgiving. As soon as we arrive at Logan Airport, I am grateful to be a nursing mother. Our morning flight is canceled. The next has mechanical problems. We are switched to another plane and spend an hour sitting at the gate before we are finally ordered to file off and return to the first plane. Around me, new mothers of bottle-fed babies worry how long their formula supply is going to hold out, where they can get water to mix it, how long their packs of blue ice will stay frozen. My heart goes out to them. I am limited only by the number of diapers in my diaper bag (ten), which is enough to carry us through for twenty-four hours.

When we finally arrive, I carry Faith, like a tiny bride, down the sidewalk and over the threshold of the house I grew up in, reenacting a scene I'd watched over and over in home movies—my own young mother bringing her newly adopted daughter home for the first time. The inside of the house looks completely different to me, even though it has not changed at all. How vast seems the distance between my old room—once my nursery—and my parents' bedroom on the opposite side of the house. By the time I had left for college, the space between them could not have been far enough. Now, I lie on the big bed in my parents' room and imagine listening down the long span of empty air—past the television set, the stairway, the piano, the bathroom door—for the sound of a baby breathing. How many steps would it take in the middle of the night to walk between these two rooms? Through all the years of my childhood, and then my sister's, how many times did my mother make this trip?

Mom laughs. "Oh, thousands, probably. I can remember making this bed and thinking, 'I should just rent my side of it out—I never get to sleep in it anyway.' "

As for distance, she claims she could hear a child cough in any room of the house, no matter where she was, upstairs or downstairs. Many jokes have been made about this aspect of motherhood—the radar ears, the proverbial eyes in the back of the head—but it's deadly serious. Some part of one's brain goes on guard duty the moment the baby is born, and never goes off again. Which means, no matter what else a mother is doing, even sleeping, part of her mind is preoccupied. I tell Mom that it is precisely this dimension of motherhood that threatens to level me. Mom says that no one can prepare you for the unrelentingness of being a parent. World Without End. Amen.

In fact, there is lots I agree with Mom about—and lots I suddenly feel I understand about her, even though we became daughters and mothers by two completely different means. Mom was the third of my grandmother's six children, all born at home on the farm, all breastfed for a year—or until the next one came along. She grew up watching the younger ones nurse at her mother's breast, infants nursing in the pews on Sunday, and farm animals nursing in the barn. But she became a mother herself when the phone rang and a stranger's voice said, "We have a baby for you." I, on the other hand, grew up in a family bound together by forces other than pregnancy and birth, and never witnessed breastfeeding. Even as an adult, I looked away politely when my own woman friends nursed babies in my presence. I learned to breastfeed my daughter without ever having seen it done. Thus, my mother is the breastfed child of a woman who gave birth to a houseful of children; I am the formula-fed child of a woman who never gave birth. We each came to this job unprepared by our own mother's experience.

Across these differences, Mom and I fuss over Faith, croon her little songs, and discuss naps and diapers. Mom watches closely as I nurse her.

"See how her lower lip just tucked in?" I point out. "It needs to flare out to create a good seal. So I pull her chin down—like this—and then the lip comes back out. See?"

"How do you know when to switch sides?"

"When her swallowing rate starts slowing down, I switch. She eats faster now. It used to take her an hour to nurse sometimes. Now she's usually finished with both sides in about twenty minutes."

Mom especially appreciates the disease-fighting properties of breast milk, which I extol to her at great length. I have always joked that my mother, when she gave up microbiology for motherhood, turned her house into a laboratory. Cooking was a chemistry experiment and housework a form of disinfection. Hands were washed with surgical scrupulousness. The sick were swiftly quarantined from the healthy and their dishes washed separately. Later, I learned that children in other families sometimes shared towels or licked their spoons before putting them into the sugar bowl. Unthinkable! Such breaches of sterile technique would never have happened in our house. Accordingly, bottles and artificial nipples seemed to my mother—as they did to many mothers of the day—clean, methodological, superior to nature. Even the word "formula" was appealing in its scientific intimations.

"I wonder now, looking back on it," Mom says, "if all the allergies you girls had might have been related to formula. Lots of kids your age had allergies. I don't remember anyone in my generation ever having them. It was just something we never heard of."

I had forgotten all about this part of my childhood, but it comes back to me in a rush—the stuffy nose, the little pills at breakfast, not being allowed to have pets or sleep on feather pillows.

"When did I develop allergies?"

"I don't remember exactly. We can look in your baby book."

Mom's idea of a baby book was not to keep track of first haircuts or baptismal gifts but to document diseases, treatments, and cures, with symptoms and dosages meticulously described, as though she were writing up results for a case study in the *New England Journal of Medicine*. So it doesn't take me too long to learn that my sister and I both developed allergies ("chronic rhinitis") by the time we were toddlers and were placed on antihistamines for the remainder of our childhoods.

But there is more. I also learn that we both suffered from mysterious digestive pains and, after a battery of x-rays and electroencephalograms, were diagnosed with abnormal brain waves ("excess electrical discharge down the vagus nerve, contributing to a spastic sphincter in the stomach"). For this disorder we were placed on Dilantin, an anticonvulsive medication, which we continued to take until adolescence. Before she was even a year old, Julie was also taking Phenobarbital, a sedative, because she woke up crying every hour of the night, seemingly because of cramping and gas. By the time I was four, I was also taking a daily dose of Thorazine, a powerful tranquilizer, because of "emotional storms." By the time I was seven, I developed a liver infection severe enough to land me in the hospital for a week.

I'm completely amazed. So is Mom, who had forgotten a lot of these episodes herself. But she is quick to defend her decisions.

"Remember that I grew up in the days of polio and penicillin. Medicines were wonder drugs. When the pediatrician wrote out a prescription, I didn't question it. I can remember when doctors couldn't do anything for a sick person except hold their hand and pray."

"Mom, nobody's blaming you. We don't know if breast milk would have made any difference. Not that it was even an option for you. I'm just glad for the chance to breastfeed Faith. Maybe she won't have allergies. Maybe she won't have stomach troubles."

"I always did think it was strange that you girls had so many of the same health problems even though you weren't related genetically."

"Well, it is."

Like the infant immune system, the digestive system is a late bloomer. The intestine is especially slow to mature after birth—probably because it has such a tricky balancing act to master. On the one hand, it needs to remain permeable to food molecules. On the other, it must stand as an unbreachable wall to hordes of disease-causing organisms. The intestine is born with permeability but it must gradually acquire its barrier against bacterial invasion. Once again, breast milk sets up a makeshift defense system even while supervising the construction of a permanent one.

To this end, breast milk acts to speed up intestinal growth. Elements in breast milk also turn on certain genes in the cells of the small intestine, which in response send protein signals to developing immune tissues. In other words, breast milk apparently helps the infant's digestive tract set up a communications network between its interior lining and the nascent immune system. The details of this association are just beginning to be worked out.

Two key contributors to the system of temporary protection are bacteria themselves. Lactobacillus and bifidobacterium are species of symbiotic one-celled organisms that set up residence in the gut of breastfeeding infants soon after birth. No one exactly knows where they come from—the interior of the intestine is completely sterile at birth—but the breast itself is the most likely source. As they colonize their new habitat, these two helpful occupants deplete the oxygen supply and make lots of acids, both of which prevent less innocuous microbes from taking root. By contrast, the intestines of bottle-fed babies develop a bacterial flora low in disease-repelling species and high in putrefactive organisms.

Special sugars in human milk called oligosaccharides fertilize the intestinal garden. These substances, which are not found in formula, are indigestible to the infant but provide food for the beneficial bacteria in the colon. Oligosaccharides also can pass through the gut. Many take up residence in the mucous membranes of the respiratory tract, where they block the attachment of ill-intentioned microbes there as well.

Interestingly, the presence of lactose, the highly digestible sugar found in breast milk, interferes with the actions of oligosaccharides. The breast compensates for this problem by allowing their concentrations to wax and wane in opposition to each other: levels of oligosaccharides in breast milk rise in the afternoon when lactose levels are low. Because these two types of sugars work at cross-purposes, adding oligosaccharides to infant formula, which is also high in lactose, is not advised by leading researchers. Moreover, human milk contains at least 130 oligosaccharides; their variety cannot be matched by the manufacturing process. In experiments, oligosaccharide-enriched formula failed to produce the bumper crop of bifidobacteria that human milk yields. The investigators concluded, "Human milk oligosaccharides remain 130 reasons to breastfeed."

Let us speak now of baby poop. Faith's poop is the color and consistency of French mustard. It does not smell. Or rather, it smells ever so faintly of warm yogurt. I feel quite confident that this is an objective truth and not just the demented opinion of new parents. Jeff and I use cloth diapers—even when we travel—which means their contents have plenty of time to reveal any aromatic properties. Also, my mother says Faith's poops don't smell, and she does not suffer fecal matter gladly.

By contrast, the stools of formula-fed babies are reputed to be quite stinky, owing to all those putrefying organisms in the gut. In addition, because formula is less digestible, there is a lot more of it. Breast milk, on the other hand, is utilized so completely that not much is left over at the end of the pipe. Small blessings.

I'm told this will all change once Faith starts eating solid food—especially proteins—but for now, on this Thanksgiving Day, I offer praise for breast-milk poop. A not-unpleasant substance at all. Like something a plant would extrude. Making the changing of diapers no big deal. Really.

When Faith is three months old, she begins to give me The Look. When I walk into the room, her eyes widen and meet mine in a gaze that rivals anything John Donne ever tortured into a sonnet ("Our eyebeams twisted, and did thread / Our eyes upon a double string . . . "). As I unbutton my blouse, she coos excitedly and begins to wave her hands above her head like an Andalusian flamenco dancer. As she feeds, she strokes the skin of my chest with the palm of her hand and moans with pleasure. Lest you imagine these to be the romantic projections of a besotted mother, consider this description of the nursing infant from *The New England Journal of Medicine*, a periodical scarcely known for overblown flights of fancy: "The total body shows signs of eagerness—rhythmic motions of the hands, feet, fingers, and toes may occur along with the rhythm of suckling.

Erection of the penis is common in male babies. After feeding there is often a relaxation that is characteristic of the conclusion of satisfactory sexual response."

As for me, The Look makes the top of my head feel like it is going to fly off. My hands tremble, and all ambient sound fades away. I learn a new kind of love, forged in the crucible of those first early days. It's rooted in the knowledge that I would empty my bank account for her. That I would lay down my life for her. That I would pick up arms for her. That I will defend her against all evil. It's a kind of love so primal and all-encompassing that it would necessitate psychiatric intervention if it involved another adult. Jeff says—only half jokingly—that it's a kind of fatal attraction, which, when directed at infants, should be called *natal* attraction. He feels it, too, so I know that breastfeeding is not its sole source, but feeding her from my own body is, for me, its supreme physical manifestation.

Again, lest you suspect I exaggerate, here are the thoughts of one of the nation's foremost experts on lactation, Ruth Lawrence, M.D., professor of pediatrics and director of the Breastfeeding and Human Lactation Study Center at the University of Rochester Medical Center in New York: "In addition to the clinically proven medical benefits, breastfeeding empowers a woman to do something special for her child. The relationship of a mother with her suckling infant is considered to be the strongest of human bonds. Holding the infant to the mother's breast to provide total nutrition and nurturing creates an even more profound and psychological experience than carrying the fetus in utero."

During the first year of life, the human brain more than doubles its weight. It makes sense to suppose that breast milk might have something special to contribute to this remarkable growth spurt.

Certainly, an impressive battery of studies suggests it does. For example, in a laboratory setting, three-month-old babies who were breastfed exhibited more activity, especially in their arms, than those fed on formula. At age three and a half, children who were breastfed at least six weeks showed more fluency of movement—in swinging their arms while walking, in rotating their trunk while standing, etc. Other studies report that breastfed children are more mature, secure, and assertive, and score higher on developmental tests. They are somewhat less likely to suffer from learning disabilities and have higher IQs when tested as seven- and eight-year-olds.

But are these differences really attributable to breast milk? Perhaps mothers who breastfeed are simply more likely to possess superior parenting skills or value education more highly or have more money and time to spend on brain-enhancing activities for their children. Indeed, at least one study found that differences in IQ scores disappeared once socioeconomic factors were corrected for. But in most studies, significant differences remain.

Turning a critical eye on such claims, a recent study reanalyzed the results of all studies that professed to find a link between intelligence and breastfeeding. There are about twenty such studies. After controlling for factors such as family size, birth order, father's education, mother's education, and social class, the investigators still found that breastfed children had IQ scores three to five points higher than their formula-fed counterparts. This difference persisted even among fifteen-year-olds, the oldest cohort tested. The same researchers also substantiated differences in cognitive abilities among six-month-olds. Most convincingly, the trend across all age groups was dose-dependent: the longer the duration of breastfeeding, the greater the difference in intelligence scores between breast- and formula-fed children. And more than just cognition is apparently affected. Breastfed children also exhibited more rapid development of vision, earlier mastery of motor skills, and suffered fewer emotional and behavioral problems.

Other recent studies support these findings. In New Zealand, an eighteen-year study followed more than 1,000 children from birth. Researchers found that breastfeeding was a significant predictor of later cognitive and educational outcomes, even after adjusting for differences in socioeconomic and health status. Most dramatically, children who had been nursed for eighteen months or longer had mean test scores significantly higher than those of children not breastfed. They also received higher grades in reading and math, and dropped out of school less often.

Another study examined premature infants who received their early feedings by tube rather than by breast or bottle. Preterm babies who received mother's milk were more advanced developmentally at eighteen months, and then again at eight years old, than those who received formula in their feeding tubes. This is an important study because it controls for the method of feeding—which other studies cannot—leaving the type of food, breast milk or formula, as the only variable.

So what is that special something that breast milk offers to the infant brain? No one is exactly sure, but there is a short list of candidates. One is a sugar called sialic acid, needed by the neuron's branching dendrites. It is also used to form the connecting synapses between neurons. The body can manufacture sialic acid on its own, but breast milk is a particularly rich source of it, containing five times more sialic acid than infant formula. Two other candidates are polyunsaturated fats: docosahexaenoic acid and arachidonic acid. Both are substances common in breast milk and absent, or nearly so, in infant formula. The strongest evidence for their possible direct involvement in brain development comes from a sad source: autopsies of babies who died. Those who had been breastfed during their short lives had much higher levels of these fatty acids in their brain tissues than those who had been formula-fed.

When Faith is four months old, I go back to work. For me, this means a patchwork of teaching, writing, research, travel, and lecturing. For now, Jeff takes over most of the domestic chores. Neither of us feels exactly prepared for the roles we are playing. Every day we improvise. When I am in the library, I walk home every few hours to breastfeed. When I am teaching a three-hour class that extends through one of Faith's prime feeding times, Jeff brings the baby to me, and I take a fifteen-minute nursing break in the foyer of the biology building. When I attend science meetings in Los Angeles, Jeff comes along, and I return to the hotel room in between seminars. When I lecture in Salt Lake City, I travel alone with Faith and rely on the assistance of colleagues. When Jeff flies again to L.A. for college art meetings, I stay home alone with Faith for five days. At a conference in downtown Manhattan, Faith comes to the podium with me. At a conference in downtown Boston, Faith sits in the back of the room with her father. At home, I write at night with Faith and Jeff sleeping behind me. Some of these arrangements work beautifully and others are huge mistakes. Some of them work beautifully one day and become huge mistakes the next.

Throughout it all, I make three observations that seem to hold true for more than a few days at a time. One is that sharing a bed with the baby makes everything much easier. If motherhood is an exercise in multi-tasking, then bed sharing is its most luxurious incarnation. It indulges simultaneous sleeping, cuddling, and eating. It permits symbiosis. If we have been apart all day, sleeping together provides us hours of time together. If Faith is going through a growth spurt, it allows her to feed through the night with neither of us fully waking up. If we are sleeping in hotel rooms, it means not being dependent on possibly unsafe cribs.

There are plenty of books that extol the practice of co-sleeping: It fosters trust, intimacy, and self-assuredness. It prevents Sudden Infant Death Syndrome. And there are plenty that condemn it: It fosters dependency, bad sleep habits, and poor limit-setting. It contributes to accidental suffocation. There are very few books that provide practical advice on how to do it. My method, which I invented myself, is for Jeff and me to turn our pillows lengthwise, which creates a pillow-free space between our upper bodies. Faith sleeps on her back within this space, covered with her own baby blanket. (If in a hotel, I also wedge a towel into the crack between mattress and headboard.) When she stirs and wants to eat, I pull her down to my breast and then push her back up when she's finished. If she stirs and doesn't want to eat, I pat her gently, and she goes back to sleep.

And so do I. All night she and I fall and rise through the various stages of sleep together—up and down the hills and valleys of consciousness on a bicycle built for two. No one cries alone at the end of the hall. No one trudges down the cold hallway toward the sound of crying. No one sits, half crazed, in a rocking chair at 3 A.M. trying to stop the crying. Everybody spends the night lying down.

My second observation is that, in spite of rumors to the contrary, most people are friendly toward breastfeeding mothers in public places. Not a single soul questions my presence in restaurants, convention centers, art galleries, public parks, bookstores, airport terminals, or libraries. If Faith and I provoke any reaction at all it's smiles of encouragement from other women. Most men just ignore us. (One teenage boy, passing us on his way out of a breakfast diner, turned around for a second look and ran headlong into a coat rack.) The siren sound of an infant bawling, on the other hand, elicits all kinds of harrumphing. Happily, nothing works better to hush a baby than a breast stuffed into her mouth.

My third observation is that, in spite of the apparent cheerfulness of individual people toward nursing mothers, the culture itself is largely unaccommodating. Being in a breastfeeding relationship with another human being is not an officially recognized association in the same way that, say, being married, incorporated, employed—or even pregnant—is. The idea that there are women walking around in the world whose bodies are the sole sustenance for other living beings has not inspired new working, travel, urban planning, or business arrangements. Even though breastfeeding saves lives, prevents illness, and makes children smarter, there are few special protections to safeguard it or public policy provisions to encourage it. In a nation that venerates autonomy, breastfeeding is a largely unacknowledged ecological bond between interdependent individuals.

This last observation I reach while trying to express breast milk in an airplane. It is one thing to breastfeed a baby in public; it is quite another to pump your breasts. I am traveling back home from a speaking engagement, having been separated from Faith overnight for the first time. My first flight is late taking off, and I barely make my connection, which leaves me no time to pump milk in the restroom. Now, air turbulence prevents me from unbuckling my seat belt and seeking refuge in the tiny airplane toilet. Hours have passed since I last expressed milk; my breasts have hardened into porcelain lumps; and shooting pains radiate down my arms. Sitting in first class by some strange fluke, I glance over at my seat partner, a gray-haired man in a gray suit, his face buried deeply in the pink pages of the *Financial Times*. The flight attendant hands out coffee. Overhead, the video monitor offers tips for improving one's putting skills on the golf course. My electric breast pump is inside my checked luggage. My hand-held pump is inside the overhead bin. I am in the window seat.

I decide it is time to try something recommended to me by Jill Stein, a mother and a Harvard-trained physician: manual expression of breast milk. It's almost a lost art, she said, but you need to know how to do it, otherwise you are forever dependent on technological contraptions whenever you are apart from your baby. Jill described the proper technique over the phone to me last week. The trick, she emphasized, is to keep your fingers wet with milk; the butterfat minimizes the friction.

So I finish my coffee and pretend to go to sleep, pulling my overcoat up around my shoulders. Under the coat I unbutton my shirt and go to work, holding the empty coffee cup with one hand and massaging my breasts with the other. I try to relax into the letdown. I conjure up Faith's sweet face in my mind's eye. The smell of her breath. Her toes kneading my arm while she nurses. I imagine the overhead video offering tips for how to breastfeed babies on the putting green. The milk starts to flow.

Six ounces later I glance over at Gray Man. Still reading his pink paper. And, as far as I can tell, none the wiser.

In 1997, the American Academy of Pediatrics released a new policy statement on infant feeding. Recognizing the superior value of human milk over infant formula, it officially recommends that all babies breastfeed for at least one year. Had this resolution been passed at the turn of the twentieth century, the majority of American mothers would have been in compliance. Today, the United States has one of the lowest breastfeeding rates in the world: only half of all mothers attempt to initiate nursing at birth, and less than 20 percent continue to six months. The proportion who dutifully persist until their child's first birthday doesn't even register a statistic. In this, breastfeeding has actually *declined* in popularity since the 1980s, when the initiation rate was 60 percent and duration at six months was 24 percent. Nonetheless, today's dismal rates are still a distinct improvement over 1958, when only one in five U.S. newborns left the hospital nursing.

I suspect that few mothers, if given accurate, complete information and a real choice in the matter, would opt to feed their babies an inferior food source that retards development, carries with it the risk of death and disease, and costs them an additional $1,000 a year. And yet, a mother in the United States who chooses to follow the AAP's laudable recommendation faces a daunting array of obstacles.

It starts forty-eight hours after the birth, when most health insurance policies require that mothers and babies leave the hospital and go home. On average, the milk comes in seventy-two hours after birth. In biological terms, this means a new mother is driven from her place of birth just after her placental relationship to her baby has been severed but before her mammary relationship is established. Given that breastfeeding is a learned art and that few new mothers have lactation specialists waiting in their homes to assist them, this forced expulsion leaves new mothers in the same position as captive chimpanzees who give birth in zoos and don't have a clue how to nurse their offspring. For me, getting help meant negotiating toll booths, parking garages, and rush-hour Boston traffic with a newborn in the backseat and tears streaming down my face because every time I pushed the clutch in, my episiotomy stitches dug deeper into tender flesh and trickles of urine ran down the seat. Fortunately for us, Faith had the good sense to be born on a Friday. We went home from the hospital on Sunday, and by Monday I knew we needed help. Tuesday is the only day of the week that free lactation assistance is available at Beth Israel.

Once breastfeeding is established, further problems await. Doctors and nurses have little training in lactation and often project an attitude that nursing is more trouble than it is worth. When problems arise—mastitis or newborn jaundice or teething—uninformed practitioners too often recommend a switch to infant formula instead of offering assistance in finding solutions. A 1995 study found that only one third of practicing physicians were able to describe how to manage common breastfeeding problems. Most characterized their clinical experience with breastfeeding as profoundly inadequate.

Not surprisingly, then, in spite of the AAP recommendation, most doctors fail to promote breastfeeding to their patients as a form of preventive medicine on par with infant car seats, smoking cessation, and sobriety. Indeed, the greatest predictor of physician self-confidence in helping patients breastfeed successfully is whether they themselves (or their wives) had ever nursed a baby. Again, I was lucky. Faith's regular pediatrician is a breastfeeding mother. She was consistently encouraging to me in the early days and regularly corresponded with my lactation consultant at Beth Israel. She rejoiced with me when Faith gained back her birth weight. And at exactly the right moment she said, "I think you're both doing great."

When a mother returns to work, she faces huge hurdles to surmount if she is resolved to continue with breastfeeding. Paid maternity leaves are brief, if they exist at all. With on-site childcare a rarity, nursing babies and lactating mothers are forced to spend their days miles from each other. Private areas for pumping milk that do not also double as toilet stalls are also hard to come by. Compare this situation with that of Norway, where mothers receive full pay for ten months of maternity leave, breast milk production is included in statistics on annual food production (19.2 million pounds in 2000), and breastfeeding rates are among the highest in the industrialized world. The mean duration of breastfeeding in Norway is 9.5 months, with 80 percent of infants still nursing at six months and 70 percent at one year.

All the while, nursing mothers and their infants in the United States are surrounded by popular media that present bottle-feeding as normal and breastfeeding as . . . well, nonexistent. Recent television advertisements promoting breastfeeding—paid for by the manufacturers of a breast pump—were pulled off the air by several TV stations because of "content," even though they bared no flesh, flashed no nipples, and were described by the trade magazine *Adweek* as tasteful and funny.

Of course, the formula-filled bottle as an icon of infancy goes way beyond traditional media. In the weeks after Faith was born, Jeff and I received baby gifts swathed in baby-bottle wrapping paper, cards with pictures of baby bottles and pacifiers on the front, and even a pink, glittery Christmas ornament shaped like a bottle. (Imagine gifts for new babies sent in wrapping paper festooned with pictures of lactating breasts and accompanied by cards that showed infants suckling.) Even children's books promote bottle-feeding. One of the most progressive books in Faith's library—featuring multiracial characters, nontraditional gender roles, and ecological themes—nevertheless depicts an infant waking in the night and being fed with a bottle. Another popular board book for the very young offers simple black-and-white silhouettes for identification: a rocking horse, a banana, a rubber duck, a button, and a baby bottle.

Faith's six-month birthday is a warm day in March. To celebrate we stroll down to the neighborhood playground and watch the older kids climb around on the monkey bars. I have reached my lactational peak. Faith has doubled her birth weight, and I have at least doubled my milk output. Now that she sits up, has cut two bottom teeth, and is beginning to enjoy solid food, I know my milk supply will slowly wane as more and more of her calories come directly from the rest of natural world, unfiltered through my body. I'm beginning to perceive motherhood as a long, slow letting go, of which birth is just the first step.

In the meantime, Faith remains such an enthusiastic breast-feeder that it's hard to remember she ever once seemed indifferent to it. Finished with watching children, she roots around on my chest for a snack. I unzip my jacket and turn around to keep the wind out of her ears. This attracts the attention of a wild-haired, shoelace-less six-year-old, who runs over from the slide to see what we are doing. Transfixed, she stares for a long time.

"Is that a baby?" she asks.

I assure her that it is.

"Hey!" she says loudly. "She thinks your boob is a bottle!"

12

The View from the Top

Two years before I was born, the Soviet Union sent into space *Sputnik 1*, the world's first human-made satellite. It was quickly followed by *Sputnik 2*, which contained in its payload a live dog. *Sputnik 3* contained a live man. The United States rushed to replicate these feats—founding the National Aeronautics and Space Administration along the way—and thus the Cold War entered the Space Age. Five years later, the American biologist Rachel Carson published *Silent Spring*, a best-selling book that warned about the ecological consequences of human technology, particularly chemical pesticides. I had just turned three.

Even though I'm too young to remember the launching of either *Sputnik* or *Silent Spring*, both profoundly influenced my education. In my tiny public elementary school, science became the subject of first priority. Even art classes had planetary themes, as when we were all put to work drawing the Solar System to scale. Our reading and social studies books might be taped and worn, their inside front covers bearing the names of their many previous owners, but our science books were spine-cracking new. Their first chapters invariably focused on the structure of atoms and molecules, and their final chapters were always devoted to ecology. I don't believe we ever actually made it to the end of our science books before the end of the school year, so I was left to explore the back pages on my own, during the dull moments of a spelling drill or a rained-out recess.

What fascinated me most were the elegant black-and-white diagrams representing ecological food chains. One year, the arrows of energy flowed from sunlight to grass, from grass to cows, and from cows to milk. Another year, it was sunlight to diatoms, diatoms to crustaceans, crustaceans to smelt, smelt to mackerel, mackerel to tuna. In each of these diagrams, it was man, as a drinker of milk and an eater of tuna fish, who occupied the top slot. At some point—I don't remember when exactly—the idea of biomagnification was introduced. This was Rachel Carson's big point, of course—that long-lived toxic chemicals, such as chlorinated pesticides, do not remain diluted when they are broadcast out into the environment. Instead, they magnify—are concentrated—inexorably as they move up the food chain. Smelt to mackerel. Mackerel to tuna. Tuna to man.

It was not until I studied ecology in college, however, that the underlying cause of this phenomenon became clear to me. Biomagnification follows from two laws of physics that appear in the front chapters of most elementary science books: the idea that matter can neither be created nor destroyed, and the contrasting proposition that some amount of usable energy is always lost whenever it is transformed from one type to another. Taken together, these principles mean that fewer and fewer individuals can occupy each ascending link of the food chain because fewer and fewer calories (energy) are available to feed them. The total amount of a persistent pollutant (matter), however, doesn't change. Thus, as the rarer members of the higher links dine upon the commoners below them, poisons dispersed among the many are drawn up into the bodies of the few. This process of concentration can be described mathematically, and I spent a lot of hours working out such equations. As a general rule, persistent toxic chemicals concentrate by a factor of 10 to 100 with every link ascended.

By the time I was teaching premedical biology as a graduate student, food chains and other topics of ecology were once again relegated to the back of the book—and we almost never made it there by the end of the spring semester. My remaining connection to the concept of biomagnification was a yellowing poster displayed in a glass case outside the laboratory where I taught. It depicted the flow of DDT in a marine estuary, and at the top of poster all the arrows ended, once again, with man, who was shown as a muscular male silhouette. But then a passing comment during an ecology seminar made me look at that poster more closely. "*Man*," a visiting professor intoned wryly, "is not at the top of the food chain. His breastfed infants are."

Of course! After the tuna sandwiches and glasses of cow's milk are all consumed, there still remains one more chance for the contaminants they carry to magnify, and that takes place inside the breasts of nursing mothers, where the calories gleaned from food are transferred into human milk. The human food chain depicted on the bulletin board was missing an entire trophic level—as was every other diagram I'd studied, from grade school to graduate school. The absent link was the last one, the top one, the one occupied by nursing babies.

Why was the final link in the chain left out?

As a nursing mother, I still wonder about this. Twenty years later I have yet to find a poster or textbook that places a picture of a suckling child at the pinnacle of a human food chain, one full link above adult men and women. The reason for this omission eludes me. Perhaps it reflects a larger cultural denial of breastfeeding. In any case, a failure to acknowledge the unique position of the breast fed infant within the ecological world prevents us from having an informed public conversation about a very real problem: the biomagnified presence of persistent toxic chemicals in breast milk.

When it comes to persistent organic pollutants (POPs), breast milk is the most contaminated of all human foods. It typically carries concentrations of organochlorine pollutants that are ten to twenty times higher than those in cow's milk. Indeed, prevailing levels of chemical contaminants in human milk often exceed legally allowable limits in commercial foodstuffs. One leading researcher concluded in 1996, "Breast milk, if regulated like infant formula, would commonly violate Food and Drug Administration action levels for poisonous or deleterious substances in food and could not be sold."

The hard fact of biomagnification means that breastfed babies have greater dietary exposures to toxic chemicals than their parents. On average, in industrialized countries, breastfed infants ingest each day fifty times more PCBs per pound of body weight than do their parents. The same is true for dioxins, a special class of chlorinated contaminants (discussed below in more detail). These exposures typically exceed the maximum recommended limits for adults, as determined by the World Health Organization. For example, breastfed infants in Great Britain receive seventeen times the so-called tolerable amount of PCBs and dioxins in their daily diets.

Breastfed babies also experience greater dietary exposures to certain toxic chemicals than their formula-fed counterparts. Infant formula carries significantly lower levels of persistent organic pollutants than breast milk. It is also less contaminated than whole milk from cows. All the fats in infant formula derive from plant oils such as sesame, corn, palm, and coconut, and these plants are further down on the food chain than either nursing mothers or milk-producing cows. Indeed, a 1998 study of eleven-month-olds in Germany found that organochlorine contaminants are ten to fifteen times higher in the bodies of nursed babies than of formula-fed babies. Another study found a twentyfold difference in organochlorine intake between breast- and bottle-fed infants.

The stubbornly long lives of persistent organic pollutants mean that these differences persist beyond infancy. In the Netherlands, researchers examined PCB levels among three-and-a-half-year-old Dutch children. Those who had been breastfed at least six weeks as infants had nearly four times more PCBs in their blood serum than children who had been bottle-fed. And the longer they breastfed, the higher their body burden. Other studies consistently show that the more mother's milk children consume, the higher the concentration of organochlorines in their tissues. Even at twenty-five years of age, men and women who were breastfed as infants have elevated levels of organochlorines. Dutch researchers estimate that between 12 and 14 percent of the body burden of organochlorine chemicals comes from breast milk.

None of these studies is in dispute. Indeed, their results have been corroborated by many other studies, some published years and years ago. The very first report of breast-milk contamination came in 1951, when DDT was discovered in the milk of black mothers living in Washington, D.C. The presence of PCBs in breast milk was first discovered in 1966, when, after finding traces of these chemicals in the tissues of a dead eagle, a Swedish researcher thought to test the milk of his own wife. By 1981, researchers had already identified 200 different chemical contaminants in the milk of U.S. mothers. Today, DDT (in the form of DDE, a metabolic breakdown product of DDT) still remains the most widespread contaminant in human milk around the world, and PCBs remain the most prevalent contaminant in the milk of mothers living in industrialized countries. In addition to DDT and PCBs, common contaminants of breast milk include flame retardants, fungicides, wood preservatives, termite poisons, mothproofing agents, toilet deodorizers, cable-insulating materials, dry-cleaning fluids, gasoline vapors, and the chemical by-products of garbage incineration.

My office shelves contain stacks and stacks of published reports documenting the presence of environmental chemicals in human milk. All together they would fill a couple of large suitcases. But seldom do nursing mothers hear about them. Not only are our breast-fed children omitted from popular depictions of the human food chain, but we ourselves are excluded from discussions of breast-milk contamination. Some researchers, public health officials, and lactation advocates argue in their defense that publicizing the problem would only serve to frighten women away from breastfeeding. But keeping secrets is seldom a good public health strategy, for how will we solve a problem whose existence we don't acknowledge?

Here, in the back pages of my own book, I begin to cast about for a way to make visible the final ecological link of the human food chain. I am searching for words that will provoke courage instead of fear, conversation instead of silence. On the one hand we have the chemical adulteration of human milk. On the other is the bodily sacrament between mother and child. Can we speak of them both in the same breath? Can we look at one without turning away from the other?

When Faith is nine months old, we move from our crowded apartment at the top of Somerville's Prospect Hill to a log cabin tucked into a wooded hollow just outside Ithaca, New York. The move offers me affiliation to a research university and its libraries. It offers Jeff cheap studio space and a five-hour bus trip to Manhattan. It offers Faith room to crawl, a pursuit she has just begun to consider. But beyond all this reasonableness is a deeper yearning—to live closer to the source of things.

Even though I've happily lived in cities for most of my adult life, they remain for me a kind of confusing movie, a thrilling but complicated show with an excess of characters and subplots. By contrast, I can decipher most countrysides. With a little time, I can make sense out of the placement of drainage tiles, windbreaks, orchards, wood lots, and wellheads. I can read something into the architecture of trees and the direction of the prevailing wind. My intuition works better in the rural world. I enjoy coming upon a clearing in the woods and thinking, say, *perfect goldfinch habitat*, and then, a second later, glimpsing a bobbing flash of gold among the branches. Or sensing, half consciously, that this particular grove of firs would be a great place for deer to bed down—and then looking down and seeing bowls of flattened grass. Or wondering why there are no blackberries in a sunny spot near a tree fall—and then, suddenly, there are blackberries. I wish my daughter similar insights.

In the woods behind our rented cabin there are blackberries. And deer. And goldfinches. Our wellhead is by the maples. The drainage flows east toward the swamp, out of which rise the occasional heron and great-horned owl, and around which crowd beech and basswood. Cherries and white pine prefer the higher ground nearer the house. You can estimate the age of a white pine by counting the number of its lateral branches. Cherry bark looks like layers of potato chips. Young beeches hang on to their leaves all winter. Honeybees are notably fond of basswood flowers.

Faith's first word is "tree."

While nursing on a blanket in the backyard, she points at the sun-splintered pines and leafy maples, mouthing "tree tree" into my breast. Sometimes I take this as an invitation to issue a small lecture on the wonders of photosynthesis—explaining how leaves spin sunlight, air, and water into food for all to eat. Sometimes I just laugh.

Within a week of our move to the cabin, Faith attempts and then masters the art of crawling. And thus begins the Era of Relentless Exploration. Our first act of housewarming is to install barriers, bars, locks, and latches throughout the cabin. Jeff and I get down on the floor and crawl, too. We peer at cabinets, stairwells, electrical outlets, toilet bowls, and window sills from Faith's perspective, trying to anticipate accidents, hoping to prevent and forestall harm. "Better safe than sorry," we say with a sigh to each other, as we notice yet another potential hazard that needs attention.

The farther Faith voyages away from me under her own power, the more interested she becomes in nursing when she returns. Nursing, in turn, fuels her courage for more daring forays. She and I are no longer one body, nor even two intertwined, symbiotic organisms. I have become a harbor, a destination point, a launching pad, a rest stop along the highway. Still, the milk threads connect us, one to the other, as powerfully as gravity.

It is June 1999. Each morning I carry Faith out to the road to fetch the newspaper from its crooked plastic box. A food crisis in Belgium is making international headlines. Dioxin- and PCB-tainted eggs have been pulled from supermarket shelves and sent to incinerators. No one knows exactly how they became contaminated, but the problem has been traced back to a batch of animal feed. According to the leading theory, someone dumped used industrial oil into a recycling vat for used frying oil sometime last winter. A fat-rendering company then sold the contaminated oil to makers of animal feed, who mixed it with grain and sold it to farms throughout the country. By March, Belgian chicken farmers began noticing that eggs weren't hatching, chicks had nervous disorders, and hens were dying. Lab tests showed PCB contamination and dioxin levels that were 1,500 times the legal limit. But the government delayed taking action for six weeks, withholding information from the public and offering false reassurances.

Each day the newspaper brings announcements of new recalls. Chickens join eggs on the condemned list. Then hogs. Then veal, beef, milk, and cheese. Then milk chocolate, mayonnaise, cookies, egg noodles, aged hams, and anything made with butter. An investigation reveals that some of the tainted animal feed was distributed also in France and the Netherlands. The United States moves to ban imports of meat, eggs, and poultry products from all of Europe. By mid-June, the scandal brings down the Belgian government. But even these drastic measures are too little too late. Most of the contaminated food has already been eaten. Researchers call for those exposed as fetuses, infants, and young children to be followed for at least ten years, calculating that a single egg could contribute as much as 20 percent of the dioxin burden of a three-year-old. Immunological, neurological, and behavioral effects in infants and children are "to be expected but cannot be quantified."

While I am screwing on outlet covers, Faith circles me like a satellite. I think about all the eggs I ate during my pregnancy. I wonder about the imported cheese we bought last month. But mostly, I think about nursing mothers in Belgium.

Dioxin is a paradox. It has been called the most toxic chemical on earth, and yet there is no consensus on what a dioxin molecule is or what it does exactly inside the human body. It is an industrial substance, but it's never manufactured intentionally (except for use in laboratories), and it has no known purpose.

Dioxins can be defined two ways—in terms of chemical makeup or of biological reactivity. Chemically speaking, there are seventy-five dioxins. They're all built like bicycles, with two sturdy carbon wheels held together by a frame of oxygens and a varying number of chlorine flags flying out from the fenders.

But not all chemical dioxins are dioxins. And some chemicals that are not dioxins are dioxins. That's because there is another definition that is based on function rather than form. Biologically speaking, a dioxin is any foreign substance capable of combining with, and thereby activating, a molecule inside the body called the Ah (aryl hydrocarbon) receptor. By this definition, only seven of the seventy-five chemical dioxins qualify—but in addition, 12 of the 209 PCBs and 10 of the 135 chemicals known as furans qualify. (Furans look a lot like chemical dioxins but have one less atom of oxygen holding their carbon wheels together.) Thus, from a biological point of view, there are twenty-nine dioxins.

They are not all equally potent. Toxicity depends on how tightly they can bind to the Ah receptor. The most tenacious by far is a particular dioxin called TCDD. This is the one spoken of in hushed tones as the most poisonous molecule ever synthesized, the one generally meant when people speak of dioxin. Through its unwavering attraction for the Ah receptor, TCDD is capable of altering physiological processes inside the human body at levels so minute as to be nearly undetectable—at levels of parts per trillion. Just testing a single biological sample for the presence of this dioxin requires two days of work and a piece of expensive equipment called a high-resolution mass spectrometer. There are only a handful of laboratories in the United States capable of doing it.

The Ah receptor itself was only discovered in 1976, but it has apparently been around a very long time. This protein complex has been identified in monkeys, whales, ferrets, gerbils, ducks, alligators, newts, trout, and lampreys. The last common ancestor of both vertebrate and invertebrate animals—which lived more than 540 million years ago—clearly had a gene from which the present Ah receptor genes have descended.

What this receptor actually does is not known, but researchers have identified a few of its key activities. We know that certain cellular signals are propagated through it. And we know that it regulates several genes, including those that oversee the metabolism of harmful chemical substances. Thus, dioxin, through its liaison with the Ah receptor, disrupts our body's detoxification system.

Dioxin is capable of wreaking other kinds of havoc. Exposure in laboratory animals reduces fertility, exacerbates endometriosis, induces birth defects, damages the liver, alters the development of genitals, slows growth, affects thyroid functioning, triggers learning deficits, and decreases the responsiveness of immune cells. Less is known about its effects in humans because controlled experiments are not possible. But evidence is emerging that dioxin tampers with the human thyroid, depresses the immune system, causes birth defects, and interferes with glucose metabolism, thereby contributing to diabetes. Dioxin perturbs every hormone system investigated. Oh, and it also causes cancer. In 1997, the World Health Organization declared TCDD a proven human carcinogen.

Adding to dioxin's mysteries is the fact that no one knows exactly where it all comes from. About twice as much currently rains down from the atmosphere onto the earth than can be accounted for by its known sources on the earth. Waste incinerators, especially those that burn chlorinated plastics, are known to be a leading producer. Dioxin is also a by-product of manufacturing certain chemicals, such as pesticides. Some is also generated during metal smelting, especially from scrap operations that burn plastic coatings off old copper wire. Backyard trash burning is another likely source. Some researchers suspect the atmosphere itself is creating dioxin out of the evaporated vapors of common wood preservatives.

However it is made, dioxin reaches us when it falls from the sky. Blades of grass absorb it, are eaten by cows, and then by us. Oceanic algae absorb it, are eaten by crustaceans, are eaten by fish, and then by us. The crusty fronds of lichens absorb it, are eaten by caribou, and then by us.

And then we feed our babies.

Nunavut is Canada's newest province. It sits at the top of the world. Entirely treeless, the political entity of Nunavut was carved from the Northwest Territories in 1999. It includes most of the frozen islands of Canada's vast polar archipelago and reaches across the Hudson Bay, stopping only at Greenland. Nunavut is the traditional home of the Inuit people, and its name in their language means, simply, "Our

Land." There are no known sources of dioxin within Nunavut nor within 300 miles of its borders. And yet the breast milk of Inuit mothers who live there contains on average twice the amount of dioxin as Canadian mothers living in the south. This fact in and of itself is not particularly puzzling. As we saw earlier, persistent organic pollutants often concentrate in the northern latitudes because they are carried there in the jet stream and because temperatures are cold enough to encourage them to condense and fall.

At the Center for the Biology of Natural Systems in Queens College, New York, the director, Dr. Barry Commoner, and his collaborators recently traced this dioxin in Nunavut back to its various sources in Canada, the United States, and Mexico. More precisely, they mapped the emissions from over 44,000 known dioxin sources in North America and followed them over time and space until they arrived in Nunavut. They were able to do this using a computer program that is designed to simulate the path of radiation after a nuclear accident. In the lingo of atmospheric science, the model has "source-to-receptor tracking capability." This program allowed them to combine data on toxic releases with meteorological records and other kinds of variables that reliably predict transport and dispersal of airborne substances. The computer tracked the emissions every hour for a year.

The results surprised everyone. Only 600 of the 44,000 sources accounted for most of the contamination in Nunavut. In one community in the Hudson Bay, more than one third of its dioxin arrived from only nineteen sources in the south. About three quarters of all the dioxin falling over Nunavut originated from the United States, mostly from facilities in the East and Midwest. Among the leading contributors are three municipal waste incinerators, an iron sintering plant, and a secondary copper smelter. They are located in places whose names I recognize: Ames, Iowa; Harrisburg, Pennsylvania; Red Wing, Minnesota; Gary, Indiana; Hartford, Illinois.

Hartford is located near the Mississippi River in Madison County. It is home to the copper smelter, which is a well-known polluter in Illinois. Most recently, several of its employees and at least one manager pleaded guilty to felony charges following their admission that they conspired to build a secret pipeline that discharged toxic chemicals into a tributary of the Mississippi. The pipe operated for ten years before they were caught.

The mothers of Nunavut say they plan to contact the various facilities whose dioxin emissions now lodge in their breast milk. If they choose to call the manager of the Illinois copper smelter, they shouldn't have much trouble finding him. At this writing, he is sentenced to home confinement.

Breast-milk contamination has been documented around the world. I possess reports from, among others, Australia, Canada, Hong Kong, India, Jordan, New Zealand, Saudi Arabia, Scandinavia, Uganda, Ukraine, the United States, and Zimbabwe; from Paris, Madrid, Rio de Janeiro; from villages near the Caspian oil fields. Comparisons are difficult to make; different labs use different methods for measuring contaminants, and these methods have changed over time. Nevertheless, some broad geographic patterns emerge as consistent.

One is that—apart from the northward migration just described—dioxin and PCB concentrations tend to be highest in the milk of women living in industrialized areas. The more polluted the industrial area, the higher the level of dioxins. PCB concentrations are highest in countries where they have been both manufactured and used extensively; are lower where they have been imported but not manufactured—such as Australia; and often are not detectable at all in the breast milk of women living in rural developing countries. In Europe, the lowest levels of PCBs and dioxins in breast milk are found in Hungary and Albania.

In general, residues of chlorinated pesticides, such as DDT, tend to be higher in the breast milk of women living in nonindustrial nations, although not necessarily in farming areas. As DDT use has shifted from agriculture to mosquito control, DDT contamination in the breast milk of urban mothers in developing nations has surpassed that of their rural counterparts. Within Europe, the Ukraine reported the highest levels of chlorinated pesticides in breast milk. In the 1980s, within the United States, mother's milk in the southeastern states carried higher levels of pesticides used for termite control (chlordane, heptachlor, dieldrin) than milk from other regions. (These pesticides are now banned for use, but they remain in soil for up to twenty years.)

Local ecology plays an important role, too. The highest levels of furans in Scandinavian breast milk were found near a magnesium factory in Norway known for producing this kind of pollution. And in Canada, elevated levels of PCBs were found in the milk of a mother who lived close to a municipal incinerator for five years. In Hawaii, concentrations of the pesticide heptachlor tripled in mother's milk between 1979 and 1983 after heptachlor-treated pineapple leaves were fed to dairy cows. The more dairy products a woman consumed during the period of contamination, the higher the heptachlor levels in her breast milk.

Even household-level ecology plays a role in breast milk contamination. In Australia, home termite treatment is predictive of how much dieldrin and heptachlor is found in breast milk. In the United States, levels of chlordane were found elevated among mothers living in military housing that had been treated for termites five years earlier.

In addition, of course, there are the long-distance effects. Not only do Nunavut women have higher levels of dioxin than women further south, but milk from mothers in Canada's Northwest Territories has ten times more toxaphene (an insecticide used on cotton) than milk collected from mothers further south. Toxaphene residues are also detectable in Swedish breast milk. Similarly, the termite poison, chlordane, has been found in breast milk in Finland, although it has never been used inside that country's borders.

September 1999. Shortly before Faith's first birthday, I pass a jar of my own breast milk around an auditorium filled with somewhat startled United Nations delegates. This is how it happened.

Right before the Labor Day weekend, Jeff, Faith, and I leave for Geneva, where the U.N. treaty on POPs is being negotiated. Specifically, we are traveling to the Third Session of the Intergovernmental Negotiating Committee for an International Legally Binding Instrument for Implementing International Action on Certain Persistent Organic Pollutants. Well, I am going to the conference. Jeff and Faith have other plans, involving art museums, outdoor cafés, and the Swiss National Circus.

Faith quickly adds croissants and crème brulée to her diet and "Voilà!" to her vocabulary. Meanwhile, I prepare to give an invited presentation to U.N. delegates from 122 nations. I also attend meetings of the International POPs Elimination Network, a coalition of citizen groups from around the world who are observing the negotiations and lobbying for a strong treaty. What unites this group is the conviction that persistent organic pollutants are, by their very nature, dangerous, unmanageable, and disrespectful of political boundaries and therefore should no longer be manufactured nor used anywhere in the world. Elsewhere in the city, chemical industry trade groups are holding their own strategy meetings, hoping to lengthen timelines, add exemptions, and soften the treaty's language. I attend workshop after workshop, listening to presentations by Inuit mothers, Native American fishers, Filipino activists, Dutch pediatricians, an American biologist, and a Russian chemist. Pamela K. Miller of Alaska is here to press the issue of contaminated military bases. We have not seen each other since I was seven months pregnant and the treaty negotiations had just completed their first round in Montreal.

At a strategy meeting of the women's caucus group, participants describe what they will be looking for in the final treaty. A representative from Women in Europe for a Common Future suggests we keep three questions in mind when we meet with delegates: Is the treaty going to protect reproductive health? Is it going to end the contamination of breast milk? Will it protect our children from harm by POPs?

Meanwhile, I fret over the text of my formal remarks to the delegates and tear up draft after draft. I have never been so nervous about a lecture. My task is a simple one, really. I am the third in a panel of three speakers presenting a summary of recent scientific research on the reproductive health effects of POPs. My colleagues on the panel, two esteemed researchers, both men, will present state-of-the-art slide shows filled with graphs, charts, and references. I have been invited to speak more specifically, and more personally, if I wish, about the issue of breast-milk contamination.

I know that I want to speak as a nursing mother. I know also that I want to speak dispassionately, as an ecologist, about the evidence. But how to strike the right balance between the intimate and the empirical?

The morning of the forum I am still unsure what I will say. I am still unsure at breakfast. I am still unsure in the taxi cab. I'm still unsure when I open the big door of the auditorium where dark-clothed men and women wait in glass booths, ready to provide simultaneous translation of whatever it is I am going to say into one of several languages, which will then be piped into the headsets that rest on the deeply polished tables.

Fortunately, I'm early. My breasts are aching because I haven't nursed Faith since dawn, so I head for the women's room to pump. Before I pour the half cup of expressed milk into the toilet, I hesitate, as I always do. Breast milk may be the most contaminated human food on the planet, but it's still Holy Water to a mother. That's when it occurs to me: probably most of those drafting this treaty have never before seen human milk. I screw the lid on the jar and put it back in my book bag.

When it's my turn to speak, I send the jar around the room and watch as delegate after delegate holds it briefly in his or her hands. Some study it closely. Some avert their eyes. Some smile with recognition.

Then I begin talking about the food chain.

Many factors besides geography influence the level of chemical contamination in a mother's milk. Her age is of paramount significance. So is the number of previous children she has breastfed and the total accumulated period of breastfeeding. Weight gain and loss before and after delivery also play a role. So does dietary history.

In order to understand why these factors are important, we first need to look more closely at how chemical pollutants are carried within breast milk. Heavy metals, such as mercury and lead, bind to milk proteins. Other chemicals become trapped inside the milk fat globules, which are carried within the liquid fraction of milk like so many bath-oil beads. It is these fat-soluble contaminants— including all of the POPs—that appear to pose the greatest threat to infant health.

At least 60 percent of the fat in milk-fat globules is drawn from adipose reserves scattered throughout the mother's body—from belly, hips, thighs, buttocks, etc.—and only 30 percent comes from the mother's daily diet. (The remaining 10 percent is manufactured on the spot within the mammary gland.) This ratio holds true even if a mother is well nourished and is consuming plenty of daily calories to meet both her own and her infant's energy requirements. What this means is that a lifetime burden of long-lived, fat-soluble contaminants becomes mobilized when adipose tissue is called upon to supply fat for breast-milk production. Some of the chemicals lodged in a mother's fat depots may have been transferred to her through the milk of her own mother.

Once they are released into the bloodstream, molecules of body fat, along with whatever POPs are dissolved in them, travel to the breast. Here the newly freed contaminants slip through the cellular barrier that stands between the blood and the breast's glandular tissue. Once on the other side, they concentrate in the developing milk-fat globules. This transfer of contaminants from blood to milk is far more efficient than the transfer across the placenta. For example, about ten to twenty times more organochlorines are passed into milk than into umbilical cord blood. Once in the milk, organochlorines are easily absorbed by the digestive tract of the baby. Analyses of infant diapers show that very little comes out the other end. Experiments on lab animals support these findings. Newborn mice breastfed for only ten hours had five times more DDT in their blood than newborn mice tested before being allowed to suckle.

We accumulate POPs in our body fat faster than we can break them down. Thus, the older the mother, the higher the concentration of POPs in her breast milk. All other things being equal, a forty-year-old first-time mother has significantly more contaminants in her milk than a twenty-year-old first-time mother.

The accumulated period of past breastfeeding also helps to determine the POP levels in breast milk. The longer a woman nurses, the more she depletes her body fat of chemical contaminants, and the purer her milk becomes. After six months of breastfeeding, levels of organochlorines in breast milk are 20 percent lower than those at the beginning. By eighteen months, they are half what they are at birth. One study monitored the milk of a U.S. mother who nursed twins for three years. By the time of weaning, she had lowered her own body burden of dioxin by 69 percent. Which is another way of saying that, during the course of nursing, she delivered to each one of her two children a third of her own lifetime exposure to dioxin.

Firstborn children thus receive more chemical contaminants in breast milk than their younger siblings. One study from Finland found that the third-born child was exposed to only 70 percent of the PCBs and dioxins as the firstborn. The eighth, ninth, and tenth children received only 20 percent as much. Thus, the more children a woman has nursed, the lower the concentrations of POPs in her breast milk. All other things being equal, a forty-year-old mother of one has more contaminants in her milk than a forty-year-old nursing her fourth child.

A mother's diet during the period of lactation appears to play a minor role in contributing to the contaminants her milk carries, but her lifetime dietary habits are quite predictive. In general, women who are longtime fish and seafood eaters have the highest levels of contaminants, with meat-eating mothers somewhat lower, and long-time vegetarians lower still. In short, the higher on the food chain you eat, the higher your milk contamination. For example, women eating fish from Lake Ontario have significantly higher levels of PCBs in their milk than women living in the same upstate New York communities who don't eat the local fish. Similar patterns were seen among mothers living in the coastal city of New Bedford, Massachusetts. Swedish researchers have also found a strong relationship between organochlorine contamination in breast milk and diets high in food of animal origin—butter, milk, eggs, meat, cheese.

December 1999. My Christmas present to Faith is a backyard bird feeder, which I fill with thistle, sunflower seeds, and suet. During meals, I park the highchair in front of the picture window for inspiration. Faith likes to eat when the chickadees eat.

"Dee dee!" she cries and lifts another chunk of sweet potato to her mouth.

The chickadees are her favorites. For a fifteen-month-old, she's a pretty good birder, easily able to distinguish dee-dee's from ha-ha's (nuthatches). They travel in mixed flocks, chickadees and nuthatches, but are apparently different enough in their appearance and personality to warrant separate names from an almost-verbal toddler. My personal favorites are the slate-colored juncos, shy and elegant, who flutter silently on the ground beneath. Faith has no word for them yet. Nor for the downy woodpeckers who arrive stiffly at the suet basket. She heralds their arrival, however, by tapping an index finger on the crown of her head in staccato imitation of their pecks.

Washing dishes at the sink, I hear Faith cry out. When I rush over, she points out the window, and I look just in time to see the blur of a hawk banking sharply away. Is it carrying one of Faith's beloved dee-dee's in its talons? It's gone before I can tell. Faith begins to sob.

"What did you see?" I implore, but she has no words to tell me.

"Num!" she finally says emphatically, her word for nursing.

And so I unbutton my sweater, and we sit on the rocking chair together until I feel her body melt into my own. Outside, snow begins to fall. The little birds have all scattered and won't be back anytime soon. Day by day, language is forging a new bond between Faith and me. But this is a moment even I have no words for. I could say, "Mommy hawks have to feed their babies, too," but that is a lesson for another day. So I offer the other breast and keep rocking as the winter afternoon darkens toward dusk.

In order to ask whether breast milk contaminants are rising or falling over time, one needs a breast-milk monitoring program. Ideally, it would be one that routinely collects, analyzes, and archives breast milk from the population at large, using standardized methods. Many European nations, as well as New Zealand, have such programs. The United States does not. It did, but the National Human Milk Monitoring Program was mothballed in 1978. What we know about contaminant trends in the United States comes from scattered individual studies. Canada has conducted six major breast-milk surveys since 1967, so we do have some good information from there.

Of all the monitoring programs, the Mothers' Milk Centre in Stockholm is the gold standard. It has been systematically collecting breast milk for three decades, and it offers plenty of good news. Its surveys show that when persistent organic pollutants are banned, their levels begin falling in breast milk swiftly and dramatically. The Swedish surveys show a clear downward trend in organochlorine contamination of breast milk between 1972 and 1992, a period characterized by widespread European restrictions on the use and manufacture of PCBs and many pesticides. Other nations show similar trends. In Germany, between 1986 and 1997, organochlorine contaminants fell 80 to 90 percent for pesticides and 60 percent for PCBs, with corresponding declines reported in the Netherlands, Denmark, and the United Kingdom. These trends parallel the decline in organochlorine contamination in human foodstuffs over the same period. The Canadian data show a fall in pesticide residues in breast milk between 1967 and 1992. The U.S. data are considered too ambiguous to draw conclusions from.

As for dioxin, the trends look hopeful here as well. Tight restrictions on dioxin emissions in the late 1980s in Europe have already resulted in cleaner breast milk there. Average dietary intake of dioxins in 1997 was half of what it was in 1989, and dioxins in breast milk have fallen in almost every area for which good data exist, with the possible exception of Italy and Lithuania. Between 1988 and 1993, the average dioxin concentration in breast milk from European Union states decreased by about 8 percent a year, for a total drop of 35 percent. Once again, the data available on dioxins in U.S. breast milk are too sketchy to analyze, forcing researchers to assume that breast milk levels of dioxins are probably falling in tandem with the declines now seen in Europe.

There is also troubling news, however. Some declines show signs of leveling off and may be plateauing. Furthermore, concentrations of some persistent organic pollutants are still rising in breast milk. One group is the polybrominated diphenyl ethers (PBDEs), a class of flame retardants widely used in both Europe and the United States. PBDEs are found in computers, TV sets, foams, upholstery, rugs, draperies, and car interiors. Over the lifetime of the product, they gradually seep out, enter the general environment, and work their way up the food chain. Once again, fish consumption is our main route of exposure. PBDEs are similar to PCBs in their chemical architecture, except that their carbon frames are studded with bromine rather than chlorine atoms, and they have an oxygen atom stuck between their carbon wheels. These differences do not prevent them from mimicking PCBs toxicologically. Like PCBs, PBDEs are known to interfere with thyroid functioning and neurological development and may cause cancer. According to Swedish surveys, concentrations of PBDEs in breast milk have been doubling every five years, meaning that they are rising exponentially. PBDEs percentages are presumably also rising in the breast milk of U.S. mothers, but without a monitoring program no one knows for sure.

Just as ominously, in 1999 Canadian researchers discovered a whole new class of industrial chemicals in breast milk: aromatic amines. Used in photography and in the manufacture of dyes, plastic foams, vulcanized rubber, pesticides, and pharmaceuticals, aromatic amines all contain nitrogen, as well as a circular ring of carbons (hence, "aromatic") and are all derived from ammonia (hence, "amine"). Aniline is a well-known member of the group. Although their concentrations in Canadian breast milk are comparable to present-day levels of POPs, aromatic amines have much shorter half-lives, meaning that they are broken down and excreted from our bodies much more quickly. This implies that our exposures must be recent and ongoing. But exactly what the source is—and how and when exposure happens—remain unsolved mysteries. Aromatic amines are carcinogens.

I never thought I'd be nursing a toddler, but I never thought I wouldn't be, either. In the early, chaotic days of learning how to breastfeed, I had no firm idea one way or the other about how long I'd continue. I do remember sitting next to the mother of a nursing two-year-old once when Faith was still a flannel-wrapped bundle. "Other side!" the boy commanded his mother at one point, his furious face popping out from under her blouse. I wouldn't say I was horrified, but I did make a mental note to myself along the lines of "As soon as they can talk about it, it's time to stop."

But then, everything that toddlers do seems alarming and grotesque to first-time parents of infants. Compared to one's own sweet babe, who coos and waves her hands so delicately in the air, toddlers are a tribe of dangerous giants. As though your child would never ever become one of *them*. The feelings that the parents of toddlers have for tiny babies aren't exactly reciprocal—although I confess feeling vague pity for the proud parents of one newborn in the pediatrician's office recently. She just looked so puny and uninteresting.

July 2000. After months of sleeping through the night, or maybe stirring only once in the predawn hours, Faith begins waking every few hours and nursing for long stretches. And rather than lulling her back to sleep, the act of breastfeeding seems to wake her up further, so that at 3 A.M., a small child is jumping on my bed, demanding dance music and a book to read. After running through the usual checklist—teething? illness? stress? growth spurt?—and eliminating each possible cause, I decide it is time for some mother-centered guidance. The new policy is: no nums at night. Nighttime is for sleeping.

The next night, as I'm putting her to bed, I explain the rules. At night, the sun goes down, and everyone goes to sleep—Mommy, Daddy, baby, chickadees, woodpeckers—and we stay asleep until morning time. Even nums go to sleep at night. Faith seems agreeable.

All that changes at 2 A.M. when she nuzzles me and I remind her that the mommy milk is asleep.

"Wake up, nums! Wake up!" she cries in a panic.

"Remember? Nighttime is for sleeping."

Wild flailing. Shrieks of anger. Faith sits bolt upright and demands that the sun rise and the birds sing. Now what? I try singing, massage, rocking, walking the floors with her. The shrieking grows louder. Finally, an endless hour or two later, I remember the method of last recourse for inconsolable crying. *Take the baby outside.* I wrap us both in a blanket and step out onto the balcony, intending to show her the slumbering earth.

Tricked again. Nothing out here is asleep. A full moon rides high in the sky. Fireflies advertise in the grass. Bullfrogs boom in the swamp. A screech owl warbles, ghostlike. Eyes glint. Trees drip. Twigs snap. The whole world is out cruising for dinner, sex, or both.

But all this drama has the opposite effect on Faith. She stares, mesmerized, at the nighttime sky.

"Moon sleeping?" she asks.

Yes, I say quickly.

"Frogs sleeping?" she asks.

Let's say yes.

"Rain sleeping?"

Yes, I suppose it is.

And then she lays her head on my shoulder and falls fast asleep.

I have never felt more surprised, more humbled, more blessed, more sad, more happy, more in love. Wide awake, I lean against the door and slide slowly down into a sitting position, watching the night's carnival, waiting, amazed, for the sun to rise.

It is one thing to document the presence of contaminants in breast milk. It is another to document evidence of harm. The latter kind of study is much more difficult to conduct, for ideally it would require comparing breastfed infants receiving contaminated milk with breastfed infants receiving uncontaminated milk, which does not exist. The best we can do is to compare breastfed infants receiving highly contaminated milk with those receiving less-contaminated milk. Unfortunately, for purposes of scientific inquiry, infants who receive highly contaminated breast milk tend also to receive more contaminants via their umbilical cords before birth, so we need study designs that try to tease apart the relative effects of prenatal exposures and breast-milk exposures. Such investigations are rare—but there are some, as we shall see.

Animal studies, which can be more carefully controlled, consistently show that POP-contaminated breast milk contributes to structural, functional, and behavioral problems in offspring. Furthermore, these effects can be triggered at levels of contamination that approach levels now seen in human milk. For example, monkeys exposed as infants to PCB mixtures typical of that found in human breast milk had a decreased ability to learn and master new tasks, as compared to unexposed controls. The exposed monkeys ended up with blood and fat levels of PCBs that were within the range now seen in human populations living in industrialized nations, whereas the higher-performing control monkeys had body burdens below the human average.

Popular guidebooks on breastfeeding, if they acknowledge the presence of breast-milk contamination at all, are dismissive of the potential for harm. Of the three I have in my personal library, one says, "The quantities of pollutants received through mothers' milk are so minute as to be biologically trivial." Another says, "Not one case has been reported in which environmental contaminants in mother's milk have injured children." The third says simply, "No untoward effects observed." Statements in the biological literature are not so sanguine. For example, one researcher wrote in 1998, "Biochemical, immunological, and neurological alterations have been observed in infants fed breast milk in countries with relatively low TEQ levels in human milk." (TEQ, or "toxic equivalents," is a measure of dioxin toxicity.) Let's look now at the human evidence.

A number of U.S. studies have investigated the health effects of breast-milk contaminants at background levels. These have documented few problems—at least in the short term. For example, the North Carolina Breast Milk and Formula Project studied 930 children born between 1978 and 1982. Researchers measured PCBs and DDT metabolites in mothers' blood, cord blood, and breast milk. They then tested the mental and physical development of children from infancy to ten years. Though there was some evidence of temporary developmental lags with prenatal exposure, the authors found no evidence for harm from breast-milk exposure. Similar results were found in New York and Massachusetts, where prenatal exposures, but not postnatal exposures, were associated with poorer performance on tests of development. Thus, even though exposures that occur during prenatal development are much smaller, they are more accurate predictors of early-childhood performance than later, and much larger, breast-milk exposures.

Studies conducted among the Inuit people living in northern Quebec reached similar conclusions. In this population, high prenatal exposures to POPs correlated with a high incidence of middle-ear infections. That is, ear infections were most common among one-year-olds whose umbilical cords carried the highest levels of POPs. This is not surprising, since many POPs are known immune suppressors and Inuit children are born with some of the highest POP body burdens ever recorded. Unknown before the 1940s, now chronic ear infections are a major pediatric health problem among the Inuit, with a quarter of all children suffering hearing loss in one or both ears because of it.

On the other hand, when breastfed babies were compared to bottle-fed babies, their risks of contracting infectious diseases were not higher, even though their body burdens of toxic chemicals were. Thus, breast-milk exposure to chlorinated chemicals did not increase susceptibility of Inuit children to infections—at least not when compared to their formula-fed counterparts. Of course, no one knows whether Inuit breast milk might offer more complete protection against disease if it were not also carrying a load of immune-suppressive chemicals in it, as there are no uncontaminated Inuit mothers to enroll in a study.

An ongoing series of studies in the Netherlands tells a different story. Begun in 1989, this investigation focuses specifically on PCBs and dioxins and has been following more than 400 infants born between 1990 and '92. Half were breastfed and half formula-fed. In this way researchers could compare a group of children who were exposed only prenatally with a group exposed both before and after birth through breast milk. The mothers' blood levels of PCBs were measured in the last month of pregnancy. Then, at birth, umbilical cord blood was collected. Breast milk was also collected and analyzed. The children were then tested in various ways, from two weeks after birth through early childhood.

In both breast- and bottle-fed babies, prenatal exposures to PCBs produced lots of deficits. The higher the cord blood levels, the poorer the neurological condition, the lower the psychomotor scores, the lower the cognitive abilities, the slower the reaction times, and the more signs of hyperactive behaviors and attention problems.

The effects of lactational exposures, however, were more subtle. At eighteen months, breastfed babies, in spite of their higher exposure level, scored higher than formula-fed babies on neurological tests. Lactation exposures were also not related to cognitive performance. Indeed, three-and-a-half-year-olds breastfed as infants performed better on tests of, for example, verbal recognition than formula-fed children. But among seven-month-old breastfed babies whose mothers had the *highest* levels of PCBs and dioxins in their milk, scores on movement and muscular activity were compromised—and were comparable to the scores of their formula-fed counterparts. These deficits eventually faded with time. However, at three and a half years old, the children with the highest total body burden of PCBs had correspondingly poorer attention spans. The finding indicates that lactational exposures as well as prenatal ones may diminish a child's ability to pay attention.

The Dutch researchers also looked at immunological development. Here they did find a clear effect. When the children were eighteen months old, researchers began to notice subtle changes in the immune cells of some of the breastfed children, indicating that they might be less able to fight off infections. At eighteen months, their chances of contracting diseases were not affected. However, by three and a half years old, this had changed. Children with high PCB body burdens were eight times more likely to have contracted chicken pox and three times more likely to have suffered multiple ear infections. The authors concluded, "The positive effect of breastfeeding on recurrent middle-ear infections was counteracted by the negative effect of PCB exposure." In other words, the breast milk of some Dutch women contain levels of PCBs high enough to compromise its famed immune-boosting powers.

Some careful sleuthing in Finland is also worthy of mention here. In the early 1980s, a Finnish dentist began noticing an increasing number of children in her practice with soft, mottled molars. These teeth had not been damaged mechanically or by decay but seemed instead to have emerged from the gums with holes in their enamel already, as though created that way. The dentist set out to learn why. The medical literature reports that early dioxin exposure can disrupt tooth development in both humans and animals, so she tracked down six- and seven-year-olds whose mothers' breast milk had been analyzed when the children were infants, as part of a World Health Organization study. She found a striking pattern: the children exposed to the most dioxin in breast milk had the most tooth problems. But the investigation went further. Animal studies of embryonic tooth tissue revealed that dioxin interferes with the receptor site for a protein called epidermal growth factor. In teeth, this substance helps guide the formation of enamel coatings. By altering the number of receptors, dioxin can apparently prevent the growth factor from sending its message, resulting in a tooth that is not fully mineralized.

The Dutch study also investigated tooth development. In contrast to the Finnish study, it uncovered no such abnormalities. However, the period of breastfeeding was much shorter in the Dutch children, who were breastfed, on average, for about three months, than among their Finnish counterparts, who were breastfed, on average, for 10.5 months. The Finnish results are especially significant because the researchers there were able to eliminate prenatal dioxin exposure as a possible confounding factor: the elements of the teeth that were affected are all formed well after birth, at about six to twelve months of age.

Summer 2000 in upstate New York is one of the coldest and wettest on record. Even by August, the area lakes haven't warmed up enough for swimming. So when a hot, sunny Saturday finally arrives, Faith and I head for the county 4-H fair. It's one of my better ideas.

When I was a kid, I loved 4-H Club ("I pledge my Head to clearer thinking, my Heart to greater loyalty, my Hands to larger service, and my Health to better living") and had a fairly illustrious career as a member. I received blue ribbons for both my rock collection and my sewing project—a princess-style minidress complete with hand-sewn buttonholes and flat fell seams. But I always knew that, whatever my achievements in geology and sewing, they could not compete with the prestige of the agricultural projects. The annual 4-H fair was, first and foremost, a showcase for the farm kids, whose projects had titles like "Feeding and Fattening for Market a Beef Steer."

Little has changed. A trickle of visitors is viewing the tables of wood carvings and canned peaches, while crowds are to be found at the pole barn at the end of the fairgrounds. The building's *moo*-ing sounds immediately attract Faith, so we walk there ourselves. Plenty of cows, sheep, and even the occasional llama graze the pastures near our cabin, but Faith has never met them up close. She's ecstatic. What she notices first about the cows is their Big Poops. The next thing she notices is even more exciting: Big Nums. Big Big Big Nums! The goats are similarly equipped, as are a couple of the sheep. Soon she's checking all of the animals for mammary glands.

"Bunny nums?" she asks as we peruse the ribbon-adorned rabbit hutches.

I assure her that mommy rabbits do have them, but they're very small.

"Chicken nums?" she asks at the poultry display.

I hesitate, and then launch into a quick discussion of vertebrate taxonomy, introducing the concept of *mammals*. She looks bewildered. I've explained too much. Meanwhile, the proud preadolescent owner of three champion hens asks if we want to feed them some cracked corn. Faith watches silently as they frantically peck up the kernels.

"No nums," she finally says in a whisper.

We make another loop around the stalls where the large animals are quartered. Suddenly, she stops.

"Mammal?" she asks, pointing at a brown Jersey named Daisy. "Mammal?" she asks again, pointing at her calf.

"Mammal?" she inquires of the goats.

Her eyes light up. "Mommy a mammal!" she declares, pointing at me.

Then, in a moment of epiphany, like Helen Keller learning the word "water," she looks down her own shirt.

"Faith a mammal!" she announces triumphantly to all within earshot. "Faith a mammal!"

Any discussion of breast-milk contamination, either in the popular press or in the scientific literature, is almost invariably followed by a reassuring statement to the effect that breastfeeding is, nevertheless, the best method of infant nourishment. In other words, if you piled up all the positive, health-promoting virtues of mother's milk, as described in Chapters 10 and 11 of this book, and balanced them against all the known and possible dangers created by its burden of toxic chemicals, as described in this chapter, the scales of health would still tip in favor of the breast. If forced to agree or disagree with this statement, I would agree: I believe that, in most cases, breastfeeding is better than not breastfeeding. Were this not my credo, I would not have nursed my daughter for two years.

I also believe these kinds of risk/benefit analyses are an unhelpful approach to the problem of chemical contaminants in breast milk. They offer no solutions. The usual recommendation that follows from them—"Just keep nursing because the benefits outweigh the risks"—means that we nursing mothers should take no action until our milk becomes so contaminated as to pose as many risks as formula. In other words, until breast milk, like formula, kills 4,000 U.S. infants a year. (This figure is the experts' best estimate of the annual number of infant deaths—from infectious diseases and other causes—attributable to lack of breastfeeding.) Risk/benefit analyses imply that as long as one danger (breastfeeding) is less than another (failure to breastfeed), we should accept the lesser danger—even though it still necessitates endangering our children. The narrow duality of the equation leaves no room for the proposition that feeding our infants industrial poisons is unacceptable. Period.

Furthermore, the scientific knowledge on which risk/benefit assessments rest is scanty. One of the earliest risk assessments compared lives saved from infectious diseases with an estimate of the number of additional cases of cancer that might be caused by the exposure to carcinogenic chemicals in breast milk. Lacking data on other health endpoints—immune functioning, hormone disruption, altered brain development—the authors considered no other health risks besides cancer. Their conclusion was that fewer children would die from breast milk–induced cancers than from formula-induced infections; therefore breast is best. A noble effort at quantifying lives saved and lost, this study is still widely cited. However, it has been wrongly interpreted by many as meaning that breast milk is perfectly safe, which was neither the intent nor the conclusion of the study.

Later risk assessments tried to account for problems other than cancer, but they assumed that the high levels of exposure during the brief period of breastfeeding would be counterbalanced by lower levels of exposure later in life. These assumptions have now been questioned. One recent report states: "Consideration must also be given to whether the effects of short periods of very high exposure differ from those of prolonged periods of much lower exposure, particularly when the former occur during a critical period for infant neurological, physical, and intellectual development."

The more variables scholars attempt to incorporate into their analyses, the more uncertain the outcome of the analysis becomes. Thus, recent researchers who attempt to balance risks against benefits come to much more troubled conclusions than their predecessors: "Arguments for ignoring contaminated breast milk are no longer valid," says one. "Officially, it is said that breast milk is safe. However, there are still many unknown factors regarding the effects of dioxin on growth and development," says another. Of course, in the United States, where we keep no systematic records on breast-milk contaminants, risk/benefit assessments cannot even be attempted. A 2001 review of the situation came to the following conclusion: "Although we can draw inferences from breast milk data from other countries, the paucity of breast milk data from the United States limits the confidence in our ability to access infants' exposures, risks, and benefits from breast-feeding . . . [and] to compare these risks and benefits to formula-feeding."

Beyond the lack of simple monitoring data lie further complications. For example, an emerging body of evidence suggests that some common chemical contaminants interfere with human milk production (possibly by inhibiting prolactin). In studies conducted in both North Carolina and Mexico, women with the highest levels of DDT in their breast milk had "poorer lactation performance," meaning that they weaned their infants sooner than mothers whose pesticide levels were lower. Similar findings come from the Netherlands, where mothers with high levels of PCBs in their breast milk had significantly lower volumes of milk during the first critical three months of nursing. Further supporting these studies are animal experiments showing that PCBs interfere with the ability to lactate.

How would we include poor lactational performance in a risk/benefit equation? The problem here is not that the contaminants pose a direct, quantifiable toxic threat to the infant (which they might also do), but that the contaminants threaten to deprive the infant of mother's milk altogether. I think most nursing mothers would find any threat to our ability to make milk a serious threat indeed—whether risk assessments can account for it or not. And so far, they have not.

The question is not whether we should feed our babies chemically contaminated, yet clearly superior, breast milk or chemically uncontaminated, yet clearly inferior, formula. The question is, what do we need to do to get chemical contaminants out of clearly superior breast milk? There are two basic approaches to answering it. One focuses on changes that individual mothers can make in their own lifestyles. The other focuses on political action.

The problem with the lifestyle approach is that it shifts responsibility from those who created it—makers and users of breastmilk-accumulating chemicals—onto the shoulders of new mothers, who are already overwhelmed with responsibilities. It's also not very effective. For example, eating lower on the food chain should, theoretically, lower one's levels of contaminants. Vegetarianism, then, could be recommended to new mothers as a milk-protecting lifestyle. But the data offer only scant support for this idea. Though life-long vegetarians do enjoy lower levels of some contaminants in their milk, switching diets during the period of lactation appears to provide little benefit. Dietary studies from Germany, Uganda, the United States, and the Netherlands all consistently indicate that vegetarianism must be strictly plant-based and longstanding to result in meaningful declines in contamination. This is not completely surprising. Remember that most of the fat in breast milk arises from previously deposited fat depots, not from food consumed during lactation.

Even if one were foresightful enough to embrace absolute vegetarianism a decade or more before commencing reproduction, it may not be a practical choice during pregnancy. I myself was a happy vegetarian before becoming pregnant—but then could not look at grains, beans, nuts, and vegetables to save my life during the first trimester. Weeks went by during which time the only protein sources I could tolerate were eggs and milk and pork chops. I did not need a lecture on the glories of tofu. I needed to know that dioxin levels in eggs, milk, and pork were safe for pregnant and soon-to-be lactating mothers.

Mothers concerned about breast-milk contamination are sometimes advised not to lose weight while nursing. The rationale here is that weight loss during lactation mobilizes fat-soluble contaminants, which are released into the bloodstream as fat is burned. It's a sensible hypothesis, but, once again, the data do not fully support it. One study did find a connection between weight loss and contaminant level. But others did not.

Even more drastic is the suggestion to pump and discard early milk as a way of depleting its contaminants. In this case, the data consistently show that contaminant levels drop steadily as more milk is removed from the breast, but in real-life terms, this recommendation is impractical to the point of being sadistic. In between feedings, a new mother would spend hours expressing and dumping milk rather than sleeping and taking care of other needs. The nipple pain would be intense, the extra pumping would ratchet up her milk supply far beyond the baby's needs, and the psychology of treating her own milk as toxic waste would be unbearable. Of course, I did both pump and breastfeed in the early days of motherhood as a means to increase my milk supply until Faith was ready to participate more enthusiastically. The experience remains in my memory as the most extreme of all the extremities motherhood has so far demanded of me. I would never advise it as a method of detoxification.

Some women wonder whether they should hedge their bets by breastfeeding in the early weeks and then switching over to formula before body burden levels build too high. There are a number of drawbacks to this strategy as well. One is that breast milk is most contaminated at the beginning of nursing and becomes less so as lactation continues, with the biggest decrease in the early weeks. Also, even though formula is less contaminated with POPs, it tends to be more contaminated with lead. (Remember that heavy metals bind to milk proteins, not to fat.)

Moreover, even though the formula itself may be free of organic chemical contaminants, the water in which it is mixed may not be. In many areas of the Midwest, bottle-fed infants are exposed to high doses of weed killers and nitrate fertilizers when powdered formula is mixed with tap water. Conventional water treatment plants cannot filter these contaminants out. The breast can. (Ready-to-drink liquid formula has been specially filtered to remove agricultural chemicals but is far more expensive to purchase than powder.) Consider also the container. Human skin is made of nontoxic materials. By contrast, plastic baby bottles, particularly those constructed of polycarbonate, have been shown to leach hormone-disrupting plasticizers into the liquid they hold. Thus, in real-life situations, bottle-feeding is not as contaminant-free an operation as the ingredients in the box would imply.

One method does hold real promise for detoxifying breast milk: have babies early in life, have a lot of them, and have them in rapid succession. The data quite clearly indicate that this is a lifestyle choice capable of bringing about dramatic reductions in breast milk contaminants across the board. I suspect I am not alone in finding this strategy too high a price to pay for accommodating myself to the ongoing pollution of the food chain.

So let's look at political action as an alternative approach to purifying breast milk. All the biological evidence indicates that it works. The dramatic declines in certain key breast-milk contaminants from the 1970s to the turn of the twenty-first century are a direct consequence of DDT-style bans, tighter regulations, incinerator closings, emission reductions, permit denials, right-to-know laws, recycling initiatives, and tough environmental enforcement at both local and national levels. Here is how leading breast-milk researchers account for these successes:

From the United States: *"It would appear bans of the type placed on DDT can successfully reduce the population burdens of these compounds and produce a noticeable decline, albeit after several years."*

From Germany: *"Efforts to reduce emissions in the industry have notable effects."*

From Sweden: *"The data show that restrictions on the use of DDT and PCBs have led to decreased levels . . . in human milk."*

From the Netherlands: *"One might maintain relatively low levels by means of life-long dietary measures . . . but major effects can only be expected from a world-wide decline in environmental levels."*

In short, we nursing mothers owe a great debt to thousands of anonymous citizens from all around the world who have worked over the past three decades to stop toxic pollution at its source. These include public interest lawyers, public health workers, journalists, doctors, elected officials, scientists, environmental policy makers, environmental engineers, and organic farmers. They also include plain ordinary folks who cared enough to organize, agitate, write letters, publish articles, testify at pubic hearings, file law suits, sign petitions, talk to their neighbors, march in the streets, stage sit-ins, and generally raise awareness about toxic chemicals. Because of their past efforts, the milk we feed our babies today is purer.

The way we repay this debt—and continue the process of detoxi-fication—is to continue the struggle. The most urgent need is to de-mand nontoxic alternatives to chemicals such as PBDE flame retar-dants whose levels are still rising in breast milk. We must also ensure that persistent organic pollutants are banned worldwide so that the breasts of northern mothers don't continue to become their final repositories. We must take a close look at the 44,000 facilities in North America known to generate dioxin. We need to remind every-one—friends, neighbors, and political leaders—that all toxic chemi-cals capable of accumulating in the human food chain will, sooner or later, reach their highest concentrations in the milk of human moth-ers. In the same breath, we also need to insist that breastfeeding is a sacrament of motherhood that cannot be reduced to a risk/benefit equation—even if we did have all the data to create one. By placing breastfeeding in a human rights context, we avoid stultifying breast-versus-bottle discussions that urge us to either shut up and nurse or switch to formula if we're so worried about toxic chemicals.

In this last effort, we are assisted by a few powerful legal prece-dents. For example, the Convention on the Rights of the Child, which was adopted by the United Nations General Assembly in 1989, recognizes breastfeeding as an essential component of the right of the child to "the enjoyment of the highest attainable standards of health." Many states, including the one in which I live, also consider the right of a woman to breastfeed a civil right.

Consider, too, the case of Janet Dike, a kindergarten teacher in Orange County, Florida. Dike was a new mother who wished to continue breastfeeding her son after her maternity leave ended. Her principal, however, forbade her from leaving school grounds during her lunch period and also refused to allow her husband to bring the child onto the premises. When her baby began suffering distress during bottle feedings and developed an allergy to formula, she was forced to take an unpaid leave for the rest of the year. She then sued the school board, claiming that breastfeeding is a fundamental right, entitled to constitutional protection under the Ninth and Fourteenth amendments, which govern the right to privacy. The district court disagreed, but the appellate court thought otherwise. In the end, Dike received back pay and reinstatement to her job. The appellate court's decision included the following statement: "Breastfeeding is the most elemental form of parental care. It is communion between mother and child that, like marriage, is 'intimate to the degree of being sacred. . . .' We conclude that the constitution protects from excessive state interference a woman's decision respecting breastfeeding her child."

Surely, then, the toxic contamination of breast milk—to the degree that it routinely violates laws governing contaminant levels in commercial foodstuffs and threatens a woman's ability to produce sufficient milk to feed her child—is also a violation of this sacred communion. The presence of toxic chemicals in breast milk compromises its goodness and lowers its capacity to heal, promote brain growth, and orchestrate the development of the immune system. Even if, thus compromised, the benefits of breastfeeding still outweigh the risks of not breastfeeding, the contamination of breast milk infringes nevertheless on a child's right to attain its full capacity as a human being and to enjoy the right to safe food and security of person.

Barnegat is a Dutch word that refers to the treacherous shoals that sometimes line the narrow passages between barrier islands. The

Barnegat Lighthouse stands at the northern tip of one such island off the coast of New Jersey, and it helps guide boats through a breaker-filled inlet and into the quiet waters of Barnegat Bay. A week after Faith's second birthday, we move into a shingled house just south of that lighthouse. For the next two months, Jeff is serving as an artist-in-residence at a local art foundation. I have no official role other than full-time mother, housekeeper, and beachcomber.

It's quiet here. The island's summer residents have all gone for the season, leaving only commercial fishermen and their families, a few barkeepers and bait-shop owners, some hardy retirees, and a handful of devoted year-rounders. In early October, the salt-spray roses are still blooming, and the berry bushes are filled with restless warblers. The beaches' sandy slopes blaze with seaside goldenrod to which migrating monarch butterflies flock.

I have never lived by the ocean. Maritime ecology is as new to me as it is to Faith, so we set out each morning to learn it together. Our destination is entirely dictated by the wind. If it is blowing off-shore, we head over the dunes to the open ocean, where we collect seashells along the high-tide line. The white plaster saucers are clams. The delicate blue-black canoes, mussels. Caught among the heaps of seaweed are hollow, leathery pillows with long tails curling out from each corner. These are the egg cases of sea skates, and their common name, according to the field guides, is mermaid's purse. After storms, we find whelks the size of beer steins, great spiraling moon snails, and scatterings of translucent gold coins called jingle shells.

If the wind is blowing onshore, we stay away from the stinging sand and pounding surf and walk instead along the bay. Here we learn to distinguish the pelicans from gulls and low-swimming cormorants from the higher-bobbing Brandt geese. In the lapping, waveless water, we find other treasures: orange crab claws and limpet shells shaped like a girl's tiny slippers. Behind us, the wind-shielding phragmites reeds whisper a continuous *sssssshhhhhh* that sounds all the world to me like the white noise of a cornfield in August.

If, however, the wind blasts straight out of the north, neither dunes nor reeds offer shelter, and we bundle up and point the stroller toward Barnegat Lighthouse State Park, where a small remnant of maritime woods rebuffs even 25 mph breezes. We call this the Magical Forest. Its canopy consists of a spiky armor of holly leaves and splintering cedar branches. Beneath these are the twisted, snaky trunks of black cherry trees and the warm, brown branches of sassafras, which pelt us with their yellow mitten leaves. Here I learn to identify bayberry, whose waxy fruits are used for making the famous candles, and shadbush, so called because its flowers open when shad run in the spring. In the fall, flame-red Virginia creeper vines trail along the ground and climb the great blond trunks of holly trees. Faith always brings with her an assortment of stuffed animals so she can feed them holly berries, creeper berries, and rose hips. Scarlet, deep blue, and orange. Poison ivy also offers fruit, its berries white as pearls. I point them out.

"Never eat white berries, Faith," I say. It's a botanical rule to live by.

"Nev eat why berries," she solemnly instructs her bunnies in turn.

Other than learning the names of the various species who share this island with us, there is another agenda to all this exploration. I am trying to help Faith learn how to fall asleep without nursing. It's a skill many children acquire far sooner than toddlerhood, but, for whatever reason, she hasn't mastered it yet. Probably the ease of breastfeeding her down—which takes ten minutes, tops—has prevented me from considering other methods. Because of breastfeeding, I have a child who loves to go to sleep. Thus, Jeff and I have never had to endure nightly battles over bedtime or endless requests for one more story, one more drink of water, one more trip to the potty. Since my work day largely begins once Faith is asleep and the household settled, this arrangement not only spares us all conflict but offers me precious writing time. And besides the practical advantages, there is a philosophical dimension to what is officially known as "prolonged breastfeeding." As expressed by the sociologist Robbie Pfeufer Kahn, extended nursing offers a model of human development based on affiliation rather than separation. The breastfed child gains independence within an embodied connection to its mother rather than through an act of expulsion from her.

What I am feeling now, though, is a growing desire to transfer some of this connectedness from me to the natural world. My hope is that the sound of waves, whistling buoys, and crying gulls might take over from my body the power to lull my daughter to sleep. I sense a new flexibility and eagerness in Faith, too. So, one morning, rather than return home for nap time, we keep walking.

I learn two things quickly. A sleepy child wants to be carried. And carrying a thirty-pound sleepy child on sand is not easy. I change my strategy. After a morning walk and a snack, we take a stroller ride down a paved cul-de-sac behind the lighthouse. I call it the Road of Sleep. The long *husssshhhh* of the stroller's wheels rolling over dry sassafras leaves does the trick—especially if I also sing "Clementine," whose chorus Faith finds strangely comforting ("You are lost and gone for-ev-er, dreadful sor-ry, Clementine!"). Soon the eyes close and the head slumps forward. I thought I would find the breast-free nap a poignant achievement, but I confess it feels liberating. I guess we were both more ready than I realized.

A mother. A stroller. A dozing child. To all outward appearances, this must seem a perfectly ordinary scene. It occurs to me that there should be some kind of ceremony for the commencement of weaning, as there is for birth, marriage, and other rites of passage. So I whisper a little prayer of commemoration. *Sleeping girl, I release you from my breast into the world, where the tides run with fish and berry bushes flutter with migrating birds.*

Out on the breakwater, fishermen wave to us as we roll by, and I wave back. They are angling for bluefish and striped bass. Both are species the state of New Jersey considers too contaminated for children, women of childbearing age, pregnant women, and nursing mothers to eat. Dioxin. PCBs. Chlordane.

May the world's feast be made safe for women and children. May mothers' milk run clean again. May denial give way to courageous action. May I always have faith.

Afterword

A CALL TO PRECAUTION

*I*n January 1998, two days after learning that I was pregnant with Faith—when she was a two-week-old embryo and I was still in shock about it—I traveled by train from downstate Illinois to Racine, Wisconsin, where the first U.S. conference on the Precautionary Principle was being convened at the Frank Lloyd Wright–designed Wingspread Center. The principle itself has been around a long time, probably as long as human mothers, for at its core it simply means that we should err on the side of caution whenever a situation seems potentially dangerous. It's the credo that prompts us to buckle seat belts, get out of the pool when lightning flashes, and throw away mysterious leftovers discovered in the back of the refrigerator. It's why we keep plastic bags and books of matches away from young children. "An ounce of prevention is worth of pound of cure" is one of the principle's more recognizable incarnations.

As a tool to direct environmental decision-making, the Precautionary Principle has been in existence since at least the 1970s, when it was introduced into West German environmental law. In this hemisphere, however, it was little known until the 1992 Earth Summit in Brazil identified precaution as a key principle to guide policies ranging from chemical regulation to climate change: "Where there are threats of serious or irreversible damage, lack of full scientific certainty shall not be used as reason for postponing cost-effective measures to prevent environmental degradation."

At the Wingspread conference, we participants tried to articulate the essential elements of precaution and make them practical. The burden of proof, we agreed, should rest with those seeking to conduct possibly harmful activities—not with the public in demonstrating that harm has already occurred. Environmental decision-making should be open, informed, and democratic. It should also examine all possible alternatives to harmful technologies.

Finally, reaffirming the Earth Summit definition, we were unanimous in the belief that precautionary measures should be taken even if some cause-and-effect relationships are not yet fully established scientifically. The scientists in the group, in particular, knew from direct experience that it is never possible to assess all possible cause-and-effect relationships. The reasons are many: there are no populations free from toxic exposures that can serve as control groups; conducting controlled experiments on human beings is unacceptable; and real-life variables are infinite because some individuals are more sensitive than others, because chemicals exert multiple effects, and because chemicals interact in unpredictable ways with other chemicals. Most important, the idea of precaution recognizes that science, even at its finest, is fundamentally a slow process. Before science was able to demonstrate conclusively exactly how the citizens of Minamata were being poisoned by methylmercury, two generations of children had been permanently brain-damaged, and a new word had been introduced into the Japanese language: *kogai*. It means "destruction of the public domain."

Since that 1998 convention, the Precautionary Principle has spread like a prairie fire. Breast cancer activists have invoked the Precautionary Principle to focus attention on preventing breast cancer rather than betting the farm on elusive cures. Public school districts have adopted it in their approach to pesticide use in schools. In New England, a coalition of health and environmental groups has formed the Massachusetts Precautionary Principle Project, which seeks to incorporate into state laws, regulations, and policies a "better safe than sorry" approach to child health. Meanwhile, in Europe, the environment minister of Sweden, Kjell Larsson, has called for a ban on all chemicals that build up in human tissues over time on the grounds that they are inherently dangerous, whatever else we do or don't know about their health effects. In addressing the European

Parliament's environment committee, he specifically mentioned the need to rid the world of bio-accumulative chemicals found in breast milk. "Children don't create their environment," he said. "We do."

Most dramatic, the precautionary principle was incorporated into the language of the United Nations treaty on persistent organic pollutants. This convention was finalized in Johannesburg, South Africa, in December 2000 and was formally signed by representatives of 122 nations—including the United States—in Stockholm in May 2001. The treaty is a strong one. It immediately abolishes from worldwide production and use eight toxic pesticides and severely restricts the use of two others. Beginning in 2025, it prohibits the use of PCBs in electrical transformers. (Until then, PCBs are allowed to be used only if the equipment does not leak.) Dioxins and furans are to be reduced immediately and eventually eliminated "where feasible," and DDT is allowed only on a limited basis and strictly for malaria control. The treaty, now officially called the Stockholm Convention, provides money to help poor nations phase in new alternatives. And when chemicals are being chosen to be added next to the treaty's list of banned substances, precaution—not just the accumulation of scientific evidence—is to play a role. Obvious candidates include chemicals that cross placentas and accumulate in breast milk.

At this writing, the treaty has not yet gone into effect. Its activation requires ratification by at least fifty countries. The Stockholm Convention certainly has not yet been endorsed by the U.S. Congress.

It is time for mothers around the world to join the campaign for precaution, which is fundamental to our daily lives as parents or expectant parents and about which we are all experts. Precaution lies at the heart of our own private decision-making, in which we engage every day in our unrelenting efforts to keep our children safe from harm. We need to ensure that it is enacted in political decision-making as well.

Precaution requires setting firm goals and then figuring out the steps required for achieving them. Again, this is something mothers have long experience with. If the goal is to teach a child how to cross a street safely, the first step might be to demonstrate how to stop and look both ways. Many steps later, the child is finally permitted to cross alone. Suppose our goal is that every child should be born free of toxic chemicals. How do we get there? What steps do we need to take? In what order do we take them? When do we want to arrive?

When mothers make their voices heard in the political arena of environmental policy-making, the effect is powerful—even when they are silent. In November 2000, twenty women traveled to Washington, D.C., where the EPA's Science Advisory Board was meeting to evaluate its latest assessment on dioxin, which includes new evidence that birth defects and reproductive abnormalities may be occurring at levels of contamination close to those now seen in the general population. The women said nothing. Instead each wore over her clothes a plaster-of-paris belly cast from a real-life pregnant mother. Lining both sides of a narrow corridor and filling the front row of seats, the women displayed on their plaster bellies signs reminding the panelists that dioxin is toxic to unborn babies. Some panelists were visibly uncomfortable. But others, particularly the women scientists, were moved. One later said to one of the participants that the "corridor of bellies" served to remind her that debates like these are about more than dose-response curves, models, and data points. Real lives are at stake.

And one of the women activists, moved both by the proceedings—which endorsed the major findings of the draft report—and by the act of holding up a plaster belly for hours on end, decided she was ready for the real thing. She went home and became pregnant.

Source Notes

Author's Note: A full citation is provided for each source the first time it appears in each chapter. Thereafter in that chapter only author and title are given.

The following abbreviations are used in the notes:

AAP = American Academy of Pediatrics
EHP = Environmental Health Perspectives
JAMA = Journal of the American Medical Association
NEJM = New England Journal of Medicine
sup. = supplement
Am. = American
J. = Journal
Intl. = International

PREFACE

ix Moon names: Some are Native American names, and others were used by European colonists. R. E. Guiley, *Moonscapes: A Celebration of Lunar Astronomy, Magic, Legend, and Lore* (New York: Prentice Hall, 1991).

x Katsi Cook: See W. LaDuke, "Akwesasne: Mohawk Mothers' Milk and PCBs," *All Our Relations: Native Struggles for Land and Life* (Cambridge: South End Press, 1999), pp. 9–23.

PART I

4 Migrational patterns: S. Weidensaul, *Seasonal Guide to the Natural Year* (Golden, Colo.: Fulcrum Publishing, 1993), pp. 208–10.

CHAPTER ONE: OLD MOON

6 Aschheim-Zondek pregnancy test: Selmar Aschheim and Bernhard Zondek, both Jewish gynecologists, were forced to flee Germany in 1933. See P. Schneck [Selmar Aschheim (1878–1965) and Bernard Zondek (1891–1966), On the Fate of Two Jewish Physicians and Researchers at the Berlin Charité Hospital], *Zeitschrift für Ärztliche Fortbildung und Qualitätssicherung* 91(1997):187–94 (in German). The variation of their method using rabbits was called the Friedman test. For more on the history of pregnancy testing, see A. Frye, "Pregnancy Testing," in B. K. Rothman, ed., *Encyclopedia of Childbearing: Critical Perspectives* (Phoenix: Oryx Press, 1993), pp. 327–28.

7–9 Description of menstrual cycle and ovulation: B. M. Carlson, *Human Embryology and Developmental Biology*, 2d ed. (St. Louis: Mosby, 1999), pp. 10–20; P. Shuttle and R. Redgrove, *The Wise Wound: Myths, Realities, and Meanings of Menstruation* (New York: Grove Press, 1986), pp. 34–38. For a thorough discussion of the biology of menstruation and ovulation see Natalie Angier's eloquent and witty account in *Woman: An Intimate Geography* (Boston: Houghton Mifflin, 1999), pp. 90–119 and 176–92.

8 Textbook case: Carlson, *Human Embryology*, pp. 24–25.

8 Fallopian tubes move: K. L. Moore and T. V. N. Persaud, *Before We Are Born: Essentials of Embryology and Birth Defects*, 5th ed. (Philadelphia: Saunders, 1998), p. 30.

8 Movement of egg down fallopian tube: Carlson, *Human Embryology*, pp. 24–25.

9 Sans fertilization: Ibid. p. 26; Moore and Persaud, *Before We Are Born*, pp. 29–30.

9–10 Description of fertilization and implantation: Carlson, *Human Embryology*, pp. 24–58; Y. W. Loke and A. King, *Human Implantation: Cell Biology and Immunology* (Cambridge, U.K.: Cambridge University Press, 1995), pp. 1–33; D. A. Fisher, "Endocrinology of Development," in J.

D. Wilson and D. W. Foster, eds., *Williams Textbook of Endocrinology*, 8th ed. (Philadelphia: Saunders, 1992), pp. 1049–77; P. W. Nathanielsz, *Life Before Birth: The Challenges of Fetal Development* (New York: W. H. Freeman, 1996), p. 28.

10 Human chorionic gonadotropin: M. L. Casey et al., "Endocrinological Changes of Pregnancy," in Wilson and Foster, *Williams Textbook of Endocrinology*, pp. 977–1005.

10 Immunological basis of pregnancy test kits: R. J. Mayer and J. H. Walker, *Immunological Methods in Cell and Molecular Biology* (San Diego: Academic Press, 1987); FDA Center for Devices and Radiological Health, *Review Criteria for Assessment of Professional Use of Human Chorionic Gonadotropin (hCG) In Vitro Diagnostic Devices (IVDs)* (Washington, D.C.: Food and Drug Administration, 1996; www.fda.gov/cdrh/ode/phcg.html).

CHAPTER TWO: HUNGER MOON

11–12 Two different systems for dating pregnancy: B. M. Carlson, *Human Embryology and Developmental Biology*, 2d ed. (St. Louis: Mosby, 1999), p. ??

15 Formation of three-layered disc: W. J. Larsen, *Human Embryology* (New York: Churchill Livingstone, 1993), pp. 47–63.

14–15 Description of organogenesis: Carlson, *Human Embryology*, pp. 75–105; Larsen, *Human Embryology*, pp. 65–130; K. L. Moore and T. V. N. Persaud, *Before We Are Born: Essentials of Embryology and Birth Defects*, 5th ed. (Philadelphia: Saunders, 1998), 81–100.

15 Genesis of tooth enamel: Carlson, *Human Embryology*, p. 103.

15 Like a detail on a stair banister: See Carlson, *Human Embryology*, pp. 100, and Larsen, *Human Embryology*, pp. 328–29.

15–16 Migration: Carlson, *Human Embryology*, pp. 60–64.

16 Journey of primordial sperm cells: Ibid., p. 142.

16 Induction: Ibid., pp. 59–105; Larsen, *Human Embryology*, pp. 47–92.

16 Restriction points: Carlson, *Human Embryology*, pp. 70–71.

16 Sonic hedgehog: Ibid., pp. 80–82, 89. Sonic hedgehog also refers to the glycoprotein governed by this gene. It is the protein that directly regulates gene expression during embryogenesis. For a brief review of its many functions, see J. M. Britto et al., "Life, Death and Sonic Hedgehog," *Bioessays* 22(2000):499–502.

16–17 DiGeorge syndrome: M. Hagmann, "A Gene That Scrambles Your Heart," *Science* 283(1999):1091–93; H. Yamagishi et al., "A Molecular Pathway Revealing a Genetic Basis for Human Cardiac and Craniofacial Defects," *Science* 283(1999):1158–61.

17 Ptyalism: A. Eisenberg et al., *What to Expect When You're Expecting* (New York: Workman, 1996), p. 107.

18 Progesterone slows metabolism: E. Davis, "Common Complaints of Pregnancy," in B. K. Rothman, ed., *Encyclopedia of Childbearing: Critical Perspectives* (Phoenix: Oryx Press, 1993), p. 79.

19 Morning sickness: The average onset is at six weeks. Symptoms typically peak at the ninth week and often stop suddenly at week fourteen (R. Gadsby, "Pregnancy Sickness and Symptoms: Your Questions Answered," *Professional Care of Mother and Child* 4[1994]:16–17; F. D. Tierson et al., "Nausea and Vomiting of Pregnancy and Association with Pregnancy Outcome," *Am. J. of Obstetrics and Gynecology* 155[1986]:1017–22). Descriptions in the popular literature often trivialize the problem. In telephone interviews with pregnant women, duration and severity were greater than generally believed. Many women said they were forced to leave work; others expressed anxiety about where to throw up at work (B. O'Brien and S. Naber, "Nausea and Vomiting During Pregnancy: Effects on the Quality of Women's Lives," *Birth* 19[1992]:138–143). Some women have chosen to end their pregnancies, or have seriously considered elective abortion, because of the debilitating nature of their symptoms (P. Mazzotta et al., "Nausea and Vomiting in Pregnancy: the Motherisk Experience," *Teratology* 55[1997]:101).

19 Percentage of women suffering from morning sickness: M. A. Klebanoff et al., "Epidemiology of Vomiting in Early Pregnancy," *Obstetrics and Gynecology* 66(1985):612–16; O'Brien and Naber, "Nausea and Vomiting During Pregnancy"; I. D. Vellacott et al., "Nausea and Vomiting in Early Pregnancy," *Intl. J. of Gynaecology and Obstetrics* 27 (1988):57–62. See also Gadsby, "Pregnancy Sickness and Symptoms" and Tierson, "Nausea and Vomiting of Pregnancy and Association with Pregnancy Outcome."

19 Morning sickness in other cultures: P. Andrews and S. Whitehead, "Pregnancy Sickness," *News in Physiological Sciences* 5(1990):5–10; K. Karasawa and S. Muto, "Taste Preference and Aversion in Pregnancy," *Japanese J. of Nutrition* 36(1978):31–37; L. Minturn and A. W. Weiher, "The Influence of Diet on Morning Sickness: A Cross-Cultural Study," *Medical Anthropology* 8(1984):71–75; K. A. O'Connor et al., "Reproductive Hormones and Pregnancy-Related Sickness in a Prospective Study of Bangladeshi Women," *Am. J. of Physical Anthropology* 105(1998, sup. 26):172; I. L. Pike, "Pregnancy Sickness and Food Aversions During Pregnancy for Nomadic Turkana Women of Kenya," *Am. J. of Physical Anthropology* 104(1997, sup. 24):186; M. Shostak, *Nisa: The Life and Words of a !Kung Woman* (Cambridge: Harvard University Press, 1981), pp. 178, 190; A. R. P. Walker et al., "Nausea and Vomiting and Dietary Cravings and Aversions During Pregnancy in South African Women," *British J. of Obstetrics and Gynaecology* 92(1985):484–89.

19 Ancient descriptions of morning sickness: Andrews and Whitehead, "Pregnancy Sickness"; B. O'Brien and N. Newton, "Psyche Versus Soma: Historical Evolution of Beliefs About Nausea and Vomiting During Pregnancy," *J. of Psychosomatic Obstetrics and Gynecology* 12(1991)91–120; O. Tempkin (trans.), *Soranus' Gynecology* (Baltimore: Johns Hopkins University Press, 1956), p. 51.

19 Waning of sympathy with rise of psychological theories: M. Erick, *No More Morning Sickness* (New York: Plume, 1993); A. S. Kaspar, "Nausea of Pregnancy: An Historical Medical Prejudice," *Women and Health* 5(1980):35–44; Minturn and Weiher, "The Influence of Diet on Morning Sickness."

19 Forbidden visitors and vomit bowls: H. B. Atlee, "Pernicious Vomiting of Pregnancy," *J. of Obstetrics and Gynaecology* 41(1934):750–59. See also Erick, *No More Morning Sickness*, p. 69.

19–20 Morning sickness and mother attachment: G. G. Robertson, "Nausea and Vomiting of Pregnancy," *Lancet* 251 (1946):336–41.

20 Quote from the nursing literature: O'Brien and Naber, "Nausea and Vomiting During Pregnancy," p. 141.

20 No correlation with feelings about being pregnant: S. A. Whitehead et al., "Pregnancy Sickness," in A. L. Bianchi et al., eds., *Mechanisms and Control of Emesis* (London: John Libbey, 1992), pp. 297–306.

20 Morning sickness does not vary with sociological factors: Vellacott, "Nausea and Vomiting in Early Pregnancy." It also appears to be relatively independent of psychosocial factors such as depression, anxiety, stress, social support, and work load (K. M. Paarlberg et al., "Psychosocial Factors as Predictors of Maternal Well-Being and Pregnancy-Related Complaints," *J. of Psychosomatic Obstetrics and Gynaecology* 17[1996]:93–102.

20 More common in urban areas: C. N. Broussard and J. E. Richter, "Nausea and Vomiting of Pregnancy," *Gastroenterology Clinics of North America* 27(1998):123–51.

20 More common if mother also suffered from it: R. Gadsby et al., "Pregnancy Nausea Related to Women's Obstetric and Personal Histories," *Gynecologic and Obstetric Investigation* 43(1997):108–11.

20 Women with morning sickness have better birth outcomes: R. S. Boneva et al., "Nausea During Pregnancy and Congenital Heart Defects: A Population-Based Case-Control Study," *Am. J. of Epidemiology* 149(1999):717–25; M. A. Klebanoff et al., "Epidemiology of Vomiting in Early Pregnancy," *Obstetrics and Gynecology* 66(1985):612–16; F. D. Tierson et al., "Nausea and Vomiting of Pregnancy and Association with Pregnancy Outcome," *Am. J. of Obstetrics and Gynecology* 155(1986):1017–22.

21 Slow-wave disruption: J. W. Walsh et al., "Progesterone and Estrogen Are Potential Mediators of Gastric Slow-Wave Dysrhythmias in Nausea of Pregnancy," *Am. J. of Physiology* 270(1996):G506-14.

21 HCG: Boneva, "Nausea During Pregnancy and Congenital Heart Defects"; Walsh, "Progesterone and Estrogen."

21 Progesterone/estrogen: Broussard and Richter, "Nausea and Vomiting of Pregnancy"; J. Hawthorne, *Understanding and Management of Nausea and Vomiting* (Oxford: Blackwell, 1995), p. 66–68; A. Järnfelt-Samsioe et al., "Nausea and Vomiting in Pregnancy—A Contribution to Its Epidemiology," *Gynecologic and Obstetric Investigation* 16(1983):221–29; Walsh, "Progesterone and Estrogen."

21–22 Thyroid and other hormones: Andrews and Whitehead, "Pregnancy Sickness"; Walsh, "Progesterone and Estrogen."
22 Hormonal transport: Andrews and Whitehead, "Pregnancy Sickness."
22 Area postrema: Ibid. See also H. L. Borrison et al., "Phylogenic and Neurological Aspects of the Vomiting Process," *J. of Clinical Pharmacology* 21(1981):23S–29S.
22 Grand unifying hypothesis: Andrews and Whitehead, "Pregnancy Sickness."
22–23 Miriam Erick: Erick, *No More Morning Sickness.*
22 Hyperemesis gravidarum: Because its incidence is higher in multiple pregnancies, at least one researcher has suggested that HCG must be the culprit in pregnancy nausea. Estrogens and progesterones are not any higher among women with hyperemesis gravidarum. For more on this condition, see M. Hod et al., "Hyperemesis Gravidarum: A Review," *J. of Reproductive Medicine* 39(1994):605–12. More recently, a Swedish study reports that women hospitalized with hyperemesis gravidarum in early pregnancy were significantly more likely to have girls. They note that a female fetus is associated with higher levels of HCG at birth than is a male fetus—although levels in early pregnancy are unknown. They also, therefore, suspect that HCG is the culprit behind morning sickness (J. Askling et al., "Sickness in Pregnancy and Sex of the Child," *Lancet* 354 [1999]:2053).
22 Charlotte Brontë: G. Weis, "The Death of Charlotte Brontë," *Obstetrics and Gynecology* 78(1991):705–8.
23 Studies from space program: In spite of them, the causes of vomiting are still not well understood. There appears to be no one single place in the brain responsible for the vomiting reflex. For example, people with injuries to certain parts of the brain stem will not vomit in response to vomit-inducing drugs. However, they will still throw up in response to motion sickness. On the other hand, people missing a part of their inner ear called the vestibular apparatus do not suffer from motion sickness, nor do they vomit in response to vomit-inducing drugs (A. D. Miller, "Physiology of Brain Stem Emetic Circuitry," in Bianchi, *Mechanisms and Control of Emesis*, pp. 41–50).
23–25 Margie Profet: M. Holloway, "Margie Profet: Evolutionary Theories for Everyday Life," *Scientific American* 274(1996):40; ibid., *Protecting Your Baby-to-Be: Preventing Birth Defects in the First Trimester* (Reading, Mass.: Addison-Wesley, 1995); Ibid., "The Evolution of Pregnancy Sickness as Protection to the Embryo Against Pleistocene Teratogens," *Evolutionary Theory* 8(1988):177–90.
24 "Reversal of a mistake": Hawthorne, *Understanding and Management of Nausea and Vomiting*, p. 4.
24 Profet's predictions not borne out: Curiously, all the foods reputed to help alleviate morning sickness are strongly flavored plant-based ones. They include raw almonds, watermelon, and citrus (G. Bennett, "Queasy No More!" *Parenting* 11[Oct. 1997]:144–48). On the other hand, Profet seems to have a good point about coffee. A more recent study reports that more than 93 percent of pregnant women experience an aversion to coffee (C. C. Lawson et al., "Coffee Aversion Patterns of Early Pregnancy," *Am. J. of Epidemiology* 147[1998, sup. 11]:S18).
24 No link between vegetable intake and vomiting: J. E. Brown et al., "Profet, Profits, and Proof: Do Nausea and Vomiting of Early Pregnancy Protect Women from 'Harmful' Vegetables?," *Am. J. of Obstetrics and Gynecology* 176(1997):179–81.
25 Animals species that can and cannot vomit: Miller, "Physiology of Brain Stem Emetic Circuitry," pp. 41–50.
25 Revision of Profet's hypothesis: S. M. Flaxman and P. W. Sherman, "Morning Sickness: A Mechanism for Protecting Mother and Embryo," *Quarterly Review of Biology* 75(2000):113–48.
25 Other factors known to trigger vomiting: Hawthorne, *Understanding and Management of Nausea and Vomiting*, pp. 1–4; B. O'Brien et al., "Diary Reports of Nausea and Vomiting During Pregnancy," *Clinical Nursing Research* 6(1997):239–52; and O'Brien and Naber, "Nausea and Vomiting During Pregnancy." Interestingly, women who suffer from motion sickness are far more likely to vomit during pregnancy (Whitehead, "Pregnancy Sickness").
26 I have gained four pounds: Studies show significant changes in body composition, as well as cardiopulmonary and metabolic functions, by the ninth week of pregnancy. These include an increase in skin-fold thickness, body fat, blood plasma volume, heart rate, ventilation, and oxygen consumption. The increased rate of fat deposition appears to be preparatory for late pregnancy

and lactation (J. F. Clapp et al., "Maternal Physiologic Adaptations to Early Pregnancy," *Am. J. of Obstetrics and Gynecology* 159[1988]:1456–60).

CHAPTER THREE: SAP MOON

30 Mysteries of sugar maples: R. Archibald, "How Sweet It Is!" *American Forests* 100(1994):28–34; J. W. Marvin et al., "New Research Findings at the University of Vermont's Proctor Maple Research Farm," *Proceedings of the Seventh Conference on Maple Products* (Philadelphia: USDA, 8–9 Oct. 1968), pp. 16–19.

30–31 Description of placenta: D. A. Fisher, "Endocrinology of Development," in J. D. Wilson and D. W. Foster, eds., *Williams Textbook of Endocrinology*, 8th ed. (Philadelphia: Saunders, 1992), pp. 1049–77; K. L. Moore and T .V. N. Persaud, *The Developing Human: Clinically Oriented Embryology*, 5th ed. (Philadelphia: Saunders, 1993), pp. 113–141; P. W. Nathanielsz, *Life Before Birth: The Challenges of Fetal Development* (New York: W.H. Freeman, 1996), pp. 65–82; J. R. Scott et al., eds., *Danforth's Obstetrics & Gynecology*, 8th ed. (Philadelphia: Lippincott Williams & Wilkins, 1999), p. 37–38.

31–32 Placental hormones: The placenta secretes at least twenty different hormones. The function of most are not yet known (M. L. Casey and P. C. MacDonald, "Placental Endocrinology," in C. W. G. Redman et al., eds., *The Human Placenta* [Oxford: Blackwell, 1993], pp. 237–72). See also Fisher "Endocrinology of Development," pp. 1049–77, and Nathanielsz, *Life Before Birth*, pp. 65–82.

32 Loosens joints: This hormone is called, appropriately enough, relaxin (D. Bani, "Relaxin: A Pleiotropic Hormone," *General Pharmacology* 28[1997]:13–22).

32 Placenta and immune function: Nathanielsz, *Life Before Birth*, pp. 65–82.

32–33 Placental comparative anatomy: E. M. Ramsey, *The Placenta: Human and Animal* (New York: Praeger, 1982); Scott, *Danforth's Obstetrics & Gynecology*, p. 37.

33 Description of human placenta: Moore and Persaud, *The Developing Human*, pp. 113–41; D. D'Alessandro, "Placenta," in B. K. Rothman, ed., *Encyclopedia of Childbearing: Critical Perspectives* (Phoenix: Oryx, 1993); Scott, *Danforth's Obstetrics & Gynecology*, p. 37.

33 We are the only mammal that does not eat it: Nevertheless, in most human cultures the expelled placenta is treated with great regard. The contemporary culture of the industrialized West is unusual in discarding and incinerating the expelled human placenta as medical waste. In some societies, the placenta is considered the infant's twin or double and is believed to be intimately involved in the well-being of the infant, mother, and community. In the Hmong language, for example, the word for placenta means "jacket," as it is understood to serve as the first garment for the infant. After death, the placenta is believed to clothe the soul once again as it journeys to be with the other ancestors. The geographic site of placental burial thus defines the ancestral home (W. M. Birdsong, "The Placenta and Cultural Values," *Western J. of Medicine* 168[1998]:190–92). I chose to bury Faith's placenta in my parents' backyard.

33–34 Placental barrier: Moore and Persaud, *The Developing Human*, pp. 119–20.

34 Placenta keeps out pathogens: Nathanielsz, *Life Before Birth*, pp. 65–82.

34 Hofbauer cells: Ibid., pp. 65–82; E. J. Popek, "Normal Anatomy and Histology of the Placenta," in S. H. Lewis and E. Perrin, eds., *Pathology of the Placenta*, 2d ed. (New York: Churchill Livingston, 1999), pp. 49–88.

34 Deactivation of adrenal hormones: Nathanielsz, *Life Before Birth*, p. 79.

34 Chemicals sorted by size, charge, and solubility: E. Reynolds, "Drug Transfer Across the Term Placenta: A Review," in A. Carter et al., eds., *Trophoblast Research, vol. 12: The Maternal-Fetal Interface* (Rochester, N.Y.: University of Rochester Press, 1998), pp. 239–55; J. Stulc, "Placental Transfer of Inorganic Ions and Water," *Physiological Reviews* 77(1997):805–36.)

34 Passage of pesticides and methylmercury through placenta: R. G. Gupta, "Environmental Agents and Placental Toxicity: Anticholinesterases and Other Insecticides," in B. V. Rama Sastry, ed., *Placental Toxicology* (Boca Raton: CRC Press, 1995), pp. 257–78; L. W. Chang and G. L. Guo, "Fetal Minamata Disease: Congenital Methylmercury Poisoning," in W. Slikker, Jr., and L. W. Chang, eds., *Handbook of Developmental Neurotoxicology* (San Diego: Academic Press, 1998), pp. 507–15.

34 Nicotine's effects: A. Pastrakuljic et al., "Maternal Cocaine Use and Cigarette Smoking in Pregnancy in Relation to Amino Acid Transport and Fetal Growth," *Placenta* 20(1999):499–512.

34 PCBs' effects: These experiments were carried out on minks (C. J. Jones et al., "Environmental Pollutants as Aetiological Agents in Female Reproductive Pathology: Placental Glycan

Expression in Normal and Polychlorinated Biphenyl [PCB]-exposed Mink [*Mustela vison*]," *Placenta* 18[1997]:689–99).

34–35 Nickel's effects: E. Reichrtova et al., "Sites of Lead and Nickel Accumulation in the Placental Tissue," *Human and Experimental Toxicology* 17(1998):176–81.

35 Ancient ideas: R. Jaffe et al., "Maternal Circulation in the First Trimester Human Placenta—Myth or Reality," *Am. J. of Obstetrics and Gynecology* 176(1997):695–705.

35 Wedding nights in Carthage: A. Dally, "Thalidomide: Was the Tragedy Preventable?," *Lancet* 351(1998):1197–99.

35 Injecting wax: Jaffe, "Maternal Circulation in the First Trimester Human Placenta."

35–36 Ann Dally's historical analysis: Dally, "Thalidomide."

36 Gregg's 1941 report rocked the world of medicine: M. A. Burgess, "Gregg's Rubella Legacy, 1941–1991," *Medical J. of Australia* 155(1991):355–7; N. M. Gregg, "Congenital Cataract Following German Measles in the Mother," *Transactions of the Ophthalmological Society of Australia* 3(1941):35–46.

37 Rubella's injuries to eyes, heart, brain, and ears: Burgess, "Gregg's Rubella Legacy, 1941–1991."

37 1964 rubella outbreak: Ibid."; K. Ueda and K. Tokugawa, "Gregg's Rubella Legacy," letter, *Medical J. of Australia* 157(1992):282.

37 Abortions: R. Rapp, *Testing Women, Testing the Fetus: The Social Impact of Amniocentesis in America* (New York: Routledge, 1999), p. 35.

37 First vaccine marketed in 1969: Burgess, "Gregg's Rubella Legacy, 1941–1991."

38 Quote by Gregg on other toxic influences: Gregg, "Congenital Cataract."

39 Rich's poem: A. Rich, *Diving into the Wreck: Poems 1971–1972* (New York: W. W. Norton, 1973).

39 History of thalidomide: "A Stubborn FDA Inspector Saves the Day," *The CQ Researcher* 7(1997):493; Dally, "Thalidomide"; Insight Team of the Sunday Times of London, *Suffer the Children: The Story of Thalidomide* (New York: Viking Press, 1979); C. Marwick, "The Drug That Changed US Pharmaceutical History," *JAMA* 278(1997):1136; E. Roskies, *Abnormality and Normality: The Mothering of Thalidomide Children* (Ithaca, N.Y.: Cornell University Press, 1972).

39 8,000 children affected: G. J. Annas and S. Elias, "Thalidomide and the Titanic: Reconstructing the Technology Tragedies of the Twentieth Century," *Am. J. of Public Health* 89(1999):98–101.

39 Reduction limb deficits: T. V. N. Persaud et al., *Basic Concepts in Teratology* (New York: Wiley-Liss, 1985).

39 Wrecked lives: Insight Team of the *Sunday Times* (London), *Suffer the Children.*

40 Thalidomide and nerve damage: Marwick, "The Drug that Changed US Pharmaceutical History."

40 Quote from FDA: H. Burkholz, "Giving Thalidomide a Second Chance," *FDA Consumer* 31(Sept.–Oct. 1997):12–14.

40 Phocomelia in Germany: In November 1961, Widukind Lenz correctly concluded that thalidomide was the cause of an epidemic of congenital limb malformations in Germany. See "Stubborn FDA Inspector"; and W. Lenz and K. Knapp, "Foetal Malformations due to Thalidomide," *German Medical Monthly* 7(1962):253–58.

40 Letter by McBride: W. G. McBride, "Thalidomide and Congenital Abnormalities," *Lancet* 2(1961, no. 721):1358–63.

40 Reports streamed in: "Stubborn FDA Inspector."

40 Marketed in Canada after banned in Europe: A. Elash, "Thalidomide Is Back," *Maclean's* 110(10 Mar. 1997):48.

40 Inklings of evidence for harm: Dally, "Thalidomide," p. 1197.

40–41 Story of Francis Kelsey: "Stubborn FDA Inspector"; Burkholz, "Giving Thalidomide a Second Chance."

41 Mechanism of thalidomide damage: Ibid.

42 Thalidomide's window of vulnerability: Persaud, *Basic Concepts in Teratology*, pp. 10–11.

43 Fetal events of third month: Moore and Persaud, *Developing Human*, p. 106.

43 Smith's photoessay: W. E. Smith and A. M. Smith, *Minamata: Words and Photos* (New York: Holt, Rinehart & Winston, 1975).

44 Aristotle and alchemists: T. W. Clarkson, "The Toxicology of Mercury," *Critical Reviews in Clinical Laboratory Sciences* 34(1997):369–403.

44 History of Minamata poisoning: S. Nomura and M. Futatsuka, "Minamata Disease from the Viewpoint of Occupational Health," *J. of Occupational Health* 40(1998):1–8.; C. Watanabe and H. Satoh, "Evolution of Our Understanding of Methylmercury as a Health Threat," *EHP* 104(1996, sup. 2):367–79.

44 Three clues argued against an infectious cause: Ibid.

44–45 Progression of maladies: M. Harada, "Minamata Disease: A Medical Report," in Smith and Smith, *Minamata*, pp. 180–92; Watanabe and Satoh, "Evolution of Our Understanding."

44–45 Previous observations ignored: Harada, "Minamata Disease."

45 1956 report: Ibid.

45 Opposition of local government: Watanabe and Satoh, "Evolution of Our Understanding."

45 Chisso refused to change: Smith and Smith, *Minamata*, pp. 28–33.

45 Announcement of university research team: Harada, "Minamata Disease"; Nomura and Futatsuka, "Minamata Disease."

45 Chisso said it used only metallic mercury: Nomura and Futatsuka, "Minamata Disease."

45–46 Secret finding: Harada, "Minamata Disease."

46 Diversion of water, cerebral palsy, recommended abortions: Watanabe and Satoh, "Evolution of Our Understanding."

46 "Cerebral palsy" is Minamata disease: Clarkson, "Toxicology of Mercury"; Watanabe and Satoh, "Evolution of Our Understanding." In three of the most profoundly affected villages, "cerebral palsy" afflicted almost 8 percent of all newborns (K. Kondo, "Congenital Minamata Disease: Warnings from Japan's Experience," *J. of Child Neurology* 15[2000]:458–64).

46 Those born with the disease had worse symptoms: Watanabe and Satoh: "Evolution of Our Understanding."

46 29 percent of children mentally deficient: Harada, "Minamata Disease."

46 1962 discovery of forgotten bottle: Nomura and Futatsuka, "Minamata Disease."

46 Chisso continued dumping until 1968: Ibid.

46–47 1969 lawsuit: Harada, "Minamata Disease."

47 The beating of Smith: Smith and Smith, *Minamata*, p. 95.

47 Photo of Tomoko before the officials: Ibid., p. 44–45.

47 1973 Ruling: Ibid., p. 129.

47 Translated thesis: K. Tsurumi, "New Lives: Some Case Studies in Minamata," Ph.d. diss., Sophia University, Institute of International Relations, Sophia University, 1988.

47 Mercury to decline by 2011: A. Kudo et al., "Lessons from Minamata Mercury Pollution, Japan—After a Continuous 22 Years of Observation," *Water Science and Technology* 38(1998):187–93.

47 Fish and shellfish safe to eat: Dr. Tomohiro Kawaguchi, University of South Carolina, personal communication.

48 Formation of methylmercury: In the case of Chisso, the methylating process occurred inside the factory. But inorganic mercury released from industrial sites, paper mills, or coal-burning power plants will also methylate once it drifts into open water. See Nomura and Futatsuka, "Minamata Disease from the Viewpoint of Occupational Health," and Clarkson, "Toxicology of Mercury."

48 Principle of biomagnification: Persistence is not synonymous with biomagnifiability, however. Some pollutants, such as phthalate plasticizers, are persistent in the environment but do not biomagnify.

48 One million times higher: Clarkson, "Toxicology of Mercury."

49 Brain cell migration: K. Eto, "Pathology of Minamata Disease," *Toxicologic Pathology* 25(1997):614–23. Mercury also has other mechanisms of toxicity within the fetal brain. It disrupts synaptic transmission, microtubule formation, and amino acid transport. Mercury also contributes to oxidative stress and mitochondrial disfunction, and has adverse effects on enzymes, membrane function, and neurotransmitter levels (T. Schettler et al., *In Harm's Way: Toxic Threats to Child Development* [Cambridge: Greater Boston Physicians for Social Responsibility, 2000], p. 67).

49 Dose makes the poison: M. A. Gallo, "History and Scope of Toxicology," in C. D. Klaassen et al., eds., *Casarett and Doull's Toxicology: The Basic Science of Poisons,* 5th ed. (New York: McGraw Hill, 1996), pp. 3–11.

49 Umbilical cords saved in boxes: H. Akagi et al., "Methylmercury Dose Estimation from Umbilical Cord Concentrations in Patients with Minamata Disease," *Environmental Research* 77(1998):98–103.

50 *A Healthy Baby Girl:* Helfand's film appeared on PBS television on June 17, 1997. It is currently distributed through Women Make Movies, 462 Broadway, #500, New York, NY 10013 (www.wmm.com).

52–54 History of DES: R. J. Apfel and S. M. Fisher, *To Do No Harm: DES and the Dilemmas of Modern Medicine* (New Haven, Conn.: Yale University Press, 1984); R. Mittendorf, "Teratogen Update: Carcinogenesis and Teratogenesis Associated with Exposure to Diethylstilbestrol (DES) In Utero," *Teratology* 51(1995):435–45; National Research Council, *Hormonally Active Agents in the Environment* (Washington, D.C.: National Academy Press, 1999), pp. 10–12, 399–406. For a highly readable account see T. Colborn et al., *Our Stolen Future: Are We Threatening Our Fertility, Intelligence, and Survival? A Scientific Detective Story* (New York: Dutton, 1996), pp. 47–57. For a taste of the original argument promoting DES supplementation in pregnancy, see O. W. Smith, "Diethylstilbestrol in the Prevention and Treatment of Complications of Pregnancy," *Am. J. of Obstetrics and Gynecology* 56(1948):821–34; For interviews with DES-exposed families, see M. L. Brown, *DES Stories: Faces and Voices of People Exposed to Diethylstilbestrol* (Rochester, NY: Visual Studies Workshop Press, 2001).

52 Quote from NAS report: National Research Council, *Hormonally Active Agents in the Environment*, p. 11.

53 Studies from 1930s: C. F. Geschickter, "Mammary Carcinoma in the Rat with Metastasis Induced by Estrogen," *Science* 89(1939):35–37; R. Greene et al., "Experimental Intersexuality: Modification of Sexual Development of the White Rat with a Synthetic Estrogen," *Proceedings of the Society for Experimental Biology and Medicine* 41(1939):169–70.

53 Studies from the 1950s showing DES did not prevent miscarriages: For example, W. Dieckmann et al., "Does the Administration of Diethylstilbestrol During Pregnancy Have Therapeutic Value?" *Am. J. of Obstetrics and Gynecology* 66(1953):1062–1081. These studies are vividly described in Colborn, *Our Stolen Future*, p. 54. See also J. Travis, "Modus Operandi of an Infamous Drug," *Science News* 155(1999):124–26.

53 Manufactured by more than two hundred companies: R. Meyers, *D.E.S.: The Bitter Pill* (New York: Seaview/Putnam, 1983), p. 18.

53 Doctor who listened to mothers in Boston: Ibid., pp. 93–94. See also Colborn, *Our Stolen Future*, p. 55.

53 1971 paper: A. L. Herbst et al., "Adenocarcinoma of the Vagina: Association of Maternal Stilbestrol Therapy with Tumor Appearance in Young Women," *NEJM* 284(1971):878–81.

53 DES health risks: R. M. Giusti et al., "Diethylstilbestrol Revisited: A Review of the Long-Term Health Effects," *Annals of Internal Medicine* 122(1995):778–88.

53 Reproductive tract abnormalities: Several studies document these. They are summarized in National Research Council, *Hormonally Active Agents in the Environment*, pp. 10 and 400–402. See also Giusti, "Diethylstilbestrol Revisited," and Mittendorf, "Teratogen Update."

53–54 Gene Wnt7a: C. Miller et al., "Fetal Exposure to DES Results in De-regulation of Wnt7a During Uterine Morphogenesis," *Nature Genetics* 20(1998):228–30. See also Travis, "Modus Operandi of an Infamous Drug."

54 Quote from monograph: Redman, *The Human Placenta*, p. ix.

55 1944 skepticism about Gregg's discovery: "Rubella and Congenital Malformations" [annotation], *Lancet* 246 (1944):316.

CHAPTER FOUR: EGG MOON

56 Habits of Illinois birds: Much of what I know about birds in central Illinois I learned from a 1941 guidebook authored by Virginia S. Eifert, *Birds in Your Backyard: Typical Native Birds in Their Habitats* (Springfield, Ill.: Illinois State Museum), which was reissued by popular demand in 1986. My own descriptions are undoubtedly shaped by those of this delightful writer.

58 Veery: H. D. Bohlen, *The Birds of Illinois* (Bloomington, Ind.: Indiana University Press, 1989), p. 138.

58 Songbird migration: K. P. Able, ed., *Gatherings of Angels: Migrating Birds and their Ecology* (Ithaca, N.Y.: Comstock Books, 1999); B. Wuethrich, "Songbirds Stressed in Winter Grounds," *Science* 282(1998):1791–94.

58–59 Moon watching: R. Burton, *Bird Migration* (London: Aurum Press, 1992), p. 14; J. Elphick, ed., *The Atlas of Bird Migration: Tracing the Great Journeys of the World's Birds* (New York: Random House, 1995), pp. 17, 47; see also Able, *Gatherings of Angels*.

60 Composition of amniotic fluid: R. M. Goldblum and S. Hilton, "Amniotic Fluid and the Fetal Mucosal Immune System," in P. L. Ogra et al., eds., *Mucosal Immunology*, 2d ed. (San Diego: Academic Press, 1999), pp. 1555–64.

60 Description of amniocentesis: *Gale Encyclopedia of Medicine*, s.v. "Amniocentesis," by K. R. Sternlof.

60 Alpha-fetoprotein: *Gale Encyclopedia of Medicine*, s.v. "Alpha-fetoprotein Test," by A. R. Massel.

60 Risk of miscarriage: *Gale Encyclopedia*, "Amniocentesis."

61 John Down: R. Rapp, *Testing Women, Testing the Fetus: The Social Impact of Amniocentesis in America* (New York: Routledge, 1999), pp. 295–29.

61 Risk/benefit analysis: *Gale Encyclopedia*, "Amniocentesis."

61–62 Quote from medical encyclopedia: Ibid.

62 Incapacitating knowledge: B. K. Rothman, *The Tentative Pregnancy: How Amniocentesis Changes the Experience of Motherhood* (New York: W. W. Norton, 1993), pp. 135–76.

62 Rayna Rapp: Rapp, *Testing Women, Testing the Fetus*. See also Rapp's essays "Refusing Prenatal Diagnosis: The Meanings of Bioscience in a Multicultural World," *Science, Technology, and Human Values* 23(1998):45–70, and "The Ethics of Choice," *Ms. Magazine*, April 1984, pp. 97–100. Rapp herself chose abortion at age thirty-six when an amniocentesis revealed Down syndrome.

63 Sealed adoption records: At this writing, only four states have open records: Alabama, Alaska, Kansas, and Oregon. The adoptee-rights organization at the forefront of fighting for open records in all states is Bastard Nation (www.bastards.org).

63 Quote from guidebook on prenatal screening of adoptees: K. Wexler and L. Wexler, *The ABC's of Prenatal Diagnosis: a Guide to Pregnancy Testing and Issues* (Aurora, Colo.: Genassist Publishing, 1994).

64 Mechanisms of bird migration: Elphick, *Atlas of Bird Migration*, pp. 32–34.

65 Migration of hummingbirds: Eifert, *Birds in Your Backyard*.

65–66 Amniotic fluid: B. M. Carlson, *Human Embryology and Developmental Biology*, 2d ed. (St. Louis: Mosby, 1999), pp. 106–9; Goldblum and Hilton, "Amniotic Fluid and the Fetal Mucosal Immune System."

67–68 Description of ultrasound: R. A. Bowerman, *Atlas of Normal Fetal Ultrasonographic Anatomy*, 2d ed. (St. Louis, Mo.: Mosby, 1992). Many mothers-to-be wonder whether ultrasound is safe. Clinicians presume that low-energy ultrasound does not harm fetal tissues, but there has never been a long-term study of its possible risks. Studies have found an association between exposure to prenatal ultrasound and left-handedness (B. B. Haire, "Ultrasound in Obstetrics: A Question of Safety," in B. K. Rothman, ed., *Encyclopedia of Childbearing: Critical Perspectives* [Phoenix: Oryx Press, 1993], pp. 407–9). In laboratory experiments, moreover, ultrasound has been shown to cause membrane changes of the type that could potentially affect pre- and postnatal development. It is reassuring that a large case-control study in Sweden found no association between exposure to ultrasound during pregnancy and risk of childhood leukemia (E. Naumburg, "Prenatal Ultrasound Examinations and Risk of Childhood Leukaemia: Case-Control Study," *British Medical Journal* 320[2000]:282–83).

67 History of ultrasound as a military tool: R. V. Wade, "Images, Imagination and Ideas: a Perspective on the Impact of Ultrasonography on the Practice of Obstetrics and Gynecology," *Am. J. of Obstetrics and Gynecology* 181(1999):235–39.

68 Study in England: R. H. Steinhorn, "Prenatal Ultrasonography: First Do No Harm?" *Lancet* 352(1998):1568–69.

69 Myrtle warblers: As ornithological readers of this book manuscript swiftly pointed out to me, myrtle warblers have been officially renamed yellow-rumped warblers; I will forever call them myrtles.

69 Birds and broadcast towers: Bohlen, *Birds of Illinois*, p. 158; R. Braile, "Bird Life: Towers Exacting Terrible Tolls," *Sports Afield* 222(Aug. 1999):18.

69–70 Given Harper and pesticide contamination in birds: G. Harper, personal communication; J. A. Klemens et al., "Patterns of Organochlorine Pesticide Contamination in Neotropical Migrant Passerines in Relation to Diet and Winter Habitat," *Chemosphere* 41(2000):1107–13.

72–74 Description of genetic analysis: Rapp, *Testing Women*, pp. 191–219.

72 Geneticist friend: Michael Hoffman, Dept. of Genetic Epidemiology, University of Utah, personal communication.

73–74 Types of chromosomal abnormalities: J. Barrett, "*Gale Encyclopedia of Medicine*, s.v. "Edwards' Syndrome," by J. Barrett; R. J. M. Gardner and G. R. Sutherland, *Chromosomal Abnormalities and Genetic Counseling*, 2d ed. (Oxford, U.K.: Oxford University Press, 1996).

75 Pesticides and PCBs in amniotic fluid: D. Christensen, "Pesticide Exposure Begins Early," *Science News* 156(17 July 1999):47; W. Foster, "Detection of Endocrine Disrupting Chemicals in Samples of Second Trimester Human Amniotic Fluid," *J. of Clinical Endocrinology and Metabolism* 85(2000):2954–57.

CHAPTER FIVE: MOTHER'S MOON

79 Report from Johns Hopkins. Pew Environmental Health Commission, *Healthy from the Start: Why America Needs a Better System to Track and Understand Birth Defects and the Environment* (Baltimore: Johns Hopkins School of Public Health, 1999).

79 Ancient ideas about birth defects: M. V. Barrow, "A Brief History of Teratology in the Early 20th Century," and J. Warkany, "Congenital Malformations in the Past," in T. V. N. Persaud, ed., *Problems of Birth Defects from Hippocrates to Thalidomide and After* (Baltimore: University Park Press, 1977), pp. 5–17 and 18–28.

79 Theories of inheritance did not hold up: D. T. Janerich and A. P. Polednak, "Epidemiology of Birth Defects," *Epidemiologic Reviews* 5(1983):16–37.

79 Quote from recent review: Ibid., p. 19

79 Moderate amounts of alcohol cause mental retardation: N. L. Day et al., "Effect of Prenatal Alcohol Exposure on Growth and Morphology of Offspring at 8 months of Age," *Pediatrics* 85(1990):748–52; Pew Environmental Health Commission, *Healthy from the Start*, p. 23. There is no real consensus on what constitutes "moderate." Some studies suggest that as few as two drinks a week may result in increased agitation and stressful behavior in newborns (P. W. Nathanielsz, *Life in the Womb: The Origin of Health and Disease* [Ithaca, N.Y.: Promethean Press, 1999], p. 179). It is clear that children whose mothers drink during pregnancy suffer increased attention and memory problems—even when the mothers average less than one drink per day (M. May, "Disturbing Behavior: Neurotoxic Effects in Children," *EHP* 108(2000):A262–67.) See also the note for page 105 under the key phrase "one good drunk."

79 Cigarette smoke lowers birth weight: This includes exposure to secondhand smoke among nonsmoking mothers. See J. C. Kleinman and J. H. Madans, "The Effects of Maternal Smoking, Physical Stature, and Educational Attainment on the Incidence of Low Birth Weight," *Am. J. of Epidemiology* 121(1985):843–55; Pew Environmental Health Commission, *Healthy from the Start*, p. 23; G. C. Windham et al., "Evidence for an Association Between Environmental Tobacco Smoke Exposure and Birthweight: A Meta-analysis and New Data," *Paediatric and Perinatal Epidemiology* 13(1999):35–57.

79 Quote from Johns Hopkins report: Pew Environmental Health Commission, *Healthy from the Start*, p. 23.

80 The nature of the defect doesn't indicate its origin: B. M. Carlson, *Human Embryology and Developmental Biology*, 2d ed. (St. Louis: Mosby, 1999), pp. 133–34.

80 Quote by Richard Clapp: Dr. Richard Clapp, Boston University School of Public Health, personal communication.

80 The most venerable of the lot: K. L. Jones, ed., *Smith's Recognizable Patterns of Human Malformation*, 5th ed. (Philadelphia: Saunders, 1997).

81 Far more disturbing: D. A. Nyberg et al., *Diagnostic Ultrasound of Fetal Abnormalities: Text and Atlas* (Chicago: Year Book Medical Publishers, 1990).

81 Bruce Carlson's book: Carlson, *Human Embryology*.

81 Onset of fetal movement: M. R. Primeau, "Fetal Movement," in B. K. Rothman, ed., *Encyclopedia of Childbearing: Critical Perspectives* (Phoenix: Oryx Press, 1993), pp. 151–53.

81 The picture labeled "Massive Oopharyngeal Teratoma": Carlson, *Human Embryology*, p. 4.

82 Birth defects the number one killer: Pew Environmental Health Commission, *Healthy from the Start*, p. 8.

82 Birth defect prevalence: I follow the practice of many epidemiologists who use the term "prevalence" at birth as a substitute for "incidence" when describing the frequency of birth defects. "Prevalence" acknowledges the role of fetal loss, both by spontaneous miscarriage and selective abortion, in the underestimation of the true number of fetuses afflicted by birth defects, which would be a measure of incidence (Janerich and Polednak, "Epidemiology of Birth Defects"). "Incidence," as epidemiologists use the word, refers to the cumulative number of people diagnosed with a particular health problem during a given period of time. It is usually expressed as the number of new cases per every 100,000 people per year. "Risk," by contrast, is a probability and represents the likelihood of any one individual or group of individuals becoming affected. "Excess risk," in the context of birth defects, refers to an increased chance of a particular infant's being diagnosed with a particular anomaly. Excess risk can be calculated by comparing the prevalence rates of a particular defect within a particular subpopulation (e.g., genital anomalies within DES-exposed sons) to an expected, or background, rate within the population as a whole.

83 Statistics on birth defect prevalence: M. C. Lynberg and L. D. Edmonds, "Surveillance of Birth Defects," in W. Halperin et al., eds., *Public Health Surveillance* (New York: John Wiley, 1992), pp. 157–72; Pew Environmental Health Commission, *Healthy from the Start*, p. 45. In a 2000 study, the National Research Council estimated that 3 percent of all birth defects are attributable to exposure to toxic chemicals. If so, this would mean that about 3,600 babies are born deformed each year in the United States solely as the result of toxic exposures. The council further estimated that 25 percent of birth defects might be attributable to a combination of genetic predisposition and environmental factors. If so, this would mean that about 30,000 U.S. babies are born each year with birth defects caused by a combination of hereditary and environmental factors. However, the council also noted that the causes of nearly half of major defects are so poorly understood that they cannot be classified as either environmental or genetic in origin. Presumably some fraction of these have an environmental component (National Research Council, *Scientific Frontiers in Developmental Toxicology and Risk Assessment* [Washington, D.C.: National Academy Press, 2000], pp. ix, 1, and 25).

83 No national system to track birth defects: Pew Environmental Health Commission, *Healthy from the Start*, p. 65. In late 1998, the National Toxicology Program and the National Institute of Environmental Health Sciences announced the establishment of a new research institute, the Center for the Evaluation of Health Risks to Human Reproduction, which will evaluate the role of toxic chemicals in causing birth defects and infertility (J. Stephenson, "Weighing Reproductive Threats," *JAMA* 281[1999]:600).

83 Registries founded in the 1970s: Centers for Disease Control, "Temporal Trends in the Incidence of Birth Defects," *Morbidity and Mortality Weekly Report* 46(1997):1171–76; L. D. Edmonds et al., "Congenital Malformations Surveillance: Two American Systems," *Intl. J. of Epidemiology* 10(1981):247–52; G. P. Oakley, Jr., "Population and Case-Control Surveillance in the Search for Environmental Causes of Birth Defects," *Public Health Reports* 99(1984):465–68; T. Schettler et al., *Generations at Risk: Reproductive Health and the Environment* (Cambridge: MIT Press, 1999), pp. 39–42.

83 BDMP dismantled: Lynberg and Edmonds, "Surveillance of Birth Defects"; Centers for Disease Control, "Temporal Trends in the Incidence of Birth Defects." At this writing, only the nonprofit group Birth Defect Research for Children, Inc., operates a national birth defect registry. Their contact information is provided on page 331.

83 BDMP did not aggressively pursue information: Working Group on Human Reproductive Outcomes, *Improving Assessment of the Effects of Environmental Contamination on Human Reproduction: Report of Findings and Recommendations* (Washington D.C.: Child Trends, Inc., 1986), pp. 7–8.

83 Many defects not manifested at birth: M. A. Honein and L. J. Paulozzi, "Birth Defects Surveillance: Assessing the 'Gold Standard,' " *Am. J. of Public Health* 89(1999):1238–40.

83 Few birth defects accurately reported on birth certificates: M. L. Watkins et al., "The Surveillance of Birth Defects: The Usefulness of the Revised U.S. Standard Birth Certificate," *Am. J. of Public Health* 86(1996):731–34. Similarly, researchers associated with the California Birth Defects Monitoring Program evaluated birth certificate data in the San Francisco Bay area and found that "reporting of birth defects on the birth certificate was poor for every condition" (A. C. Hexter et al., "Evaluation of the Hospital Discharge Diagnoses Index and the Birth Certificate as Sources of Information on Birth Defects," *Public Health Reports* 105[1990]:296–307). Researchers examining data from the Metropolitan Atlanta Congenital Defects Program found that birth certificates were especially poor at identifying many types of digestive system defects. They also concluded that the MACDP underestimates birth defects by 13 percent at one year after birth (Honein and Paulozzi, "Birth Defects Surveillance").

83 Limitations of Atlanta registry: Dr. Lynn Goldman, Johns Hopkins University, personal communication.

83 State registries sorely wanting: Pew Environmental Health Commission, *Healthy from the Start*, p. 9.

84 Descriptions of the California Birth Defects Monitoring Program: www.cbmp.org and Jackie Wynne, California Birth Defects Monitoring Program, personal communication.

84 Research inspired by CBDMP: G. M. Shaw et al., "Maternal Pesticide Exposure from Multiple Sources and Selected Congenital Anomalies," *Epidemiology* 10(1999):60–66.

84 Texas operates one of the best registries: Ibid., 66–67.

84–85 Anencephaly in Brownsville area: Ibid., p. 49; L. E. Sever, "Looking for Causes of Neural Tube Defects: Where Does the Environment Fit In?" *EHP* 103(1995, sup. 6):165–71.

85 How anencephaly happens: L. D. Botto et al., "Neural Tube Defects," *NEJM* 341(1999):1509–19.

85 Anencephaly and gene disruption: J. Chen et al., "Disruption of the MacMARKS Gene Prevents Cranial Neural Tube Closure and Results in Anencephaly," *Proceedings of the National Academy of Science* 93(1996):6275–79.

85 Anencephaly and paternal exposures: J. D. Brender and L. Suarez, "Paternal Occupation and Anencephaly," *Am. J. of Epidemiology* 131(1990):517–21.

85–86 Atrial septal defect: Pew Environmental Health Commission, *Healthy from the Start*, pp. 15, 59.

83–86 Interpretation of birth defect data: The relative infrequency of birth defects further frustrates their statistical interpretation. However common they are by the standards of infant health—compared to, say, cancer—birth defects are rare events. To estimate cancer rates, registrars determine the number of newly diagnosed cases per 100,000 people per year. This is also how birth defect rates are calculated. But the risk of being born with a birth defect is one tenth the lifetime risk of developing cancer, which now affects 40 percent of Americans. Lower rates mean lower statistical power when making comparisons. Information on birth defects must therefore be collected from a much larger proportion of the general population to yield enough cases to withstand the rigors of statistical testing. But this information is not collected. And without the nets cast widely, real changes in birth defect rates can disappear when the statisticians go to work on the data. Dr. Ted Schettler and his colleagues at Physicians for Social Responsibility explain this vanishing act with the following hypothetical example: Say a new birth defect–inducing chemical is introduced into the marketplace. Say it causes cleft palate, and say it is so widely used in consumer products that one out of every ten pregnant women in America is exposed to it. Suppose also that its teratogenic powers are quite potent—it raises the risk of cleft palate by a factor of five, and about half of all cases of cleft palate are caused by a biological mechanism that is potentially influenced by this chemical. Because of exposure to this new teratogen, the overall rate of cleft palates in the population will go up by 40 percent, which means that in a state registry that monitors about 40,000 births each year, the number of newborns touched by this defect will increase from 40 cases each year to 56 cases. Because the numbers are so small, this increase is not a statistically significant one.

Anyone asking whether this new chemical might be responsible for the apparent increase in cleft palates (which it is) would be told that the registry data show no statistical evidence for such an increase (which they don't). Such calculations may seem like sleight-of-hand work, but public health statistics are designed to be highly conservative so that trends deemed statistically significant can be trusted to be real. The price we pay for this kind of rigor is that some very real problems do not show up in the final analysis unless the database can be expanded to capture as much of the population as possible (Schettler et al., *Generations at Risk*, pp. 39–42).

86 Green Lull: B. P. Lawton, *A Seasonal Guide to the Natural Year: Illinois, Missouri, and Arkansas* (Golden, Colo: Fulcrum, 1994), pp. 114–20.

87 Hypospadias: A. Czeizel et al., "Increased Birth Prevalence of Isolated Hypospadias in Hungary," *Acta Paediatrica Hungarica* 27(1986):329–337; H. Dolk, "Rise in Prevalence of Hypospadias," *Lancet* 351(1998):770; A. Giwercman et al., "Evidence for Increasing Incidence of Abnormalities of the Human Testis," *EHP* 101(1993, sup. 2):65–71; J. M. Moline et al., "Exposure to Hazardous Substances and Male Reproductive Health: A Research Framework," *EHP* 108(2000):803–13; L. J. Paulozzi et al., "International Trends in Rates of Hypospadias and Cryptorchidism," *EHP* 107(1999):297–302; L. J. Paulozzi, "Hypospadias Trends in Two U.S. Surveillance Systems," *Pediatrics* 100(1997):831–34.

87–88 Anencephaly and abortion: J. D. Cragan et al., "Surveillance for Anencephaly and Spina Bifida and the Impact of Prenatal Diagnosis—United States, 1985–1994," *Teratology* 56(1997):33–49. Moreover, access to prenatal tests and abortion differs widely among geographic regions of the United States.

88 Abortion rates for anencephaly in Hawaii: M. B. Forrester, et al., "Impact of Prenatal Diagnosis and Elective Termination on the Prevalence of Selected Birth Defects," *American Journal of Epidemiology* 148(1998):1206–11.

88 Spina bifida: Centers for Disease Control, "Spina Bifida Incidence at Birth—United States, 1983–1990," *Morbidity and Mortality Weekly Report* 41(1992):497–500.

88 Abortion rates for spina bifida in Hawaii: Forrester, "Impact of Prenatal Diagnosis."

88 Hawaii registry: Ibid.

88 Anencephaly rates in California: In California between 1989 and 1991 more than half of fetuses afflicted with anencephaly and 30 percent of fetuses with spina bifida were selectively aborted (E. M. Velie and G. M. Shaw, "Impact of Prenatal Diagnosis and Elective Termination on Prevalence and Risk Estimates of Neural Tube Defects in California, 1989-1991," *American Journal of Epidemiology* 144[1996]: 473–79).

88 Similar findings from France: In France, termination of pregnancy after prenatal ultrasound was found to have a definite impact on the prevalence at birth of congenital anomalies with a low survival rate (C. Julian-Reynier et al., "Impact of Prenatal Diagnosis by Ultrasound on the Prevalence of Congenital Anomalies at Birth in Southern France," *J. of Epidemiology and Community Health* 48[1994]:290–96).

88 Most chemicals not tested for teratogenicity: Pew Environmental Health Commission, *Healthy from the Start*, pp. 34–36.

88–89 Numbers of chemicals on the market, tested and untested: Ibid., pp. 34–35.

89 Pesticides more thoroughly evaluated: Ibid., p. 35

89 Quote from Johns Hopkins report: Ibid., p. 35

89 Right-to-know laws: For a brief history of right-to-know laws, see S. Steingraber, *Living Downstream: An Ecologist Looks at Cancer and the Environment* (Reading, Mass.: Addison-Wesley, 1997), pp. 100–103. For a description of the strengths and limitations of right-to-know data with special attention to fetal toxicants, see T. Schettler et al., *In Harm's Way: Toxic Threats to Child Development* (Cambridge: Greater Boston Physicians for Social Responsibility, 2000), pp. 103–16. See Afterword (page 284) for more information on obtaining toxics release data for your community.

89 1997 data for U.S. and Illinois toxic releases: Cited in Pew Environmental Health Commission, *Healthy from the Start*, p.34–36, and accompanying Illinois Fact Sheet. An analysis of 1998 data, conducted by the National Environmental Trust, ranked states by TRI releases of developmental and neurological toxins. The top ten states, in order of releases, are Louisiana, Texas, Utah, Ohio, Alabama, Indiana, Illinois, Georgia, and North Carolina. The top ranking county in the United States is Touela County in Utah (National Environmental Trust, Physicians for Social Responsibility, and the Learning Disabilities Association of America, *Polluting Our Future: Chemical Pollution in the United States that Affects Child Development and Learning* [Washington, D.C.: National Environmental Trust, 2000], p. 10).

90–92 Superiority of European registries: Since 1967, the Medical Birth Registry of Norway has received a report on all births in Norway with a gestational age of sixteen weeks or more (R. T. Lie, "Environmental Epidemiology at the Medical Birth Registry of Norway: Strengths and Limitations," *Central European J. of Public Health* 5[1997]:57–59). Similarly, the Glasgow Register of Congenital Anomalies, founded in 1974, includes all births and induced abortions following prenatal diagnosis. Using data from this registry and comparing them to reports from England and Wales, researchers were able to document an increasing gradient in the prevalence of abdominal wall defects from the south to the north of the United Kingdom, with especially high rates within Glasgow itself, a pattern that mirrors that observed for neural tube defects within the United Kingdom (D. H. Stone et al., "Prevalence of Congenital Anterior Abdominal Wall Defects in the United Kingdom: Comparison of Regional Registers," *British Medical Journal* 317[1998]:1118–19). Comparing data from registries in Slovenia, Finland, Denmark, Hungary, Poland, and Bohemia, researchers discovered that the incidence of cleft lips and palates fluctuates in synchrony across regional areas, suggesting that environmental factors of some kind play a part in their etiology (W. Kozelj, "Epidemiology of Orofacial Clefts in Slovenia, 1973–1993: Comparison of the Incidence in Six European Countries," *J. of Cranio-Maxillofacial Surgery* 24[1996]:378–82). Making broad international comparisons within Europe nevertheless remains challenging—especially for lethal and life-threatening forms of birth defects. Rates of prenatal diagnosis vary between countries, as does availability of abortion (which was still illegal in Ireland and Malta as of 1993). When women must leave their home area to obtain abortions elsewhere, problems arise for birth defect registrars. The name of the network of centrally coordinated registries in Europe is European Registers of Congenital Abnormalities and Twins (EUROCAT). It was founded in 1979 to monitor trends in the frequency of birth defects and to assess the impact of environmental causes (M. F. Lechat and H. Dolk, "Registries of Congenital Anomalies: EUROCAT," *EHP* 101[1993, sup. 2]:153–57).

    90–91 Norway study (1994): R. T. Lie et al., "A Population-Based Study of the Risk of Recurrence of Birth Defects," *NEJM* 331(1994):1–4.

    91 Quote by *NEJM* in response to Norwegian study: J. F. Cordero, "Finding the Causes of Birth Defects," *NEJM* 331(1994):48–49.

    91 Toxic waste sites and birth defects in Europe: II. Dolk et al., "Risk of Congenital Anomalies Near Hazardous-Waste Landfill Sites in Europe: The EUROHAZCOM Study," *Lancet* 352(1998):423–27; B. L. Johnson, "A Review of the Effects of Hazardous Waste on Reproductive Health," *Am. J. of Obstetrics and Gynecology* 181(1999):S12-S16. The weakness in Dolk's study is that it did not actually measure individual exposures. In Bulgaria, researchers did measure individual exposures and were able to document a link between environmental pollutants and complications of pregnancy. Significantly higher blood levels of environmentally toxic substances—namely lead and organic solvents—were found among women who lived near metal smelters and petrochemical plants and who had pregnancy complications, such as toxemia, anemia, threatened abortion, and nephopathy. Women without such complications had lower blood levels of these contaminants. Birth defect prevalence, however, was not examined (S. Tabacova and L. Balabaeva, "Environmental Pollutants in Relation to Complications of Pregnancy," *EHP* 101 [1993, sup. 2], 27–31).

    91 Similar findings in the U.S.: S. A. Geschwind et al., "Risk of Congenital Malformations Associated with Proximity to Hazardous Waste Sites," *Am. J. of Epidemiology* 135(1992):1197–1207; Johnson, "A Review of the Effects of Hazardous Waste on Reproductive Health," *Am. J. of Obstetrics and Gynecology* 181(1999):S12-S16.

    91 Toxic waste sites and birth defects in California: L. A. Croen et al., "Maternal Residential Proximity to Hazardous Waste Sites and Risk for Selected Congenital Malformation," *Epidemiology* 8(1997):347–54; Johnson, "A Review of the Effects of Hazardous Waste on Reproductive Health"; J. Raloff, "Superfund Sites and Birth Defects," *Science News* 151(1997):391. For a discussion of the epidemiologic term "risk," see note for page 82 under the key phrase "birth defect prevalence."

    91–92 Quote from recent review: Johnson, "A Review," p. S15.

    92 Solvents and birth defects: Schettler et al., *Generations at Risk*, p. 76.

    92 Tucson study: Johnson, "A Review."

    93 New York study: E. G. Marshall et al., "Maternal Residential Exposure to Hazardous Wastes and Risk of Central Nervous System and Musculoskeletal Birth Defects," *Archives of Environmental Health* 52(1997):416–25.

    93 Women's occupational exposure to solvents: R. Edwards, "The Chips Are Down: Health Problems Among Semiconductor Industry Workers," *New Scientist*, 15 May 1999, p. 18–19; A. Ericson et al., "Delivery Outcome of Women Working in Laboratories During Pregnancy," *Archives of Environmental Health* 39(1984):5–10; P. O. D. Pharoah et al., "Outcome of Pregnancy Among Women in Anaesthetic Practice," *Lancet* 1(1977, no. 8001):34–36; J. C. McDonald et al., "Chemical Exposures at Work in Early Pregnancy and Congenital Defect: A Case-Referent Study," *British J. of Industrial Medicine* 44(1987):527–33.

93 Prospective study: S. Khattak et al., "Pregnancy Outcome Following Gestational Exposure to Organic Solvents: A Prospective Controlled Study," *JAMA* 281(1999):1106–9.

93 Quote from critical analysis of all papers: K. I. McMartin et al., "Pregnancy Outcome Following Maternal Organic Solvent Exposure: A Meta-Analysis of Epidemiologic Studies," *Am. J. of Industrial Medicine* 34(1998):288–92.

94–95 Paternal exposure and birth defects: K. J. Aronson et al., "Congenital Anomalies Among the Offspring of Fire Fighters," *Am. J. of Industrial Medicine* 30(1996):83–86; B. M. Blatter et al., "Paternal Occupational Exposure Around Conception and Spina Bifida in Offspring," *Am. J. of Industrial Medicine* 32(1997):283–91; W. H. Dimich-Ward et al., "Reproductive Effects of Paternal Exposure to Chlorophenate Wood Preservatives in the Sawmill Industry," *Scandinavian J. of Work, Environment, and Health* 22(1996):267–73; A. M. Garcia et al., "Paternal Exposure to Pesticides and Congenital Malformations," *Scandinavian J. of Work and Environmental Health* 24(1998):473–80; M. A. McDiarmid et al., "Reproductive Hazards and Firefighters," *Occupational Medicine* 10(1995): 829–41; ibid., "Reproductive Hazards of Fire Fighting II. Chemical Hazards," *Am. J. of Industrial Medicine* 19(1991):447–72; A. F. Olshan et al., "Paternal Occupational Exposures and the Risk of Down Syndrome," *American J. of Human Genetics* 44(1989):646–51; Pew Environmental Health Commission, *Healthy from the Start*, p. 22–23; D. H. Poyner et al., "Paternal Exposures and the Question of Birth Defects," *J. of the Florida Medical Association* 84(1997):323–26; P. G. Schnitzer et al., "Paternal Occupation and Risk of Birth Defects in Offspring," *Epidemiology* 6(1995):577–83.

95 Sperm-chaperoned agents: Poyner et al., "Paternal Exposures." This is an emerging area of study.

96 Vietnamese journalists report high numbers of deformities: T. Whiteside, "Defoliation," *The New Yorker*, 7 Feb. 1970, pp. 32–69.

96 Evolving purpose of clandestine program: A. H. Westing, ed., *Herbicides in War: The Long-Term Ecological and Human Consequences* (Philadelphia: Taylor & Francis, 1984); Whiteside, "Defoliation."

96 Amounts of defoliants sprayed: "Exposure to Herbicide Agent Orange is Linked to Some Forms of Cancer," *Chemical Market Reporter* 255(22 Feb. 1999):17; H. Warwick, "Agent Orange: The Poisoning of Vietnam," *Ecologist* 28(1998):264–65.

96 Disclosure that Agent Orange causes birth defects in mice: R. W. Bovey and A. L. Young, *The Science of 2,4,5-T and Associated Phenoxy Herbicides* (New York: John Wiley, 1980); B. Nelson, "Herbicides: Order on 2,4,5-T Issued at Unusually High Level," *Science* 166(1969): 977–979; Whiteside, "Defoliation."

96 Laced with dioxin: G. L. Henriksen and J. E. Michalek, "Serum Dioxin, Testosterone, and Gonadotropins in Veterans of Operation Ranch Hand," *Epidemiology* 7(1996):454–55.

96–97 Health effects of dioxin: M. J. DeVito and L. S. Birnbaum, "Toxicology of Dioxin and Related Compounds," in A. Schecter, ed., *Dioxins and Health* (New York: Plenum Press, 1994), pp. 139–42.

97 Dioxin levels still elevated in environment and human tissues: S. M. Booker, "Dioxin in Vietnam: Fighting a Legacy of War," *EHP* 109(2001):A116–17; D. Cayo, "Toxic Legacy Plagues Vietnam," *Ottawa Citizen*, 9 April 2000, pp. A1, A12; S. Mydans, "Vietnam Sees War's Legacy in Its Young," *New York Times*, 16 May 1999, sec. 1, p. 12; F. Pearce, "Innocent Victims," *New Scientist*, 3 Oct. 1998, 18–19; A. Schecter et al., "Recent Contamination from Agent Orange in Residents of a Southern Vietnam City," *Journal of Occupational and Environmental Medicine* 43 (2001): 435–43.

97 Children of American fathers: J. Stephenson, "New IOM Report Links Agent Orange Exposure to Risk of Birth Defect in Vietnam Vets' Children," *JAMA* 275 (1996):1066–67.

97 My dissertation: S. K. Steingraber, "Deer Browsing, Plant Competition, and Succession in a Red Pine Forest, Itasca State Park, Minnesota," Ph.D. diss., University of Michigan, 1989.

97–98 Clearing brush from Minnesota forests: Ibid., pp. 60–105.

98 Quote from 1995 critical evaluation: T. Nurminen, "Maternal Pesticide Exposure and Pregnancy Outcome," *J. of Occupational and Environmental Medicine* 37(1995):935–40. The evidence from the laboratory is much stronger: over 100 pesticides have been shown to cause birth defects in experimental animals in at least one test (A. S. Rowland, "Pesticides and Birth Defects," *Epidemiology* 6[1995]:6–7).

98–99 Finnish study: T. Nurminen et al., "Agricultural Work During Pregnancy and Selective Structural Malformations in Finland," *Epidemiology* 6(1995):23–30. Also described in Schettler, *In Harm's Way*, p. 119.

99 Spain: A. M. Garcia et al., "Parental Agricultural Work and Selected Congenital Malformations," *Am. J. of Epidemiology* 149(1999):64–74; J. Garcia-Rodriguez et al., "Exposure to Pesticides and Cryptorchidism: Geographical Evidence of a Possible Association," *EHP* 104(1996): 1090–95.

99 Denmark: I. S. Weidner et al., "Cryptorchidism and Hypospadias in Sons of Gardeners and Farmers," *EHP* 106(1998):793–96.

99 Norway: P. Kristensen et al., "Birth Defects Among Offspring of Norwegian Farmers, 1967–1991," *Epidemiology* 8(1997):537–44.

99 California: E. M. Bell et al., "A Case-Control Study of Pesticides and Fetal Death Due to Congenital Anomalies," *Epidemiology* 12(2001):148–56.

99–100 Vincent Garry's study: V. F. Garry et al., "Pesticide Appliers, Biocides, and Birth Defects in Rural Minnesota," *EHP* 104(1996):394–99. Garry's findings are based on records of live births only, which means they overlook birth defects among fetuses miscarried or aborted.

100 Atrazine and birth defects in Iowa: R. Munger et al., "Birth Defects and Pesticide-Contaminated Water Supplies in Iowa," *Am. J. of Epidemiology* 136(1992):959.

100 Turn on a dishwasher: C. Howard-Reed et al., "Mass Transfer of Volatile Organic Compounds from Drinking Water to Indoor Air: The Role of Residential Dishwashers," *Environmental Science & Technology* 33(1999):2266–72.

100 A ten-minute shower equals a half gallon of tap water: C. P. Weisel and W. K. Jo, "Ingestion, Inhalation, and Dermal Exposures to Chloroform and Trichloroethene from Tap Water," *EHP* 104(1996):48–51.

101 Sources of Bloomington's drinking water: K. D. Smiciklas and A. S. Moore, "Fertilizer Nitrogen Management to Optimize Water Quality," unpublished report (Normal, Ill.: Illinois State University, Dept. of Agriculture, 1999; www.cast.ilstu.edu/moore/lakeproj/IFCA99.html).

101 Contaminants found in Bloomington's water in 1996–97: The Environmental Working Group lists Bloomington's drinking water as one of thirty-three large water systems in the United States that need closer monitoring because they have reported nitrate levels in excess of nine parts per million at least once since 1993 (B. A. Cohen and R. Wiles, *Tough to Swallow: How Pesticide Companies Profit from Poisoning America's Tap Water* [Washington D.C.: Environmental Working Group, 1997], p. 35).

101 Nitrates in Bloomington's water violated standards in 1990–93: Bloomington violated the nitrate standard eight years out of ten during the period 1986–95 (Ibid., p. 1.).

101 Quote from review on health risks of nitrate-contaminated water: S. Crutchfield, "Agriculture and Water Quality Conflicts," *FoodReview* 14 (April–June 1991):12–14.

101 Nitrate and frogs: A. Marco et al., "Sensitivity to Nitrate and Nitrite in Pond-Breeding Amphibians from the Pacific Northwest, USA," *Environmental Toxicology and Chemistry* 18 (1999):2836–39.

CHAPTER SIX: ROSE MOON

104 Quote from embryology textbook: M. A. England, *Life Before Birth*, 2nd ed. (London: Mosby-Wolfe, 1996), p. 15.

105 One good drunk: The effects of ethanol on the fetal brain are not well understood. A recent German study found that a single four-hour drinking episode during the third trimester exposes human fetuses to blood ethanol levels that trigger mass neuronal die-offs (via apoptosis) in lab animals. In other words, alcohol exposure caused large numbers of brain cells to be deleted from the developing brain. In this study, these alcohol-induced deaths of developing brain cells were brought about by the simultaneous blocking and activation of two different chemical receptors during the period in which neuronal synapses are forming (C. Ikonomidou et al., "Ethanol-Induced Apoptotic Neurodegeneration and Fetal Alcohol Syndrome," *Science* 287[2000]:1056–60; J. W. Olney et al., "Environmental Agents That Have the Potential to Trigger Mass Apoptotic Neurodegeneration in the Developing Brain," *EHP* 108[2000, sup. 3]:383–88). During earlier stages of pregnancy, a single alcohol binge (more than five drinks at one sitting) may permanently alter the migration of fetal brain cells. Binge drinking during pregnancy is linked to lower IQs and increased risk of learning disabilities in school-aged children. In sheep, alcohol diminishes the amount of blood flowing to the fetal brain. Furthermore, exposure to alcohol during the first weeks of pregnancy can decrease the number of fibers in the optic nerve, thus impairing vision (P. W. Nathanielsz, *Life in the Womb: The Origin of Health and Disease* [Ithaca, N.Y.: Promethean Press, 1999], pp. 112 and 180–81). For a fine overview of recent research on drinking during pregnancy, see D. Christensen, "Sobering Work: Unraveling Alcohol's Effects on the Developing Brain," *Science News* 158(2000):28–29. See also the note for page 79 under the key phrase "moderate amounts of alcohol cause mental retardation."

105 Quotation by Voltaire: P. W. Nathanielsz, *Life Before Birth: The Challenges of Fetal Development* (New York: W. H. Freeman, 1996), pp. 158. The literal translation of the original quotation is "Abstain from an action if in doubt as to whether it is right or not" (from "Le Philosophe Ignorant," in *Mélanges de Voltaire* [Paris: Bibliothèque de la Pléiade, Librairie Gallimard, 1961], p. 920). Thanks to Dr. James Matthews, a French scholar, of Illinois Wesleyan University for tracking down the original source.

105–106 Standards for nitrates in drinking water not shown safe for fetuses: Committee on Environmental Health, American Academy of Pediatrics, *Handbook of Pediatric Environmental Health* (Elk Grove Village, Ill.: AAP, 1999), p. 164; National Research Council, *Nitrate and Nitrite in Drinking Water* (Washington, D.C.: National Academy Press, 1995), p. 2.

106 4.5 million Americans drink water with elevated nitrate levels: AAP, *Handbook of Pediatric Environmental Health*, p. 164.

106 Quote from scientific report: International Joint Commission, *Ninth Biennial Report on Great Lakes Water Quality* (Ottawa, Ont.: International Joint Commission, 1998), p. 10.

106 Quote from popular guidebook: A. Eisenberg et al., *What to Expect When You're Expecting* (New York: Workman, 1996), pp. 129–32.

107 Toxics releases in McLean County: Data on toxic emissions are measured and sent by the industries in question to the U.S. Environmental Protection Agency. These are disseminated on the Internet in a user-friendly format by the Environmental Defense (www.scorecard.org). Their contact information is provided on page 331.

107 University's use of pesticides: According to the director of the grounds crew, pesticides used in 1999 include mecoprop and bromoxynil. As of 2001 they are no longer used. Thanks to my student, Sarah Perry, for investigating this issue.

108–110 34 million pounds of reproductive toxicants released in Illinois in 1997: Toxics Release Inventory (www.scorecard.org).

109–110 Description of fetal brain development, gross anatomy: B. M. Carlson, *Human Embryology and Developmental Biology*, 2d ed. (St. Louis: Mosby, 1999) pp. 208–48; England, *Life Before Birth*, pp. 51–70.

110 Description of fetal brain development, cellular anatomy: D. Bellinger and H. L. Needleman, "The Neurotoxicity of Prenatal Exposure to Lead: Kinetics, Mechanisms, and Expressions," in H. L. Needleman and D. Bellinger, eds., *Prenatal Exposure to Toxicants: Developmental Consequences* (Baltimore: Johns Hopkins University Press, 1994), pp. 89–111; Carlson, *Human Embryology*, pp. 208–48; England, *Life Before Birth*, pp. 51–70; Victor Friedrich, "Wiring of the Growing Brain," presentation at the conference Environmental Issues on Children: Brain, Development, and Behavior, New York Academy of Medicine, New York City, 24 May 1999; Nathanielsz, *Life Before Birth*, pp. 38–42; T. Schettler et al., *In Harm's Way: Toxic Threats to Child Development* (Cambridge: Greater Boston Physicians for Social Responsibility, 2000), pp. 23–28.

110 Neuroglia modulate available glucose: Nathanielsz, *Life Before Birth*, p. 16.

111 Later brain cells follow early-migrating neurons: K. Suzuki and P. M. Martin, "Neurotoxicants and the Developing Brain," in Harry, *Developmental Neurotoxicology*, pp. 9–32.

111 Mechanisms of fetal neurotoxicity: G. J. Harry, "Introduction to Developmental Neurotoxicology," in G. J. Harry, ed., *Developmental Neurotoxicology* (Boca Raton: CRC Press, 1994), pp. 1–7.

111 More than half of TRI chemicals are neurotoxins: U.S. releases of neurotoxins into air, water, wells, and landfills totaled 1.2 billion pounds in 1997. These chemicals include heavy metals such as lead and mercury as well as methanol, ammonia, manganese compounds, chlorine, styrene, glycol ethers, and a variety of solvents, such as toluene and xylene (Schettler, *In Harm's Way*, pp. 103–5).

111–112 Interspecific differences in brain development: E. M. Faustman et al., "Mechanisms Underlying Children's Susceptibility to Environmental Toxicants," *EHP* 108(2000, sup. 1):13–21; P. M. Rodier, "Comparative Postnatal Neurologic Development," in Needleman and Bellinger, *Prenatal Exposure to Toxicants*, pp. 3–23.

112 When testing expanded to include behavior: Harry, "Introduction to Developmental Neurotoxicology"; H. L. Needleman and P. J. Landrigan, *Raising Children Toxic Free: How to Keep*

Your Child Safe from Lead, Asbestos, Pesticides and Other Environmental Hazards (New York: Farrar Straus & Giroux, 1994), pp. 11–15.

114 Historical awareness of lead poisoning: Bellinger and Needleman, "The Neurotoxicity of Prenatal Exposure to Lead: Kinetics, Mechanisms, and Expressions"; Suzuki and Martin, "Neurotoxicants and the Developing Brain."

114 Lead's migration into fetal body: Bellinger and Needleman, "The Neurotoxicity of Prenatal Exposure to Lead."

114 Awareness in the 1940s: AAP, *Handbook of Pediatric Environmental Health*, pp. 131–43; H. L. Needleman, "Childhood Lead Poisoning: The Promise and Abandonment of Primary Prevention," *Am. J. of Public Health* 88(1998):1871–77; Needleman and Landrigan, *Raising Children Toxic Free*, pp. 11–15.

115 Lowering of IQs in El Paso: Described in Needleman and Landrigan, *Raising Children Toxic Free*, pp. 11–15.

115 Studies from around the world: AAP, *Handbook of Pediatric Environmental Health*, pp. 131–43.

115 Lead levels required to affect mental acuity: Suzuki and Martin, "Neurotoxicants and the Developing Brain."

115 Mechanisms by which lead wrecks brain development: Bellinger and Needleman, "The Neurotoxicity of Prenatal Exposure to Lead"; M. K. Nihei et al., "*N*-Methyl-D-Aspartate Receptor Subunit Changes are Associated with Lead-Induced Deficits of Long-Term Potentiation and Spatial Learning," *Neuroscience* 99(2000):233–42; Suzuki and Martin, "Neurotoxicants and the Developing Brain."

115 Vulnerability of fetus to lead: The elderly are also at risk. As bone demineralizes with age, blood lead levels can rise. In seniors, even slight elevations can have adverse cognitive effects (Bernard Weiss, University of Rochester, personal communication).

115 Life-changing consequences: New research suggests that these consequences include a propensity to violent behavior, as well as a lowered IQ. See, for example, R. Nevin, "How Lead Exposure Relates to Temporal Changes in I.Q., Violent Crime, and Unwed Pregnancy," *Environmental Research* 83(2000):1–22.

115 Public health triumph of lead bans: AAP, *Handbook of Pediatric Environmental Health*, pp. 131–43.

115 75 percent decline: Nevin, "How Lead Exposure Relates to Temporal Changes."

116 One in twenty children: G. Markowitz and D. Rosner, " 'Cater to the Children': The Role of the Lead Industry in a Public Health Tragedy, 1900–1955," *Am. J. of Public Health*, 90(2000):36–46.

116 Lead not outlawed in cosmetics: T. Schettler et al., *Generations at Risk: Reproductive Health and the Environment* (Cambridge: MIT Press, 1999), p. 273.

116–117 Lead paint: Markowitz and Rosner, " 'Cater to the Children' "; E. K. Silbergeld, "Protection of the Public Interest, Allegations of Scientific Misconduct, and the Needleman Case," *Am. J. of Public Health* 85(1995):165–66; Schettler et al., *Generations at Risk*, pp. 52–57.

117 A leading toxicologist remembers: Herbert Needleman, "Environmental Neurotoxins and Attention Deficit Disorder," presentation at the conference Environmental Issues on Children: Brain, Development, and Behavior, New York Academy of Medicine, New York, N.Y., 24 May 1999.

117–118 Leaded gas: J. L. Kitman, "The Secret History of Lead," *The Nation* 270(20 March 2000):11–41; Needleman, "Childhood Lead Poisoning"; H. L. Needleman, "Clamped in a Straitjacket: The Insertion of Lead into Gasoline," *Environmental Research* 74(1997):95–103; D. Rosner and G. Markowitz, "A 'Gift of God'?: The Public Health Controversy over Leaded Gasoline During the 1920s," *Am. J. of Public Health* 75(1985):344–52; Silbergeld, "Protection of the Public Interest."

118 1979 study of Somerville children: Needleman, J. Palca, "Lead Researcher Confronts Accusers in Public Hearing," *Science* 256(1992):437–38.

119 Quote on lower lead levels in men: Schettler et al., *Generations at Risk*, p. 57.

119 Lead-induced impairments: B. P. Lanphear et al., "Cognitive Deficits Associated with Blood Lead Concentrations <10 microg/dL in US Children and Adolescents," *Public Health Reports* 115(2000):521–29; J. Raloff, "Even Low Lead in Kids has High Cost," *Science News* 159(2001):277. Furthermore, a 1992 study found that slightly elevated blood lead levels in two-year-olds were associated with deficits in academic performance at age ten (D. C. Bellinger et al.,

"Low Level Lead Exposure, Intelligence and Academic Achievement: A Long-Term Follow-up Study," *Pediatrics* 90 [1992]:855-61).

120 History of mercury: L. J. Goldwater, *Mercury: A History of Quicksilver* (Baltimore: York Press, 1972). In the nineteenth century, makers of felt hats used mercury salts as a fixative of beaver pelts and suffered severe neurological damage as a result. Hence the expression "mad as a hatter."

120–121 Mercury in the food chain: Dr. Edward Swain, Minnesota Pollution Control Agency, personal communication.

121 Concentration of mercury vapor has tripled: D. C. Evers et al., "Geographic Trends in Mercury Measured in Common Loon Feathers and Blood," *Environmental Toxicology and Chemistry* 17(1998):173–83.

121 Every year airborne mercury goes up by 1 percent: Ibid.

121 Methylmercury rising in fish and loons: Ibid.

121 Impaired reproduction in loons: In Maine 27 percent of loons contain so much mercury that their behavior, development, and ability to lay viable eggs have been disrupted (P. Evers et al., *Assessing the Impacts of Methylmercury on Piscivorous Wildlife as Indicated by the Common Loon, 1998–99* [Freeport, Me.: BioDiversity Research Institute, 2000], report submitted to the Maine Department of Environmental Protection).

121 Clear-cutting and mining: B. Weiss, "The Developmental Neurotoxicity of Methyl Mercury," in Needleman and Bellinger, *Prenatal Exposure to Toxicants*, pp. 112–29.

121 Coal plants and mercury: J. Coequyt et al., *Mercury Falling: An Analysis of Mercury Pollution from Coal-Burning Power Plants* (Washington, D.C.: Environmental Working Group, 1999).

121 Illinois is fifth biggest mercury polluter: The top four states are Pennsylvania, Texas, Ohio, and Indiana (J. Coequyt, *Mercury Falling*, p. 12).

121 The plant in my hometown: National Wildlife Federation, *Clean the Rain, Clean the Lakes: Mercury in Rain Is Polluting the Great Lakes* (Ann Arbor: National Wildlife Federation, 1999); S. Richardson, "Pekin Plant Illinois's No. 3 Mercury Polluter," *Pantagraph*, 15 Sept. 1999.

121 EPA to reduce power-plant emissions of mercury: Environmental Protection Agency, "Regulatory Finding on the Emissions of Hazardous Air Pollutants from Electric Steam Generating Units," *Federal Register* 65, 20 Dec. 2000, pp. 79825-31. See also www.epa.gov/mercury.

121–122 Consumer products and industrial operations that use mercury: AAP, *Handbook of Pediatric Environmental Health*, pp. 145–54; M. T. Bender and J. M. Williams, "A Real Plan of Action on Mercury," *Public Health Reports* 114(1999):416–20; EPA, *Mercury Study Report to Congress*, vol. 1, executive summary (Washington, D.C.: U.S. Environmental Protection Agency, 1997); Weiss, "Developmental Neurotoxicity of Methyl Mercury"; B. Weiss et al., "Human Exposures to Inorganic Mercury," *Public Health Reports* 114(1999):400–401. Wastewater from U.S. households also contributes to the mercury contamination of rivers, harbors, and bays. A 2000 study found that 80 percent of the mercury arriving at U.S. sewage treatment plants from domestic sources comes from human feces and urine. Leaching amalgam fillings are believed to be the source of mercury in human excrement (Association of Metropolitan Sewerage Agencies, Mercury Working Group, *Evaluation of Domestic Sources of Mercury* [Washington D.C.: AMSA, 2000]).

122 Chlorine industry as largest consumer of mercury: As of 1994, 14 percent of the chlorine gas produced in North America was generated through the use of mercury cells. In 1995, mercury emissions from the U.S. chlor-alkali industry totaled seven tons (R. Ayres, "The Life of Chlorine, Part I: Chlorine Production and the Chlorine-Mercury Connection," *Journal of Industrial Ecology* 1[1997]:81-94). As of 1999, 12 mercury-cell chlor-alkali plants remained in the United States (Dr. Edward Swain, Minnesota Pollution Control Agency, personal communication). For a detailed discussion on the use of mercury to make chlorine, see J. Thornton, *Pandora's Poison: Chlorine, Health, and a New Environmental Strategy* (Cambridge: MIT Press, 2000), pp. 238-45.

122 Crematoria and mercury: S. R. Maloney, "Mercury in the Hair of Crematoria Workers," *Lancet* 352(1998):1602; A. Mills, "Mercury and Crematorium Chimneys," *Nature* 346(1990):615. For a reanalysis of Mills's data, see V. J. Burton, "Too Much Mercury," *Nature* 351(1991):704.

122 Mechanism by which mercury addles the fetal brain: M. Baldini and P. Stacchini, *Mercury in Food* (Strassbourg, France: Council of European Publications, 1995), pp. 7–9; M. Kunimoto and T. Suzuki, "Migration of Granule Neurons in Cerebellar Organotypic Cultures Is Impaired by Methylmercury," *Neuroscience Letters* 226(1997):183–86; Schettler et al., *Generations at Risk*, p. 60.

122 Mercury pumped across the placenta: In Greenland, blood methylmercury concentrations in newborns were 40 percent higher than in mothers; in Sweden, methylmercury in umbilical cord blood was 47 percent higher than in maternal blood (A. Foldspang and J. C. Hansen, "Dietary Intake of Methylmercury as a Correlate of Gestational Length and Birth Weight Among Newborns in Greenland," *Am. J. of Epidemiology* 132(1990):310–17; H. E. Ratcliffe et al., "Human Exposure to Mercury: A Critical Assessment of the Evidence for Adverse Health Effects," *J. of Toxicology and Environmental Health* 49(1996):221–70.

122 Fish the most significant route of exposure: EPA, *Mercury Study Report to Congress*; A. D. Kyle, *Contaminated Catch: The Public Threat from Toxics in Fish* (New York: Natural Resources Defense Council, 1998).

123 Faroe Islands: Faroe Islanders are descended from Norwegian settlers, who colonized the islands in A.D. 800. Since 1380 the islands have belonged to Denmark. Pilot whales are the source of most meat consumption among the islands' inhabitants, and cod is the major fish species consumed (Arctic Monitoring and Assessment Programs, Arctic Pollution Issues: A State of the Arctic Report [Oslo, Norway: AMAP, 1997], p. 61).

123–124 Faroe Islands study: P. Grandjean et al., "Cognitive Deficit in 7-Year-Old Children with Prenatal Exposure to Methylmercury," *Neurotoxicology and Teratology* 19(1997):417–28; D. MacKenzie, "Arrested Development: Official Safety Limits on Mercury Are Too High to Prevent Damage Before Birth," *New Scientist*, 22 Nov. 1997, p. 4; D. MacKenzie, "Mercury Alert," *New Scientist*, 12 June 1999, p. 12; K. R. Mahaffey, "Methylmercury: A New Look at the Risks," *Public Health Reports* 114(1999):396–413. Researchers were able to separate the effects of PCB exposure from mercury exposure because these two contaminants are found in different parts of the whale. Mercury concentrates in the muscle tissue, whereas chlorinated contaminants, such as PCBs, are primarily found in the blubber. Some human subjects in this investigation ate only pilot whale meat and not the blubber (U. Steurwald et al., "Maternal Seafood Diet, Methylmercury Exposure, and Neonatal Neurologic Function," *J. of Pediatrics* 136(2000):599–605).

124 Seychelles study: P. W. Davidson et al., "Effects of Prenatal and Postnatal Methylmercury Exposure from Fish Consumption on Neurodevelopmental Outcomes at 66 Months of Age in the Seychelles Child Development Study," *JAMA* 280(1998):701–7.

124 Iraqi poisoning: In the winter of 1971–72, wheat treated with mercurial fungicides was distributed to farmers in Iraq who had experienced a severe drought the previous season. However, rather than saving the grain for planting, many families ground and baked it into bread. The results were disastrous. More than 6,500 people contracted mercury poisoning, and thousands died. In a terrible replay of Minamata disease, babies born to mothers who had eaten the tainted bread while pregnant suffered from seizures, severe mental retardation, and cerebral palsy—in short, they had contracted congenital Minamata disease (Weiss, "Developmental Neurotoxicity of Methylmercury"). More recently, Minamata disease was discovered among villagers in remote Amazonian rainforests. The source is clearly fish consumption but the underlying cause of the fish contamination is not evident. It is probably a combination of upstream mining operations, which use mercury to extract gold from ore, and deforestation, which releases naturally occurring mercury into the soil (F. Pearce, "A Nightmare Revisited," *New Scientist*, 6 Feb. 1999, p. 4).

124–125 Madeira study: K. Murata et al., "Delayed Evoked Potentials in Children Exposed to Methylmercury from Seafood," *Neurotoxicology and Teratology* 21(1999):343–48.

125 Institute of Medicine warning on swordfish: Institute of Medicine, *Seafood Safety* (Washington, D.C.: National Academy Press, 1991). The I.O.M. is a private, nonprofit organization that provides health policy advice under a congressional charter granted to the National Academy of Sciences.

125 Washington State tuna advisory: Washington State Department of Public Health, "State Issues Fish Consumption Advisory: Too Much Mercury," press release, 12 Apr. 2001. See also www.doh.wa.gov/fish. For other state advisories, see www.mercurypolicy.org.

125 Report that goes further: J. Houlihan et al., *Brain Food: What Women Should Know About Mercury Contamination of Fish* (Washington, D.C.: Environmental Working Group and U.S. Public Interest Research Group, 2001).

125 National Academy of Sciences study: National Research Council, *Toxicological Effects of Methylmercury* (Washington, D.C.: National Academy Press, 2000), pp. 7, 276.

125–126 CDC study: More specifically, 10 percent of those tested had mercury levels within one tenth of the established benchmark dose, at or above which exposure damages fetal brain development (Centers for Disease Control, "Blood and Hair Mercury Levels in Young Children and Women of Childbearing Age—United States, 1999," *Morbidity and Mortality Weekly Report* 50[2001]:140-43).

126–127 History of mercury regulation: M. Bender and J. Williams, *The One That Got Away: FDA Fails to Protect the Public from High Mercury levels in Seafood* (Montpelier, Vt.: Mercury Policy Project and California Communities Against Toxics, 2000); Bender and Williams, "Real Plan of Action"; Mahaffey, "Methylmercury."

127 Study by *Consumer Reports*: "America's Fish: Fair or Foul?" *Consumer Reports* 66 (Feb. 2001): 24-31.

127 Criticisms by the GAO: United States General Accounting Office, *Federal Oversight of Seafood Does Not Sufficiently Protect Consumers: Report to the Committee on Agriculture, Nutrition, and Forestry, U.S. Senate* (Washington D.C.: U.S. General Accounting Agency, 2001).

127 Plan by the Mercury Policy Project: Bender and Williams, "Real Plan of Action."

127 Substitutes for mercury-containing products: At this writing, the cities of Boston; San Francisco; Duluth, Minnesota; Ann Arbor, Michigan; and DeForest and Stoughton, Wisconsin, have all banned the sale of mercury fever thermometers. In addition, the state of New Hampshire has passed a law banning the sale of mercury thermometers as well as all games, toys, clothing, and ornaments that contain mercury (Mercury Policy Project; www.mercurypolicy.org).

127 Pollution control strategies for power plants: These include carbon injection, in which a stream of carbon is pumped into stack gases and attaches to mercury vapors; coal washing, in which the mercury is washed from the coal before it is burned; switching to fuels with lower mercury content (such as natural gas or oil); and conservation, which would reduce our reliance on coal as a fuel if the savings from reduced power were used to retire coal-fired plants (EPA, *Mercury Study Report to Congress*; National Wildlife Federation, *Clean the Rain*). Of course, capturing mercury from stack emissions and washing the mercury out of the coal before burning still generates mercury-laden waste that requires eternal containment. Far better is to end our reliance on coal altogether.

128 FDA's guidelines on fish consumption: See www.fda.gov.

128 Forty states released 1,675 warnings: American Public Health Association, "Policy Statement Adopted by the Governing Council of the American Public Health Association, 9910: Preventing Human Methylmercury Exposure to Protect Public Health," 10 Nov. 1999 (www.apha.org).

128 Differences between Illinois and Indiana fish advisories: Richardson, "Pekin Plant Illinois No. 3 Mercury Polluter."

128 Long Island Sound: Dr. Christopher Perkins, Environmental Research Institute, University of Connecticut, personal communication.

129 Health benefits of fish: G. M. Egeland and J. P. Middaugh, "Balancing Fish Consumption Benefits with Mercury Exposures," *Science* 278(1997):1904-5.

129 Health of indigenous women suffers: American Public Health Association, "Policy Statement"; Egeland and Middaugh, "Balancing Fish Consumption."

129 Fatty acids in fish contribute to fetal brain growth: Egeland and Middaugh, "Balancing Fish Consumption."

131 International Joint Commission: International Joint Commission, Tenth Biennial Report on Great Lakes Water Quality (Ottawa, Ont.: IJC, 2000). The IJC oversees the implementation of the Great Lakes Water Quality Agreement of 1978, signed by the United States and Canada.

CHAPTER SEVEN: HAY MOON

135 Toxic sites in Alaska: Research conducted by Alaska Community Action on Toxics (www.akaction.net).

136–140 Properties of POPs: J. Thornton, *Pandora's Poison: Chlorine, Health, and a New Environmental Strategy* (Cambridge: MIT Press, 2000), pp. 4, 31–39, 203–32.

137 No government alone can control POPs: B. E. Fisher, "Most Unwanted: Persistent Organic Pollutants," *EHP* 107(1999):A18–23.

138 Nontoxic alternatives to POPs: Ibid.; World Wildlife Fund, *Successful, Safe, and Sustainable Alternatives to Persistent Organic Pollutants* (Washington, D.C.: WWF, Sept. 1999). Phasing out

DDT is the most challenging task of POPs elimination efforts, since DDT still plays a role in controlling malaria in many developing countries. Alternatives to DDT include window screens, pesticide-impregnated bed nets, and vigilant campaigns to eliminate mosquito breeding grounds. Only two nations, India and China, still manufacture DDT. See Afterword (pp. 284–287) for an update on POPs treaty negotiations.

138 Former Air Force site: State of Alaska Division of Public Health, *Health Consultation Interim Report: Former Umiat Air Force Station, Umiat Alaska* (Anchorage: State of Alaska Division of Public Health, Section of Epidemiology, Feb. 2000).

138 DEW line sites: Arctic Monitoring and Assessment Programme, *Arctic Pollution Issues: A State of the Arctic Environment Report* (Oslo: Arctic Monitoring and Assessment Programme, 1997), p. 77

138–139 Salmon as a vector for POPs contamination: G. Ewald et al., "Biotransport of Organic Pollutants to an Inland Alaskan Lake by Migrating Sockeye Salmon (*Onchorynchus nerka*)," *Arctic* 51(1998):40–47.

139 Reproductive problems among northern wildlife: Arctic Monitoring and Assessment Programme, *Arctic Pollution Issues*, pp. 73–74; P. D. Jepson et al., "Investigating Potential Associations between Chronic Exposures to Polychlorinated Biphenyls and Infectious Disease Mortality in Harbour Porpoises from England and Wales," *Science of the Total Environment* 243–44(1999): 339–48; O. Wiig et al., "Female Pseudohermaphrodite Polar Bears at Svalbard," *J. of Wildlife Diseases* 34(1998):792–96.

139–140 Orca whales in the Kenai: D. O'Harra, "High Toxin Levels Found in Alaska Killer Whales," *Anchorage Daily News*, 5 June 1999, p. A1; C. O. Matkin et al., *Comprehensive Killer Whale Investigation*, Exxon Valdez *Oil Spill Restoration Project Annual Report* (Homer, Alaska: North Gulf Oceanic Society, Restoration Project 98012, April 1999). Also called killer whales, black and white orcas are really large dolphins. High PCB levels have also been discovered in orca whales living in the coastal waters of British Columbia (P. S. Ross et al., "High PCB Concentrations in Free-Ranging Pacific Killer Whales, *Orcinus orca*: Effects of Age, Sex, and Dietary Preference," *Marine Pollution Bulletin* 40[2000]:504–15).

140 Sea otters on the Aleutian Islands: S. L. L. Reese, "Levels of Organochlorine Contamination in Blue Mussels, *Mytilus trossulus*, from the Aleutian Archipelago," master's thesis, University of California–Santa Cruz, 1998.

140 POPs and Arctic people: P. Bjerregaard and J. C. Hansen, "Organochlorines and Heavy Metals in Pregnant Women from the Disko Bay Area in Greenland," *Science of the Total Environment* 245(2000):195–202; J. C. Hansen, "Environmental Contaminants and Human Health in the Arctic," *Toxicology Letters* 112–13(2000):119–25; J. Van Oostdam et al., "Human Health Implications of Environmental Contaminants in Arctic Canada: A Review," *Science of the Total Environment* 230(1999):1–82.

140 Why POPs accumulate in the Arctic: Arctic Monitoring and Assessment Programme, *Arctic Pollution Issues*, pp. 71–91.

143–144 History and properties of PCBs: Committee on Environmental Health, AAP, *Handbook of Pediatric Environmental Health* (Elk Grove Village, Ill.: AAP, 1999), pp. 215–22.

143 Fish pose highest exposures to PCBs: AAP, *Handbook on Pediatric Environmental Health*, p. 216.

143 No known method of detoxification: Ibid., p. 220.

144 Cooking oil incidents in Japan and Taiwan: S. T. Hsu et al., "Discovery and Epidemiology of PCB Poisoning in Taiwan: A Four-Year Follow-up," *EHP* 59(1985):5–10; W. J. Rogan et al., "Congenital Poisoning by Polychlorinated Biphenyls and Their Contaminants in Taiwan," *Science* 241(1988):334–36; F. Yamashita and M. Hayashi, "Fetal PCB Syndrome: Clinical Features, Intrauterine Growth Retardation and Possible Alteration in Calcium Metabolism," *EHP* 59(1985):41–45. Taiwanese children exposed in utero also suffered a higher incidence of middle-ear diseases than nonexposed controls, suggesting PCB-mediated suppression of the immune system (W. Y. Chao et al., "Middle-Ear Disease in Children Exposed Prenatally to Polychlorinated Biphenyls and Polychlorinated Dibenzofurans," *Archives of Environmental Health* 52[1997]:257–62).

144 Quantity of PCBs in use and in dumps exceeds amount in environment: P. de Voogt and U. A. T. Brinkman, "Production, Properties, and Usage of Polychlorinated Biphenyls," in

R. D. Kimbrough and A. A. Jensen, eds., *Halogenated Biphenyls, Terphenyls, and Naphthalenes, Dibenzodioxins and Related Products*, 2nd ed. (Amsterdam: Elsevier, 1989), pp. 3–46.

144–146 Human studies showing adverse effects of PCBs on fetal brain development: For an good overview, see National Research Council, *Hormonally Active Agents in the Environment* (Washington, D.C.: National Academy Press, 1999), pp. 134–35 and 172–85.

144 North Carolina study: B. C. Gladen et al., "Development After Exposure to Polychlorinated Biphenyls and Dichlorodiphenyl Dichloroethene Transplacentally and Through Human Milk," *J. of Pediatrics* 113(1988):991–95; J. L. Jacobson and S. W. Jacobson, "Dose-Response in Perinatal Exposure to Polychlorinated Biphenyls (PCBs): The Michigan and North Carolina Cohort Studies," *Toxicology and Industrial Health* 12(1996):435–45; W. J. Rogan et al., "Neonatal Effects of Transplacental Exposure to PCBs and DDE," *J. of Pediatrics* 109(1986):335–41.

144–145 Michigan study: J. L. Jacobson and S. W. Jacobson, "Evidence for PCBs as Neurodevelopmental Toxicants in Humans," *NEJM* 335(1996):283–89.

145 Oswego study: E. Lonky et al., "Neonatal Behavioral Assessment Scale Performance in Humans Influenced by Maternal Consumption of Environmentally Contaminated Lake Ontario Fish, *J. of Great Lakes Research* 22(1996):198–212; P. Stewart et al., "Prenatal PCB Exposure and Neonatal Behavioral Assessment Scale (NBAS) Performance, *Neurotoxicology and Teratology* 22(2000):21–29.

145–146 Quote from Dutch study: C. I. Lanting and S. Patandin, "Exposure to PCBs and Dioxins: Adverse Effects and Implications for Child Development," in S. Gabizon et al., eds., *Women and POPs: Women's View and Role Regarding the Elimination of POPs— Report on the Activities of IPEN's Women's Group During the IPEN Conference and the INC3, Geneva, September 4–11, 1999* (Utrecht: Women in Europe for a Common Future, 1999), p. 11. This study is described in more detail in Chapter 12.

148 Concept of motherselfhood: K. A. Rabuzzi, *Motherself: A Mythic Analysis of Motherhood* (Bloomington, Ind.: Indiana University Press, 1988).

148 1888 discovery of cretinism: J. H. Oppenheimer and H. L. Schwartz, "Molecular Basis of Thyroid Hormone-Dependent Brain Development," *Endocrine Reviews* 18(1997):462–75;

148–149 Thyroid gland and fetal brain development: D. A. Fisher, "The Importance of Early Management in Optimizing IQ in Infants with Congenital Hypothyroidism," *J. of Pediatrics* 136(2000):273–74; J. E. Haddow et al., "Maternal Thyroid Deficiency During Pregnancy and Subsequent Neuropsychological Development of the Child," *NEJM* 341 (1999):549–55; Oppenheimer and Schwartz, "Molecular Basis of Thyroid Hormone-Dependent Brain Development"; V. J. Pop et al., "Should All Pregnant Women Be Screened for Hypothyroidism?" *Lancet* 354(1999):1224–25.

149 PCBs' effect on thyroid hormones: AAP, *Handbook of Pediatric Environmental Health*, p. 84; R. Bigsby et al., "Evaluating the Effects of Endocrine Disruptors on Endocrine Function During Development," *EHP* 107(1999, sup. 4):613–18.

149–150 Nonstress test: C. Marshall, *From Here to Maternity: A Complete Pregnancy Guide* (Minden, N.Y.: Conmar Publishing, 1994); M. R. Primeau, "Nonstress Test," in B. K. Rothman, ed., *Encyclopedia of Childbearing: Critical Perspectives* (Phoenix: Oryx Press, 1993), pp. 283–84.

151 Loss of movements during fetal compromise: M. R. Primeau, "Fetal Movement," in Rothman, *Encyclopedia of Childbearing*, pp. 283–84.

CHAPTER EIGHT: GREEN CORN MOON

157–160 Events of childbirth: M. D. Benson, *Birth Day! The Last 24 Hours of Pregnancy* (New York: Paragon House, 1993).

162 Books on natural childbirth: The ones I consulted include S. Arms, *Immaculate Deception: A New Look at Women and Childbirth in America* (New York: Bantam Books, 1975); R. B. Dancy, *Special Delivery: A Guide to Creating the Birth You Want for You and Your Baby* (Berkeley, Calif.: Celestial Arts, 1986); R. E. Davis-Floyd, *Birth as an American Rite of Passage* (Berkeley, Calif.: University of California Press, 1992); P. S. Eakins, ed., *The American Way of Birth* (Philadelphia: Temple University Press, 1986); M. Edwards and M. Waldorf, *Reclaiming Birth: History and Heroines of American Childbirth Reform* (Trumansburg, N.Y.: Crossing Press, 1984); I. M. Gaskin, *Spiritual Midwifery* (Summertown, Tenn.: Book Publishing Co., 1980); M. Odent, *Birth Reborn* (New York: Pantheon,

1984); A. Oakley, *The Captured Womb: A History of the Medical Care of Pregnant Women* (Oxford, U.K.: Basil Blackwell, 1984); B. K. Rothman, *In Labor: Women and Power in the Birthplace* (N.Y.: W. W. Norton, 1991).

162 Cascade of interventions: R. Davis-Floyd, "Hospital Birth: An Anthropological Analysis of Ritual and Practice," in Rothman, *Encyclopedia of Childbearing*, p. 179; I. D. Graham, *Episiotomy: Challenging Obstetric Interventions* (Oxford, U.K.: Blackwell Science, 1997), pp. 51–52.

162 Complications created by obstetrical anesthetics: J. L. Hawkins et al., "A Reevaluation of the Association between Instrument Delivery and Epidural Analgesia," *Regional Anesthesia* 20(1995):50–56; P. Simkin, "Epidural Update," *Birth Gazette* 15(1999):12–16.

162–163 Continuous ultrasound monitoring does not improve outcome: C. Whitbeck, "Image Techniques," in Rothman, *Encyclopedia of Childbearing*, pp. 184–85.

163 Studies showing problems with episiotomies: R. F. Harrison et al., "Is Routine Episiotomy Necessary?" *British Medical Journal* 288(1984):1971–75; M. C. Klein et al., "Relationship of Episiotomy to Perineal Trauma and Morbidity, Sexual Disfunction, and Pelvic Floor Relaxation," *Am. J. of Obstetrics and Gynecology* 171(1994):591–98; P. Shiono et al., "Midline Episiotomies: More Harm Than Good?" *Obstetrics and Gynecology* 75(1990):765–70. See also note for pages *216–17 under the key phrase "harm created by episiotomies."

163 Study showing record of midwives: M. F. MacDorman and G. K. Singh, "Midwifery Care, Social and Medical Risk Factors, and Birth Outcomes in the U.S.A.," *J. of Epidemiology and Community Health* 52(1998):310–17.

163 Natural birth less popular: The percentage of women receiving epidural anesthesia during childbirth tripled between 1981 and 1997 (C. J. Chivers, "Devotees of No-Drug Childbirth Frustrated by Rise in Use of Anesthesia," *New York Times*, 18 Oct. 1999, B1).

163 Quote from *NYT* letter: R. LaPorta, "Should Pain Be Part of Childbirth?" letter, *New York Times*, 15 Oct. 1999, p. A34.

163 "There is no other condition. . . .": J. Hawkins, quoted in J. Ritter, "Laboring Women Opt for Pain Relief," *Chicago Sun-Times*, 13 Oct. 1999, p. A1.

163 Nonpharmaceutical methods of pain relief: M. H. Klaus et al., *Bonding: Building the Foundations of Secure Attachment and Independence* (Reading, Mass.: Addison-Wesley, 1995), pp. 23–42; ibid., *Mothering the Mother: How a Doula Can Help You Have a Shorter, Easier, and Healthier Birth* (Reading, Mass.: Addison-Wesley, 1993), pp. 23–42; A. B. Lieberman, "Pain Relief in Labor: Nondrug Methods," in Rothman, *Encyclopedia of Childbirth*, pp. 297–99.

164 1996 investigation: U. Waldenstrom et al., "The Complexity of Labor Pain: Experiences of 278 Women," *J. of Psychosomatic Obstetrics and Gynecology* 17(1996):215–28.

165 One elated columnist: M. Eagan, "Drugs Limiting Childbirth Pain Can Be Every Mother's Gain," *Boston Herald*, 14 Oct. 1999, p. 14.

165 Photos showing undrugged women: Odent, *Birth Reborn.*

165–166 Culture of the hospital: Simkin, "Epidural Update."

166 One former obstetrical nurse: J. Van Olphen-Fehr, *Diary of a Midwife: The Power of Positive Childbearing* (Westport, Conn.: Bergin & Garvey, 1998).

166 Not routinely trained in alternative methods: W. L. Larimore, "Family Centered Birthing: A Style of Obstetrics for Family Physicians," *American Family Physician* 48(1993): 725–28.

166 "Hospital settings brimming with technocrats:" Larimore, "Family Centered Birthing."

166 Laboring woman's self-confidence undermined: B. K. Rothman, *In Labor: Women and Power in the Birthplace* (New York: W. W. Norton, 1991). See also Dancy, *Special Delivery.*

166 "A woman cannot view herself as healthy. . . ": Rothman, *In Labor*, p. 15–16.

166–167 Lasting legacy of natural childbirth: Larimore, "Family Centered Birthing."

167 Data on home births: L. Remez, "Planned Home Birth Can Be as Safe as Hospital Delivery for Women with Low-Risk Pregnancies," *Family Planning Perspectives* 29(1997):141–43.

169–171 Obstetricians' view of history: D. Caton, *What a Blessing She Had Chloroform: The Medical and Social Response to the Pain of Childbirth from 1800 to the Present* (New Haven: Yale University Press, 1999); L. D. Longo, "A Millennium of Obstetrics and Gynaecology," *Lancet* 354(1999):S39.

169 Quote by obstetrical anesthesiologist: Caton, *What a Blessing*, pp. xi.
169 Life before obstetrics: J. Carter and T. Duriez, *With Child: Birth Through the Ages* (Edinburgh: Mainstream Publishing, 1988).
170 Rickets: Ibid., p. 34
170 Anesthesia: Caton, *What a Blessing*, pp. 21–37 and 58–69; Longo, "A Millennium of Obstetrics and Gynaecology."
170–171 James Marion Sims: Longo, "A Millennium of Obstetrics and Gynaecology"; D. K. McGregor, *From Midwives to Medicine: The Birth of American Gynecology* (New Brunswick, N.J.: Rutgers University Press, 1998), pp. 48–49.
171 Quote on hospitalization: N. J. Eastman and K. P. Russell, *Expectant Motherhood* (Boston: Little, Brown, 1970), p. 132.
171 Scopolamine: Caton, *What a Blessing*; J. P. Rooks, *Midwifery and Childbirth in America* (Philadelphia: Temple University Press, 1997), p. 488.
171 Introduction of spinal anesthesia: Caton, *What a Blessing*, p. 168–69.
171 Romanticizing suffering in the name of naturalness: Caton provides a particularly thoughtful critique of natural childbirth (*What a Blessing*, pp. 228–34).
171–175 Midwives' version of history: Edwards and Waldorf, *Reclaiming Birth*; M. M. Lay, *The Rhetoric of Midwifery: Gender, Knowledge, and Power* (New Brunswick, N.J.: Rutgers University Press, 2000); McGregor, *From Midwives to Medicine*; Van Olphen-Fehr, *Diary of a Midwife*.
171 Doctors thought childbirth beneath them: Rooks, *Midwifery and Childbirth in America*, p. 12.
171–172 Inquisition: Edwards and Waldorf, *Reclaiming Birth*, pp. 146–47; Rooks, *Midwifery and Childbirth in America*, p. 13
172 English midwives tightly regulated by mid-sixteenth century: McGregor, *From Midwives to Medicine*, p. 39.
172 Female midwives barred: Lay, *Rhetoric of Midwifery*, p. 53.
172 U.S. Doctors waged campaigns: A. J. Slomski, "CNMs: 'We Don't Just Catch Babies,' " *Medical Economics* 77(2000):186–89; R. Weitz, "Midwife Licensing," in Rothman, *Encyclopedia of Childbirth*, pp. 245–47.
172 Midwives had lower rates of childbed fever: McGregor, *From Midwives to Medicine*, p. 117.
172 Two famous frontier midwives: Ibid., p. 37.
172 Harm caused by forceps: Ibid., pp. 33–35; 41.
172 Sims and slavery: Ibid., p. 29.   .
172–173 Women reformers threatened to go to the press: Ibid., p. 188–89.
173 Shortage of civilian doctors during World War II: Dancy, *Special Delivery*, p. 2.
173 Ability to breastfeed compromised: Graham, *Episiotomy*, p. 51–52.
173 Ire for Joseph DeLee: See Rothman, *In Labor*, pp. 57–59.
173 DeLee's 1920 paper: J. B. DeLee, "The Prophylactic Forceps Operation," *Am. J. of Obstetrics and Gynecology* 1(1920):33–44.
173–174 Claims made for episiotomies: Edwards and Waldorf, *Reclaiming Birth*, pp. 142–43; Graham, *Episiotomy*, p. 38.
174 Harm created by episiotomies: P. G. Larsson et al., "Advantage or Disadvantage of Episiotomy Compared with Spontaneous Perineal Laceration," *Gynecologic and Obstetric Investigation* 31(1991):213–16; L. B. Signorello et al., "Midline Episiotomy and Anal Incontinence: Retrospective Cohort Study," *British Medical Journal* 320(2000):86–90. See also note for page 163 under key phrase "studies showing problems with episiotomies."
174 Midwifery techniques to avoid tearing: Dancy, *Special Delivery*, pp. 65–66.
174 Quote by Ian Graham: Graham, *Episiotomy*, p. 145.
174–175 Backlash: R. Bradley, *Husband-Coached Childbirth* (New York: Harper & Row, 1974); G. Dick-Read, *Childbirth Without Fear: The Principles and Practices of Natural Childbirth* (New York: Harper & Row, 1959); R. Lamaze, *Painless Childbirth: The Lamaze Method* (New York: Pocket Books, 1972); M. Thomas, *Post-War Mothers: Childbirth Letters of Grantly Dick-Read, 1946–56* (Westport, Conn.: Bergin & Garvey, 1998).

CHAPTER NINE: HARVEST MOON

178 Polar bears: J. U. Skaare, "POP Contamination in the Norwegian Arctic; Possible Effects of High-Level PCB Contamination in Top Predators," presentation on polar bear reproduction at the Atlantic Coast Contaminants Workshop, 2000, Jackson Laboratory, Bar Harbor, Maine, 23 June 2000.

178 Shift in birth peak for humans: T. Miura, "Recent Changes in the Seasonality of Birth," and ibid., "Secular Changes in the Seasonality of Birth," in T. Miura, ed., *Seasonality of Birth* (The Hague: SPB Academic Publishing, 1987), pp. 25–31, 33–44.

178–179 Quote on cause of labor's onset: S. H. Lewis and E. Gilbert-Barnes, "Placental Membranes," in S. H. Lewis and E. Perrin, eds., *Pathology of the Placenta*, 2nd ed. (New York: Churchill Livingston, 1999), pp. 138.

179 Initiating agent once thought to be oxytocin: G. C. Liggens, "The Placenta and Control of Parturition," in C. W. G. Redman et al., eds., *The Human Placenta: A Guide for Clinicians and Scientists* (Oxford, U.K.: Blackwell, 1993), pp. 273–90.

179 Mothers of lambs with hypothalamic defects never go into labor: P. W. Nathanielsz, *Life Before Birth: The Challenge of Fetal Development* (New York: W. H. Freeman, 1996), pp. 162–81.

179 In sheep, the fetus initiates labor: R. Smith, "The Timing of Birth," *Scientific American* 280(March 1999):68–75.

179 Anencephalic infants usually overdue: Nathanielsz, *Life Before Birth*, p. 167.

179–180 Research by Smith and McClean: Smith, "Timing of Birth."

180 Role of estrogen, progesterone, and uterine muscle fibers: Smith, "Timing of Birth."

180 Role of prostaglandins: Liggens, "Placenta and Control of Parturition."

180 Role of baby's head: Nathanielsz, *Life Before Birth*, p. 185.

181 Causes of premature labor unknown: P. Nathanielsz, *Life in the Womb: The Origin of Health and Disease* (Ithaca, N.Y.: Promethean Press, 1999), pp. 226, 230–54.

181 Prematurity a leading killer: One in every ten human births is premature (less than thirty-seven weeks' gestation); 75 percent of newborn deaths not caused by malformations are caused by prematurity (Nathanielsz, *Life Before Birth*, pp. 226, 231.) Prematurity can also affect mental development. Elementary school children born at or before 28 weeks' gestation are three times more likely to repeat grades or require special education placement (G. M. Buck et al., "Extreme Prematurity and School Outcomes," *Paediatric and Perinatal Epidemiology* 4(2000):324–31.

182 Rate of prematurity rising: Between 1989 and 1997, moderately preterm births (32–36 weeks' gestation) rose 14 percent among singletons; very preterm births (less than 32 weeks' gestation) showed no change (Pew Environmental Health Commission, *Healthy From the Start: Why America Needs a Better System to Track and Understand Birth Defects and the Environment* [Baltimore: Johns Hopkins School of Public Health, 2000], p. 55).

182 Two thirds of cases remain unexplained: Nathanielsz, *Life Before Birth*, p. 208.

182 Experiments in the 1970s: Z. W. Polishuk et al., "Organochlorine Compounds in Mother and Fetus During Labor," *Environmental Research* 13(1977):278–84.

182 Women exposed occupationally to PCBs have elevated rates of preterm birth: National Research Council, *Hormonally Active Agents in the Environment* (Washington D.C.: National Academy Press, 1999), p. 134.

182 PCBs trigger uterine contractions in strips of isolated rat tissue: J. Bae et al., "Stimulation of Pregnant Rat Uterine Contraction by the Polychlorinated Biphenyl (PCB) Mixture Arochlor 1242 May Be Mediated by Arachidonic Acid Release through Activation of Phospholipase A_2 Enzymes," *J. of Pharmacology and Experimental Therapeutics* 289(1999):1112–20.

182 Quote from recent NAS report: National Research Council, *Hormonally Active Agents in the Environment*, p. 3–4.

182 Experiments at University of Michigan: J. Bae, "Stimulation of Oscillatory Uterine Contraction by the PCB Mixture Arochlor 1242 May Involve Increased $[Ca^{2+}]_i$ through Voltage-Operated Calcium Channels," *Toxicology and Applied Pharmacology* 155(1999):261–72.

183 Incidence of low birth weight is rising: Between 1989 and 1997, low birth weight increased by 4 percent among singletons; very low birth weight increased 7 percent (Pew Environmental Health Commission, *Healthy from the Start*, pp. 55–56).

183 Health risks of low birth weight: Nathanielsz, *Life in the Womb: The Origin of Health and Disease*, pp. 56–74, 110–17, 137–63.

183 Incidence of low birth weight rising among low-risk mothers: Between 1990 and 1997, low birth weight among singleton babies born to 20- to 34-year-old mothers rose 2.2 percent; incidence of very low birth weight increased by 5.9 percent (Pew Environmental Health Commission, *Healthy from the Start*, p. 56).

183 Low birth weight associated with alcohol, smoking, and drugs: N. L. Day et al., "Effect of Prenatal Alcohol Exposure on Growth and Morphology of Offspring at 8 Months of Age," *Pediatrics* 85(1990):748–52; X. O. Shu et al., "Maternal Smoking, Alcohol Drinking, Caffeine Consumption, and Fetal Growth: Results from a Prospective Study," *Epidemiology* 6(1995): 115–20. (No relation was shown between caffeine consumption and fetal growth.)

183 German study found link to wood preservatives: W. Karmaus and N. Wolf, "Reduced Birthweight and Length in the Offspring of Females Exposed to PCDFs, PCP, and Lindane," *EHP* 103(1995):1120–25.

183–184 Several studies found a link to drinking water contamination: Colorado—M. D. Gallagher et al., "Exposure to Trihalomethanes and Adverse Pregnancy Outcomes," *Epidemiology* 9(1998):484–89; Iowa—National Research Council, *Hormonally Active Agents in the Environment*, p. 139; New Jersey—F. J. Bove et al., "Public Drinking Water Contamination and Birth Outcomes," *Am. J. of Epidemiology* 141(1995):850–62; North Carolina—Agency for Toxic Substances and Disease Registry (ATSDR), *FY 1998 Agency Profile and Annual Report*, p. iv, 26–27.

184–185 Link to toxic waste sites: ATSDR, *FY 1998 Agency Profile and Annual Report*, p. iv; M. Berry and F. Bove, "Birth Weight Reduction Associated with Residence Near a Hazardous Waste Landfill," *EHP* 105(1997):856–61; N. J. Vianna and A. K. Polan, "Incidence of Low Birth Weight Among Love Canal Residents," *Science* 226(1984):1217–19.

185 Beijing study on air pollution: X. Wang et al., "Association Between Air Pollution and Low Birth Weight: A Community-Based Study," *EHP* 105(1997):514–20.

185 L.A. study on air pollution: B. Ritz and F. Yu, "The Effect of Ambient Carbon Monoxide on Low Birth Weight Among Children Born in Southern California between 1989 and 1993," *EHP* 107(1999):17–25. Air pollution also contributes to preterm birth in Southern California (B. Ritz et al., "Effect of Air Pollution of Preterm Birth Among Children Born in Southern California between 1989 and 1993," *Epidemiology* 11[2000]:502–11.)

185 Black Triangle: So called because it is one of the largest sources of air pollution in all of Europe, caused both by a concentration of heavy industry and the burning of brown coal (R. J. S[breve]ram, "Impact of Air Pollution on Reproductive Health," *EHP* 107[1999]:A542–43).

185 Czech study: M. Bobak, "Outdoor Air Pollution, Low Birth Weight, and Prematurity," *EHP* 108(2000):173–76.

185 Study from northern Bohemia: J. Dejmek et al., "Fetal Growth and Maternal Exposure to Particulate Matter During Pregnancy," *EHP* 107(1999):475–80; J. Dejmek et al., "The Impact of Polycyclic Aromatic Hydrocarbons and Fine Particles on Pregnancy Outcome," *EHP* 108(2000): 1159–64.

186 Properties of PAHs: F. P. Perera et al., "Molecular Epidemiological Research on the Effects of Environmental Pollutants on the Fetus," *EHP* 107(1999 sup. 3):451–60.

186–187 Polish studies by Perera: Perera et al., "Molecular Epidemiological Research."

189 Interspecific differences in labor: W. R. Trevathan, *Human Birth: An Evolutionary Perspective* (Hawthorne, N.Y.: Aldine De Gruyter, 1987), pp. 72–78; 96–97.

189 Monkeys born face-up: This orientation allows the largest dimension of the fetal head—the back of the head—to press against the largest dimension of the mother's pelvis, the sacrum (W. R. Trevathan, "Evolution of Human Birth," in B. K. Rothman, *Encyclopedia of Childbearing: Critical Perspectives* [Phoenix: Oryx, 1993], pp. 131–33).

190 Attendance during childbirth in human history: Ibid.

190 Role of bipedalism in making labor difficult: Ibid.

190–191 Adaptations that allow humans to cope: M. M. Abitbol, *Birth and Human Evolution: Anatomical and Obstetrical Mechanics in Primates* (Westport, Conn.: Bergin & Garvey, 1996), p. 19.

197–198 Baby's rotation in the birth canal: Trevathan, *Human Birth*, pp. 23–25.

199 Consenting to an episiotomy: I continued to suffer from sexual discomfort and urinary and fecal incontinence for six months. Two years later, I still struggle with urinary incontinence and loss of sexual sensation. That I agreed to this procedure at all, knowing all that I knew about its risks, is, I think, a testimony to great vulnerability of laboring women and the extraordinary power of suggestion during childbirth. Were I to do it all again, I would seek out a very different kind of birthplace.

PART II

202 There was a child went forth: Readers who would like to read the whole poem will find it in Walt Whitman, *Complete Poetry and Collected Prose* (New York: Penguin Books, 1982), pp. 491–93.

CHAPTER TEN: MAMMA

204 Internal anatomy of the breast: K. G. Auerbach, "Nipples, Human," in B. K. Rothman, ed., *Encyclopedia of Childbearing: Critical Perspectives* (Phoenix: Oryx Press, 1993), pp. 281–83; M. Neville, "Physiology of Lactation," *Clinics in Perinatology* 26 (1999):251–79; M. Wolff, "Lactation," in M. Paul, ed., *Occupational and Reproductive Hazards: A Guide for Clinicians* (Baltimore: Lippincott, Williams & Wilkens, 1993), pp. 60–75.

204 Plenty of women have failed at nursing: E. A. Kaplan, *Motherhood and Representation: The Mother in Popular Culture and Melodrama* (New York: Routledge, 1992), p. 55–56; S. G. McMillen, *Motherhood in the Old South: Pregnancy, Childbirth, and Infant Rearing* (Baton Rouge, La.: Louisiana State University Press, 1990); M. Yalom, *A History of the Breast* (New York: Knopf, 1997), p. 109.

204 Apes in zoos unable to nurse: Ibid., p. 109.

204–205 La Leche League: L. M. Blum, *At the Breast: Ideologies of Breastfeeding and Motherhood in the Contemporary United States* (Boston: Beacon Press, 1999), p. 70; J. D. Ward, *La Leche League: At the Crossroads of Medicine, Feminism, and Religion* (Chapel Hill, N.C.: University of North Carolina Press, 2000).

205 Same amount of glandular material per breast: N. Angier, *Woman: An Intimate Geography* (Boston: Houghton Mifflin, 1999), p. 137.

205 Variety of breast sizes a mystery: Angier, *Woman*, pp.134–56.

205 Breast fat not used to make breast milk: S. B. Hrdy, *Mother Nature: Maternal Instincts and How They Shape the Human Species* (New York: Ballantine, 1999), pp. 126–27. Some scholars contend that humans are the only mammal whose adult females have permanent breasts, i.e., fatted mammary glands that appear as enlarged even when not engorged with milk. However, all female mammals possess mammary fat pads through which the ductal tree grows. In human women, these fat pads form discrete, visible lumps on the chest wall; in other mammals, they are simply thinner and spread throughout the body. In rodents, for example, the mammary fat pad extends over the shoulder and around the back and hips in a horseshoe arrangement (Dr. Suzanne Snedecker, Cornell University, personal communication).

206 The breast as one of few organs not developed at birth: J. Russo and I. H. Russo, "Development of the Human Mammary Gland," in M. C. Neville and C. W. Daniel, eds., *The Mammary Gland: Development, Regulation, and Function* (New York: Plenum Press, 1987), pp. 67–93.

207 Development of the breast during prenatal life, puberty, and throughout menstrual cycles: Russo and Russo, "Development of the Human Mammary Gland."

207 Breast development during pregnancy: D. C. Brack, "Breastfeeding: Physiological and Cultural Aspects," in Rothman, *Encyclopedia of Childbearing*, pp. 43–44; M. Neville, *Milk Secretion: An Overview*; Russo and Russo, "Development of the Human Mammary Gland." Estrogen also promotes gland development (G. R. Cunha et al., "Elucidation of a Role for Stromal Steroid Hormone Receptors in Mammary Gland Growth and Development Using Tissue Recombinants," *J. of Mammary Gland Biology and Neoplasia* 2[1997]:393–402; J. L. Fendrick et al., "Mammary Gland Growth and Development from the Postnatal Period to Postmenopause: Ovarian Steroid Receptor Ontogeny and Regulation in the Mouse," *J. of Mammary Gland Biology and Neoplasia* 3[1998]:7–22).

207–208 Time before onset of lactation: D. J. Chapman and R. Perez-Escamilla, "Identification of Risk Factors for Delayed Onset of Lactation," *J. of the American Dietetic Association* 99(1999):450–54.

209 Properties of colostrum: N. Baumslag and D. L. Michels, *Milk, Money, and Madness: The Culture and Politics of Breastfeeding* (Westport, Conn.: Bergin & Garvey, 1995), p. 74.

210 Edema causes engorgement: Dr. Margaret Neville, University of Colorado, personal communication.

210 Life history of milk: Russo and Russo, "Development of the Human Mammary Gland."

210 Daily volume of milk produced: Neville, "Physiology of Lactation."

210–211 Dynamics of breast milk: W. G. Manson and L. T. Weaver, "Fat Digestion in the Neonate," *Archives of Disease in Childhood* 76(Fetal Neonatal Edition) (1997):F206–11; M. F. Picciano, "Human Milk: Nutritional Aspects of a Dynamic Food," *Biology of the Neonate* 74(1998):84–93; B. Wilson, "Milky Ways," *New Statesman*, 24 May 1999, pp. 43–44.

211–212 Many functions of oxytocin: Hrdy, *Mother Nature*, 137–40.

212 Role of areola: Neville, *Milk Secretion*.

213 Mechanics of suckling: N. P. Alekseev et al., "Compression Stimuli Increase the Efficacy of Breast Pump Function," *European J. of Obstetrics & Gynecology and Reproductive Biology* 77(1998):131–39; Auerbach, "Nipples, Human."

214 Mathematical model: C. Zoppou et al., "Dynamics of Human Milk Extraction: A Comparative Study of Breast Feeding and Breast Pumping," *Bulletin of Mathematical Biology* 59(1997):953–73.

214 No machine can mimic suckling: Alekseev, "Compression Stimuli."

214 Matrotropy: D. G. Blackburn et al., "The Origins of Lactation and the Evolution of Milk: A Review with New Hypotheses," *Mammal Review* 19(1989):1–26.

215 Interspecific differences in mammae: C. A. Long, "The Origin and Evolution of Mammary Glands," *Bioscience* 19(1969):519–23.

215 Etymology of "mamma": L. Schiebinger, "Why Mammals Are Called Mammals: Gender Politics in Eighteenth-Century Natural History," *American Historical Review* 98(1993): 382–411.

215–216 Uterine autolysis: S. Kitzinger, *The Year After Childbirth: Surviving and Enjoying the First Year of Motherhood* (New York: Charles Scribner's Sons, 1994), p. 16.

216 Linnaeus's decision: Schiebinger, "Why Mammals Are Called Mammals."

216 Little known about origin of the breast: Blackburn, "The Origins of Lactation"; C. A. Long, "Two Hypotheses on the Origin of Lactation," *American Naturalist* 106(1972):141–44.

216 Male breasts: J. Diamond, "Father's Milk," *Discover*, Feb. 1995, pp. 82–87; C. M. Francis, "Lactation in Male Fruit Bats," *Nature* 367(1994):691–92.

216–217 Blackburn and Pond: D. G. Blackburn, "Evolutionary Origins of the Mammary Gland," *Mammal Review* 21(1991):81–96; C. M. Pond, "The Significance of Lactation in the Evolution of Mammals," *Evolution* 31(1977):177–99.

217 Pond's ideas on newborn food: Ibid.

217 Breasts older than placentae: Long, "Origin and Evolution of Mammary Glands."

218 Humans have most dilute milk: A. M. Prentice and A. Prentice, "Evolutionary and Environmental Influences on Human Lactation," *Proceedings of the Nutrition Society* 54(1995):391–400.

218 Human babies are fat but slow-growing: C. W. Kuzawa, "Adipose Tissue in Human Infancy and Childhood: An Evolutionary Perspective," *Yearbook of Physical Anthropology* 41(1998, sup. 27):177–209; Prentice and Prentice, "Evolutionary and Environmental Influences on Human Lactation."

218 Nursing style determines nutritional content: W. R. Trevathan, *Human Birth: An Evolutionary Perspective* (Hawthorne, N.Y.: Aldine De Gruyter, 1987), pp. 29–32.

219 Milk of Mary: Schiebinger, "Why Mammals Are Called Mammals."

219 Mother's milk's healing powers: Schiebinger, "Why Mammals Are Called Mammals." See also Angier, *Woman*, pp. 157–60.

219 *Origin of the Milky Way*: This painting is reproduced as Plate 5 in Hrdy, *Mother Nature*.

220 Sugar and protein content of human milk: Baumslag and Michels, *Milk, Money, and Madness*, pp. 68–70; B. Wilson, "Milky Ways."

220 The extremity of early motherhood: This is how Sheila Kitzinger describes it: "When she becomes a mother, it is as if a woman must go deep into the bowels of the earth, back to the elemental emotions and the power that makes life possible, losing herself in darkness. She is Euridice in the underworld. She is pulled away from a world of choices . . . to the warm chaos of love, confusion, longing, anger, self-surrender, and intense pleasure that mothering entails" (S. Kitzinger, *Ourselves as Mothers: The Universal Experience of Motherhood* [Reading, Mass.: Addison-Wesley, 1995], p. 12).

222–223 Linnaeus's decision: Schiebinger, "Why Mammals Are Called Mammals." See also Hrdy, *Mother Nature*, p. 12.

223 Wet-nursing in the U.S.: The hiring of a private wet nurse in the nineteenth-century United States usually meant that a rich baby (the employer's) lived, and a poor baby (the nurse's) died. In New York, the mortality rate of wet nurses' infants, who were farmed out to other caregivers and fed artificial food during their mothers' period of employment, reached 90 percent. By contrast, in France, nursing infants were frequently sent out to the countryside to live with wet nurses in their own homes. Deaths of employer and employee infants were frequent nonetheless (J. H. Wolf, " 'Mercenary Hirelings' or 'a Great Blessing'?: Doctors' and Mothers' Conflicted Perceptions of Wet Nurses and the Ramifications for Infant Feeding in Chicago, 1871–1961," *J. of Social History* 33[1999]:97–120; Hrdy, *Mother Nature*, pp. 351–72).

CHAPTER ELEVEN: LOAVES AND FISHES

225–226 Breastfed babies have lower rates of hospitalization and death: L. M. Gartner et al., "Breastfeeding and the Use of Human Milk," *Pediatrics* 100(1997):1035–39; L. K. Pickering et al., "Modulation of the Immune System by Human Milk and Infant Formula Containing Nucleotides," *Pediatrics* 101(1998):242–49.

226 Breastfed babies breathe differently: O. P. Mathew and J. Bhatia, "Sucking and Breathing Patterns During Breast- and Bottle-feeding in Term Neonates," *Am. J. of Diseases of Children* 143(1989):588–92.

226 Reason for fewer ear infections: R. A. Lawrence, *A Review of the Medical Benefits and Contraindications to Breastfeeding in the United States*, Maternal and Child Health Technical Information Bulletin (Arlington, Va.: National Center for Education in Maternal and Child Health, 1997), p. 4.

226 Socioeconomic differences between breastfeeding mothers and formula-feeding mothers: The highest rates of breastfeeding in the United States are found among higher-income women who are over 30, college educated, and live in the Mountain and Pacific regions (Gartner, "Breastfeeding and the Use of Human Milk").

226 New Mexico study: A. L. Wright et al., "Increasing Breastfeeding Rates to Reduce Infant Illness at the Community Levels," *Pediatrics* 101(1998):837–44.

226–227 Scottish study: A. C. Wilson et al., "Relation of Infant Diet to Childhood Health: Seven Year Follow Up of Cohort of Children in Dundee Infant Feeding Study," *British Medical Journal* 316(1998):21–25.

227 More than just infectious disease protection: A. S. Goldman, "Modulation of the Gastrointestinal Tract of Infants by Human Milk, Interfaces and Interactions: An Evolutionary Hypothesis," *J. of Nutrition* 130(2000):426S–31S; L. Maher, "Advising Parents on Feeding Healthy Babies," *Patient Care* 32(15 Mar. 1998):58–68; T. Mason et al., "Breast Feeding and the Development of Juvenile Rheumatoid Arthritis," *J. of Rheumatology* 22(1995):1166–70; W. H. Oddy et al., "Association Between Breastfeeding and Asthma in 6-Year-Old Children: Findings of a Prospective Birth Cohort Study," *British Medical Journal* 319(1999):815–19; A. Rigas et al., "Breast-feeding and Maternal Smoking in the Etiology of Crohn's Disease and Ulcerative Colitis in Childhood," *Annals of Epidemiology* 3(1993):387–92; A. Singhal, "Early Nutrition in Preterm Infants and Later Blood Pressure: Two Cohorts After Randomized Trials," *Lancet* 357 (2001): 413–39. Breastfed children also enjoy straighter teeth and fewer cavities (M. P. Degano and R. A. Degano, "Breastfeeding and Oral Health: A primer for the Dental Practitioner," *New York State Dental Journal* 59[1993]:30–32).

227 Mother's milk cures colitis in rats: C. F. Grazioso et al., "Antiinflammatory Effects of Human Milk on Chemically Induced Colitis in Rats," *Pediatric Research* 42(1997):639–43.

227 How breast milk protects against diabetes: J. Paronen et al., "Effect of Cow's Milk Exposure and Maternal Type 1 Diabetes on Cellular and Humoral Immunization to Dietary Insulin in Infants at Genetic Risk for Type 1 Diabetes. Finnish Trial to Reduce IDDM in the Genetically at Risk Study Group," *Diabetes* 49(2000):1657–65; N. Seppa, "Cows' Milk, Diabetes Connection Bolstered," *Science News* 155(1999):404–5.

227–228 Breast milk and obesity: K. G. Dewey, "Growth Characteristics of Breast-Fed Compared to Formula-Fed Infants," *Biology of the Neonate* 74(1998):94–105; R. Von Kries et al., "Breast Feeding and Obesity: Cross Sectional Study," *British Medical Journal* 319(1999):147–50.

228 Breast milk and Hodgkin's lymphoma: M. K. Davis, "Review of the Evidence for an Association Between Infant Feeding and Childhood Cancer," *Intl. J. of Cancer* 11(1998, sup. 2):29–33. Recent studies have also found an association between breastfeeding and a reduced risk of childhood acute leukemia (A. Bener et al., "Longer Breastfeeding and Protection Against Childhood Leukaemia and Lymphomas," *European Journal of Cancer* 37 [2001]:234–38; X. O. Shu et al., "Breast-Feeding and Risk of Childhood Acute Leukemia," *J. of the National Cancer Institute* 91[1999]:1765–72).

228 Breastfeeding protects the health of mothers: L. M. Gartner et al., "Breastfeeding and the Use of Human Milk"; M. H. Labbok, "Health Sequelae of Breastfeeding for the Mother," *Clinical Perinatalology* 26(1999):491–503.317

228 Breastfeeding and maternal risk of breast and ovarian cancer: S. M. Enger et al., "Breastfeeding Experience and Breast Cancer Risk Among Postmenopausal Women, *Cancer Epidemiology, Biomarkers & Prevention* 7(1998):365–69; J. L. Freudenheim et al., "Lactation History and Breast Cancer Risk," *Am. J. of Epidemiology* 146(1997):932–38; H. Furberg et al., "Lactation and Breast Cancer Risk," *Intl. J. of Epidemiology* 28(1999):396–402; L. Lipworth et al., "History of Breast-feeding in Relation to Breast Cancer Risk: A Review of the Epidemiologic Literature," *J. of the National Cancer Institute* 92(2000):302–12; K. A. Rosenblatt and D. B. Thomas, "Lactation and the Risk of Epithelial Ovarian Cancer. The WHO Collaborative Study of Neoplasia and Steroid Contraceptives," *Intl. J. of Epidemiology* 22(1993):192–97; L. Tryggvadottir, "Breastfeeding and Reduced Risk of Breast Cancer in an Icelandic Cohort Study," *American J. of Epidemiology* 154(2001):37–42; T. Zheng et al., "Lactation Reduces Breast Cancer Risk in Shandong Province, China," *Am. J. of Epidemiology* 12(2000):1129–35. The mechanism underlying the protective effect of breastfeeding on breast cancer risk is unknown and may include hormonal changes, physiological changes in breast epithelial cells, delayed onset of ovulation, and lowering of chemical carcinogen levels through their excretion in breast milk. Interestingly enough, women living in fishing villages in Hong Kong who by custom nurse only with the right breast have a significantly higher risk of developing postmenopausal breast cancer in the left, unsuckled, breast than in the right one (R. Ing and J. H. C. Ho, "Unilateral Breast-Feeding and Breast Cancer," *Lancet* 2 [1977]:124-27).

228–229 Economic advantages of breastfeeding: T. M. Ball and A. L. Wright, "Health Care Costs of Formula-Feeding in the First Year of Life," *Pediatrics* 103(1999):870–76. Total medical care expenditures for fully breastfed infants are typically about 20 percent lower than for formula-fed infants (U.S. Department of Health and Human Services, Office on Women's Health, *HHS Blueprint for Action on Breastfeeding* [Washington, D.C.: HHS, 2000], p. 11).

231 All mammals are immunological incompetent: Goldman, "Modulation of the Gastrointestinal Tract."

231 Explanation for deferred immune development: Ibid.

231 Breast milk as assassin: D. G. Blackburn et al., "The Origins of Lactation and the Evolution of Milk: A Review with New Hypotheses," *Mammal Review* 19(1989):1–26.

231 Discovery of living leukocytes in breast milk: M. Xanthou, "Immune Protection of Human Milk," *Biology of the Neonate* 74(1998):121–33.

231 Types of leukocytes and their functions: H. F. Pabst, "Immunomodulation by Breastfeeding," *Pediatric Infectious Disease Journal* 16(1997):991–95; Xanthou, "Immune Protection."

231–232 Nonliving immune elements: R. M. Goldblum and A. G. Goldman, "Immunological Components of Milk: Formation and Function"; M. Hamosh, "Protective Function of Proteins and Lipids in Human Milk," *Biology of the Neonate* 74(1998):163–76; Lawrence, *Review of Medical Benefits*, p. 9; Xanthou, "Immune Protection." Biologically active polypeptides called cytocines are also found in breast milk and also appear to play a role in immune system activation (J. M. Wallace et al., "Cytokines in Human Breast Milk," *British J. of Biomedical Science* 54[1997]:85–87).

232 Role of the gut in breast immune defenses: A. S. Goldman et al., "Evolution of Immunologic Functions of the Mammary Gland and the Postnatal Development of Immunity," *Pediatric Research* 43(1998):155–162.

233 Treating eye infections with human milk: N. Baumslag and D. Michels, *Milk, Money, and Madness: The Culture and Politics of Breastfeeding* (Westport, Conn.: Bergin & Garvey, 1995), p. 64.

233–234 How breast milk sets up infant's immune system: R. P. Garofalo and A. S. Goldman, "Cytokines, Chemokines, and Colony-stimulating Factors in Human Milk: The 1997 Update," *Biology of the Neonate* 74(1998):134–42; Goldman, "Modulation of the Gastrointestinal Tract"; Pabst, "Immunomodulation by Breast-feeding"; Wallace, "Cytocines in Human Breast Milk"; Xanthou, "Immune Protection."

237–238 Digestive tract a late bloomer: Children's Environmental Health Network, *Training Manual on Pediatric Environmental Health: Putting It into Practice* (Emeryville, Calif.: CEHN, 1999), p. 62

238 Effect of breast milk on digestive tract: Goldman, "Modulation of the Gastrointestinal Tract"; Lawrence, *Review of Medical Benefits*, p. 9; J. A. Peterson et al., "Glycoproteins of the Human Milk Fat Globule in the Protection of the Breast-fed Infant Against Infections," *Biology of the Neonate* 74(1998):143–62; Rubaltelli et al., "Intestinal Flora in Breast- and Bottle-Fed Infants," *J. of Perinatal Medicine* 26(1998):186–91; I. R. Sanderson, "Dietary Regulation of Genes Expressed in the Developing Intestinal Epithelium," *Am. J. of Clinical Nutrition* 68(1998):999–1005; Wallace, "Cytocines in Human Breast Milk"; Y. Yamada, "Hepatocyte Growth Factor in Human Breast Milk," *Am. J. of Reproductive Immunology* 40(1998):122–20.

238–239 Interference of oligosaccharides and lactose: P. McVeagh and J. B. Miller, "Human Milk Oligosaccharides: Only the Breast," *J. of Paediatrics and Child Health* 33(1997):281–86.

239 Cloth diapers: Cloth diapers offer clear health benefits. Several brands of disposable diapers emit mixtures of chemicals that are toxic to the respiratory tract. In a recent study, mice exposed to airborne emissions from disposable diapers developed breathing problems, including asthma-like reactions (R. C. Anderson and J. H. Anderson, "Acute Respiratory Effects of Diaper Emissions," *Archives of Environmental Health* 54(1999):353–58). Furthermore, cloth diapers keep skin cooler. In boys, plastic-lined disposable diapers have been shown to raise scrotal temperatures significantly—so much that the normal physiological cooling mechanism of the testes is compromised. Researchers speculate that increased testicular temperature in early childhood might be contributing to the ongoing decline in sperm count and other problems of male reproductive health (C. J. Partsch et al., "Scrotal Temperature Is Increased in Disposable Plastic Lined Nappies," *Archives of Disease in Childhood* 83[2000]:364–68.) Cloth diapers also have environmental benefits. Studies commissioned by the disposable diaper industry have claimed that disposables are no more ecologically harmful than cloth diapers (A. Swasy, *Soap Opera: The Inside Story of Procter & Gamble* [New York: Times Books, 1993]). Other studies have reached different conclusions. According to the Women's Environmental Network in London, cloth diapers use about a quarter of the energy, one eighth the nonrenewable resources, and about 1 percent of the renewable resources required by disposable diapers. They also produce about 1.5 percent of the solid waste. Both cloth and disposables require similar amounts of fossil fuel energy (A. Link, *Preventing Nappy Waste* [London: Women's Environmental Network, 1998]). Cloth diapering is almost a lost art. The best book on all practical and philosophical dimensions of cloth diapers, from diaper services to diaper wraps to diaper pails, is T. R. Farrisi, *Diaper Changes: The Complete Diapering Book and Resource Guide* [Richland, Pa.: Homekeepers Publishing, 1997]).

239 Breast-milk poop: M. J. Hill, ed., *Nitrates and Nitrites in Food and Water* (New York: Ellis Horwood, 1991), pp. 166–69; Rubaltelli "Intestinal Flora."

239–240 Quote from *NEJM* on sexuality of nursing: N. Newton and M. Newton, "Psychologic Aspects of Lactation," *NEJM*, 227(1967):1179–88.

240 Quote from Ruth Lawrence: Lawrence, *Review of Medical Benefits*, p. 5.

240 Brain doubles its weight in first year: N. Gordon, "Nutrition and Cognitive Function," *Brain & Development* 19(1997):165–70.

240–241 Breast milk and brain development: Gordon, "Nutrition and Cognitive Function"; C.I. Lanting et al., "Breastfeeding and Neurological Outcome at 42 Months," *Acta Paediatrica* 87(1998):1224–29; ibid., "Neurological Differences Between 9-Year-Old Children Fed Breast-Milk or Formula-Milk as Babies," *Lancet* 344(1994):1319–22; Lawrence, *Review of Medical Benefits*, p. 5; J. Worobey, "Feeding Method and Motor Activity in 3-Month-Old Human Infants," *Perceptual and Motor Skills* 86(1998):883–95.

241 Study finding no effect: S. W. Jacobson et al., "Breastfeeding Effects on Intelligence Quotient in 4- and 11-Year-Old Children," *Pediatrics* 103(1999):E71.

241 Study reanalyzing previous studies: J. W. Anderson et al., "Breast-Feeding and Cognitive Development: A Meta-Analysis," *Am. J. of Clinical Nutrition* 70(1999):525–35.

241 New Zealand study: L. J. Horwood and D. M. Fergusson, "Breastfeeding and Later Cognitive and Academic Outcomes," *Pediatrics* 101(1998): E9; D. M. Fergusson et al., "Breast-Feeding and Cognitive Development in the First Seven Years of Life," *Social Science & Medicine* 16(1982):1705–08.

241–242 Preterm study: Gordon, "Nutrition and Cognitive Function"; A. Lucas et al., "Breast Milk and Subsequent Intelligence Quotient in Children Born Preterm," *Lancet* 339(1992):261–64.

242 Scialic acid: McVeagh and Miller, "Human Milk Oligosaccharides."

242 Polyunsaturated fats: M. Hamosh and N. Salem, Jr., "Long-Chain Polyunsaturated Fatty Acids," *Biology of the Neonate* 74(1998):106–20.

242 Autopsies: M. Makrides et al., "Fatty Acid Composition of Brain, Retina, and Erythrocytes in Breast- and Formula-Fed Infants," *Am. J. of Clinical Nutrition* 60(1994):189–94. See also J. Farquharson et al., "Infant Cerebral Cortex Phospholipid Fatty-Acid Composition and Diet," *Lancet* 340(1992):810–13.

243 Books that extol cosleeping: For example, T. Thevenin, *The Family Bed* (Wayne, N.J.: Avery, 1987).

243 Books that discourage cosleeping: For example, R. Ferber, *Solve Your Child's Sleep Problems* (New York: Simon & Schuster, 1986).

245 AAP policy statement: Gartner, "Breastfeeding and the Use of Human Milk."

245 Past and present U.S. rates of breastfeeding: R. D. Apple, *Mothers and Medicine: A Social History of Infant Feeding, 1890–1950* (Madison: University of Wisconsin Press, 1987); Baumslag and Michels, *Milk, Money, and Madness*, p. xxi; K. K. Bell and N. L. Rawlings, "Promoting Breast-feeding by Managing Common Lactation Problems," *Nurse Practitioner* 23(1998):102–10; J. E. Brody, "Breast Is Best for Babies, but Sometimes Mom Needs Help," *New York Times*, 30 Mar. 1999, p. F7; J. D. Skinner at al., "Transitions in Infant Feeding During the First Year of Life," *J. of the Am. College of Nutrition* 16(1997):209–15.

245–246 Obstacles to breastfeeding: N. Q. Danyliw, "Got Mother's Milk? Employers Gradually Make Accommodations for Nursing Moms," *U.S. News and World Report*, 15 Dec. 1997, pp. 79–80; Gartner, "Breastfeeding and the Use of Human Milk"; G. L. Freed et al., "National Assessment of Physicians' Breast-feeding Knowledge, Attitudes, Training, and Experience," *JAMA* 273(1995):472–76. Obstacles to breastfeeding also include the aggressive marketing practices of formula companies. U.S. hospitals collect millions of dollars from exclusive contracts to give away formula samples to all maternity patients upon discharge. Studies consistently show that these promotional strategies reduce the chances of successful breastfeeding. For example, exposure of pregnant women to formula advertising in their doctors' offices contributes significantly to breastfeeding cessation in the first two weeks. In 1981, the World Health Organization developed the International Code of Marketing of Breast Milk Substitute, which restricts sales and advertising of infant formula. The code specifically prohibits the distribution of free samples to expectant and new mothers. Ten years later, the World Health Organization launched the Baby-Friendly Hospital Initiative to offer official recognition to hospitals that promote breastfeeding and prohibit the distribution of formula samples. Of the 13,000 hospitals around the world certified as baby-friendly according to WHO guidelines, only 26 are located in the United States (Baumslag and Michels, *Milk, Money, and Madness*; Y. Bergevin et al., "Do Infant Formula Samples Shorten the Duration of Breastfeeding?" *Lancet* 1[1983, no. 8334]:1148–51; T. S. Briesch, "Mother Nature's Formula, *American Medical News* 41[19 Jan. 1998]:13–15; C. Howard et al., "Office Prenatal Formula Advertising and Its Effects on Breast-Feeding Patterns," *Obstetrics and Gynecology* 95[2000]:296–303; N. G. Powers et al., "Hospital Policies: Crucial to Breastfeeding Success," *Seminars in Perinatology* 18[1994]:517–24; J. M. Sharfstein, "An Interview with Breastfeeding Advocate and Formula Fighter Bobbi Philipp, M.D.," *Health Letter*, Oct. 1999, p. 2; World Health Organization, *Intl. Code of Marketing of Breast-Milk Substitutes* [Geneva: WHO, 1981]; www.babyfriendlyusa.org).

247 Breastfeeding in Norway: Dr. Elisabet Helsing, Board of Health and University of Oslo, and Halle Margrete Meltzer, National Institute of Public Health, Oslo, Norway, personal communication. Thanks also to Michael Brady of Norway for helping me confirm these figures.

247 Breast pump ad: E. Parpis, "Got Milk?" *Adweek*, 27 Mar. 2000, p. 13.

CHAPTER TWELVE: THE VIEW FROM THE TOP

251 Organochlorine pollutants in breast milk: A. A. Jensen and S. A. Slorach, "Assessment of Infant Intake of Chemicals via Breast Milk," in A. A. Jensen and S. A. Slorach, eds., *Chemical Contaminants in Human Milk* (Boca Raton: CRC Press, 1991), pp. 215–22.

251 Levels exceed legally allowable limits in commercial food: T. Schettler et al., *Generations at Risk: Reproductive Health and the Environment* (Cambridge: MIT Press, 1999), p. 205.

251 1996 quote: W. J. Rogan, "Pollutants in Breast Milk," *Archives of Pediatrics and Adolescent Medicine* 150(1996):981–90.

251 Breastfed infants ingest fifty times more PCBs and dioxins than their parents: L. Birnbaum and B. P. Slezak, "Dietary Exposure to PCBs and Dioxins in Children," *EHP* 107(1999):1; O. Papke, "PCDD/PCDF: Human Background Data for Germany, a Ten Year Experience," *EHP* 106(1998, sup. 2):723–31. In spite of their higher rate of dioxin ingestion, infants still have lower body burdens than adults because of their young age. No one knows whether daily exposure or accumulated body burden is the better measure of dose (Dr. Tom Webster, Boston University, personal communication).

251–252 Exposures exceed WHO limits: D. Buckley-Golder, *Compilation of EU Dioxin Exposure and Health Data, Summary Report*, Report Produced for the European Commission, DG Environment, UK Department of Environment Transport and the Regions (Oxfordshire, U.K.: AEA Technology, 1999).

252 British infants receive seventeen times tolerable amount of PCBs: J. Wise, "High Amounts of Chemicals Found in Breast Milk," *British Medical Journal* 314(1997):1505.

252 Formula less contaminated: J. S. Schreiber, "Transport of Organic Chemicals to Breast Milk: Tetrachloroethene Case Study," in S. Kacew and G. H. Lambert, eds., *Environmental Toxicology and Pharmacology of Human Development* (Washington, D.C.: Taylor & Francis, 1997), pp. 95–143.

252 Fat in infant formula from plant oils: J. S. Schreiber, "Transport of Organic Chemicals."

252 1998 study of eleven-month-olds: Papke, "PCDD/PCDF."

252 Difference twenty times higher: H. Beck et al., "PCDD and PCDF Exposures and Levels in Humans in Germany," *EHP* 102(1994, sup. 1):173–85.

252 Dutch study: C. I. Lanting et al., "Determinants of Polychlorinated Biphenyl Levels in Plasma from 42-Month-Old Children," *Archives of Environmental Contamination and Toxicology* 35(1998):135–39; S. Patandin et al., "Plasma Polychlorinated Biphenyl Levels in Dutch Preschool Children Either Breast-fed or Formula-fed During Infancy," *Am. J. of Public Health* 87(1997): 1711–14.

252 Studies consistently show the more mother's milk consumed, the higher the concentration of organochlorines: See Lanting, "Determinants of Polychlorinated Biphenyl Levels in Plasma from 42-Month-Old Children."

252 Even at twenty-five years old: S. Patandin et al., "Dietary Exposure to Polychlorinated Biphenyls and Dioxins from Infancy Until Adulthood: A Comparison Between Breast-feeding, Toddler, and Long-term Exposure," *EHP* 107(1999):45–51.

252 First report of breast-milk contamination: E. P. Laug et al., "Occurrence of DDT in Human Fat and Milk," *Archives of Industrial Hygiene* 3(1951):245

252 1966 discovery: "Report of a New Chemical Hazard," *New Scientist* 32(1966):612.

252 200 chemicals discovered by 1981: E. D. Pellizzari et al., "Purgeable Organic Compounds in Mothers' Milk," *Bulletin of Environmental Contamination and Toxicology* 28(1982):322–28.

252–253 DDT and PCBs the most widespread contaminants: M. Cavaliere et al., "Polychlorinated Biphenyls and Dichlorodiphenyl Trichloroethane in Human Milk: A Review," *European Review for Medical and Pharmacological Sciences* 1(1997):63–68; A. A. Jensen "Levels and Trends of Environmental Chemicals in Human Milk," in Jensen and Slorach, *Chemical Contaminants in Human Milk*, pp. 45–198.

253 Other common contaminants of breast milk: The toilet deodorizer is *p*-dichloro-benzene. The wood preservative is pentachlorophenol. The flame retardants are polybrominated biphenyls. The insecticides include toxaphene, aldrin, endrin, and lindane. The termite control agents include heptachlor and chlordane. The by-products from trash incinerators are dioxins and furans. The cable-insulating materials are polychlorinated napthalenes. The fungicide is hexachlorobenzene, which is now banned in the United States but is generated as a by-product during the manufacture of other pesticides, such as atrazine, as well as in the production of the wood preservative pentachlorophenol and common solvents, such as perchloroethylene and carbon tetrachloride. The volatile chemicals in breast milk include benzene, styrene, chloroform, toluene, and perchloroethylene. Breast milk contains higher levels of solvents than blood because breast tissue is less efficient at clearing them (A. P. J. M. van Birgelen, "Hexachlorobenzene as a Possible Major Contributor to the Dioxin Activity of Human Milk," *EHP* 106[1998]:683–88; J. Fisher, "Lactational Transfer of Volatile Chemicals in Breast Milk," *American Industrial Hygiene Association Journal* 58(1997):425–31; Schettler et al., *Generations at Risk*, p. 216; Schreiber, "Transport of Organic Chemicals"; B. R. Sonawane, "Chemical Contaminants in Human Milk: An Overview," *EHP* 103[1995, sup. 6]:197–205).

253 Argument that ignorance is bliss: One recent review concluded, "Perhaps even the knowledge that human milk may be contaminated will result in concerns in the nursing mother that may interfere with breast-feeding" (C. M. Berlin and S. Kacew, "Environmental Chemicals in Human Milk," in S. Kacew and G. H. Lambert, eds., *Environmental Toxicology and Pharmacology of Human Development* [Washington, D.C.: Taylor & Francis, 1997], pp. 67–93). See also S. L. Hatcher, "The Psychological Experience of Nursing Mothers Upon Learning of a Toxic Substance in their Breast Milk," *Psychiatry* 45(1982):172–81.

255 Food crisis in Belgium: T. J. Allen, "Dioxin: It's What's for Dinner!" *In These Times,* 22 Aug. 1999, pp. 14–16; H. Ashraf, "European Dioxin-Contaminated Food Crisis Grows and Grows," *Lancet* 353(1999):2049; R. Clapp and D. Ozonoff, "Where the Boys Aren't: Dioxin and the Sex Ratio," *Lancet* 355(2000):1838–39; B. E. Erickson, "Dioxin Food Crisis in Belgium," *Analytical Chemistry* 71(1999):541A–43A; D. MacKenzie, "Recipe for Disaster," *New Scientist,* 12 June 1999, p. 4; C. R. Whitney, "Food Scandal Adds to Belgium's Image of Disarray," *New York Times,* 9 June 1999, p. A4.

255 Quote about effects on children: N. van Larebeke et al., "The Belgian PCB and Dioxin Incident of January–June 1999: Exposure Data and Potential Impact on Health," *EHP* 109(2001):265–73.

255–256 Toxicology of dioxin: Center for Health, Environment and Justice, *American People's Dioxin Report* (Falls Church, Va.: CHEJ, 1999); International Agency for Research on Cancer, *IARC Monographs on the Evaluation of Carcinogenic Risks to Humans, vol. 69, Polychlorinated Dibenzo-para-dioxins and Polychlorinated Dibenzofurans* (Lyons, France: IARC, 1997); D. H. Buckley-Golder, *Compilation of EU Dioxin Exposure and Health Data; Task 8: Human Toxicology,* Report Produced for European Commission on the Environment, U.K. Department of the Environment, Transport and the Regions (Oxfordshire, U.K.: AEA Technology, 1999).

256–257 Ah receptor: M. E. Hahn, "The Aryl Hydrocarbon Receptor: A Comparative Perspective," *Comparative Biochemistry and Physiology,* Part C, 121(1998):23–53.

257 Health effects in animals and humans: See series of contributions on dioxin's perinatal effects, "Workshop on Perinatal Exposure to Dioxin-like Compounds," in *Environmental Health Perspectives* 103(1995, sup. 2): G. Lindstrom et al., "Workshop on Perinatal Exposure to Dioxin-like Compounds," pp. 135–42; B. Eskenazi and G. Kimmel, "II. Reproductive Effects," pp. 143–45; M. M. Feeley, "III. Endocrine Effects," pp. 147–50; M. S. Golub and S. W. Jacobson, "IV. Neurobehavioral Effects," pp. 151–55; L. S. Birnbaum, "V. Immunologic Effects," pp. 157–60.

257 The WHO declared dioxin a known human carcinogen: International Agency for Research on Cancer, *IARC Monographs,* vol. 69.

257 Twice as much rains down: D. M. Wagrowski and R. A. Hites, "Insights into the Global Distribution of Polychlorinated Dibenzo-*p*-dioxins and Dibenzofurans," *Environmental Science and Technology* 34(2000):2952–58.

257 Sources of dioxin: J. I. Baker and R. A. Hites, "Is Combustion the Major Source of Polychlorinated Dibenzo-*p*-dioxins and Dibenzofurans to the Environment? A Mass Balance Investigation," *Environmental Science and Technology* 34(2000):2879–2886; ibid., "Siskiwit Lake Revisited:

Time Trends of Polychlorinated Dibenzo-*p*-dioxin and Dibenzofuran Deposition at Isle Royale, Michigan," *Environmental Science and Technology* 34(2000):2887–91.

257–258 Nunavut: B. Commoner et al., *Long-range Air Transport of Dioxin from North American Sources to Ecologically Vulnerable Receptors in Nunavut, Arctic Canada*, Final Report to the North American Commission for Environmental Cooperation (Flushing, N.Y.: Center for the Biology of Natural Systems, Queens College, CUNY, 2000); P. J. Hilts, "Dioxin in Arctic Circle Is Traced to Sources Far to the South," *New York Times*, 17 Oct. 2000, p. F2; J. Raloff, "Even Nunavut Gets Plenty of Dioxin," *Science News* 158(7October 2000):230.

258–259 Smelter plant in Hartford, Illinois: For more on *U.S. v. Chemetco, Inc. et al.*, refer to the EPA's enforcement database: www.epa.gov/region5/enforcement.

259 Breast-milk contamination around the world: M. A. Alawi et al., "Organochlorine Pesticide Contaminations in Human Milk Samples from Women Living in Amman, Jordan," *Archives of Environmental Contamination and Toxicology* 23(1992):235–39; I. Al-Saleh et al., "Residue Levels of Organochlorinated Insecticides in Breast Milk: A Preliminary Report from Al-Kharj, Saudi Arabia," *J. of Environmental Pathology, Toxicology and Oncology* 17(1998):37–50; R. Angulo et al., "PCB Congeners Transferred by Human Milk, with an Estimate of their Daily Intake," *Food and Chemical Toxicology* 37(1999):1081–88; N. Basu et al., "DDT Levels in Human Body Fat and Milk Samples from Delhi," *Indian J. of Medical Research* 94(1991):115–18; M. N. Bates, et al., *Organochlorine Residues in the Breast Milk of New Zealand Women: A Report to the Department of Health* (Petone, New Zealand: Dept. of Scientific and Industrial Research, 1990); O. Chikuni et al., "Residues of Organochlorine Pesticides in Human Milk from Mothers Living in the Greater Harare Area of Zimbabwe," *Central African J. of Medicine* 37(1991):136–41; J. Clench-Aas et al., "PCDD and PCDF in Human Milk from Scandinavia, with Special Emphasis on Norway," *J. of Toxicology and Environmental Health* 37(1992):73–83; A. G. Craan and D. A. Haines, "Twenty-five Years of Surveillance for Contaminants in Human Breast Milk," *Archives of Environmental Contamination and Toxicology* 35(1998):702–10; F. Ejobi et al., "Organochlorine Pesticide Residues in Mothers' Milk in Uganda," *Bulletin of Environmental Contamination and Toxicology* 56(1996):873–80; B. C. Gladen et al., "Organochlorines in Breast Milk from Two Cities in Ukraine," *EHP* 107(1999):459–62; M. J. Gonzalez et al., "Levels of PCDDs and PCDFs in Human Milk from Populations in Madrid and Paris," *Bulletin of Environmental Contamination and Toxicology* 56(1996):197–204; K. Hooper et al., "Analysis of Breast Milk to Assess Exposure to Chlorinated Contaminants in Kazakhstan: Sources of 2,3,7,8-tetrachlorobenzo-*p*-dioxin (TCDD) Exposures in an Agricultural Region of Southern Kazakhstan," *EHP* 107(1999):447–57; F. J. Paumgartten et al., "PCDDs, PCDFs, PCBs, and Other Organochlorine Compounds in Human Milk from Rio de Janeiro, Brazil," *Environmental Research* 83(2000):293–97; P. M. Quinsey et al., "Persistence of Organochlorines in Breast milk of Women in Victoria, Australia," *Food and Chemical Toxicology* 33(1995):49–56.

259 Dioxins and PCBs highest in industrialized areas: Clench-Aas, "PCDD and PCDF in Human Milk from Scandinavia"; J.-C. Dillon et al., "Pesticide Residues in Human Milk," *Food and Cosmetic Toxicology* 19(1981):437–42; Jensen, "Levels and Trends of Environmental Chemicals in Human Milk"; Quinsey, "Persistence of Organochlorines in Breast Milk of Women in Victoria, Australia." There are important exceptions, however. Rural women in southern Kazakhstan have the highest dioxin levels ever documented in the world, comparable to those recorded in Vietnam at the height of Agent Orange spraying in the 1970s. Closer examination revealed a relationship between dioxin levels in breast milk and proximity to cotton fields, which are apparently treated with defoliants (2,4,5-T) known to be contaminated with dioxin (Hooper, "Analysis of Breast Milk"). Similarly, the highest breast-milk levels of PCBs ever discovered were found among farming mothers whose silos had been painted with PCB-impregnated paint (Jensen, "Levels and Trends").

259 Lowest levels in Hungary and Albania: A. K. D. Liem et al., "Exposure of Populations to Dioxins and Related Compounds," *Food Additives and Contaminants* 17(2000):241–59.

259 Chlorinated pesticides higher in nonindustrial nations: Latin America has the highest average levels of DDT in breast milk, closely followed by Asia and the Middle East (D. Smith, "Worldwide Trends in DDT Levels in Human Breast Milk," *Intl. J. of Epidemiology* 28[1999]:179–88).

259 Chlorinated pesticides highest in urban areas in developing nations: Jensen, "Levels and Trends." As of 1989, mothers in Hong Kong had the world's most pesticide-contaminated breast milk (DDT and other organochlorines), probably because of high seafood consumption.

Mussels from Hong Kong waters are known to be highly contaminated; the source of this contamination may be elsewhere in Asia (H. M. Ip and D. J. Phillips, "Organochlorine Chemicals in Human Breast Milk in Hong Kong," *Archives of Environmental Contamination and Toxicology* 18[1989]:490–94).

259 Within Europe, Ukraine is highest: G. C. Gladen, Organochlorines in Breast Milk from Two Cities in Ukraine."

259 Termiticides in southeastern U.S.: E. P. Savage et al., "National Study of Chlorinated Hydrocarbon Insecticide Residues in Human Milk, USA," *Am. J. of Epidemiology* 113(1981):413–22.

259 Norwegian magnesium factory: J. Clench-Aas, "PCDD and PCDF in Human Milk from Scandinavia."

260 Canadian incinerator: Jensen, "Levels and Trends of Environmental Chemicals in Human Milk."

260 Heptachlor in Hawaii: W. J. Rogan and N. B. Ragan, "Chemical Contaminants, Pharmacokinetics, and the Lactating Mother," *EHP* 102(1994, sup. 11):89–95.

260 Home termite treatment in Australia: M. Sim et al., "Termite Control and Other Determinants of High Body Burdens of Cyclodiene Insecticides," *Archives of Environmental Health* 53(1998):114–121; C. I. Stacey et al., "Organochlorine Pesticide Residue Levels in Human Milk: Western Australia, 1979–1980," *Archives of Environmental Health* 40(1985):102–8.

260 Chlordane in U.S. military housing: Rogan and Ragan, "Chemical Contaminants."

260 Pesticides in northern Canada, Sweden, and Finland: W. H. Newsome and J. J. Ryan, "Toxaphene and Other Chlorinated Compounds in Human Milk from Northern and Southern Canada: A Comparison," *Chemosphere* 39(1999):519–26; Jensen, "Levels and Trends"; K. Wickstrom et al., "Levels of Chlordane, Hexachlorobenzene, PCB and DDT Compounds in Finnish Human Milk in 1982," *Bulletin of Environmental Contamination and Toxicology* 31(1983):251–56.

262 heavy metals bind to milk proteins: Jensen, "Levels and Trends."

262 Fat-soluble contaminants pose the greatest threat: Ibid.

262 Where fat in breast milk comes from: Schreiber, "Transport of Organic Chemicals."

262 Lifetime body burden is mobilized during lactation: Ibid.

263 How contaminants travel to the breast: Jensen, "Levels and Trends."

263 More contaminants in breast milk than cord blood: Ibid.

263 Diaper analyses: K. Abraham et al., "Intake, Fecal Excretion, and Body Burden of Polychlorinated Dibenzo-*p*-dioxins and Dibenzofurans in Breast-fed and Formula-fed Infants," *Pediatric Research* 40(1996):671–79; K. Abraham et al., "Intake and Fecal Extraction of PCDDs, PCDFs, HCB and PCBs (138, 153, 180) in a Breast-fed and Formula-fed Infant," *Chemosphere* 29(1994):2279–86.

263 DDT in newborn mice: Jensen, "Levels and Trends."

263 Breast-milk contamination rises with maternal age: J. M. Albers et al., "Factors That Influence the Level of Contaminations of Human Milk with Polychlorinated Organic Compounds," *Archives of Environmental Contamination and Toxicology* 39(1996):285–91; M. Schlaud et al., "Organochlorine Residues in Human Breast Milk: Analysis Through a Sentinel Practice Network," *J. of Epidemiology and Community Health* 49(1995, sup. 1):17–21.

263 Contamination falls with cumulated period of nursing: Rogan and Ragan, "Chemical Contaminants"; Schettler et al., *Generations at Risk*, pp. 225–26.

263 Study of nursing twins: A. Schecter et al., "Decrease in Levels and Body Burden of Dioxins, Dibenzofurans, PCBs, DDE, and HCB in Blood and Milk in a Mother Nursing Twins over a Thirty-eight Month Period," *Chemosphere* 37(1998):1807–16.

263 Firstborn children receive the most: T. Vartianen et al., "PCDD, PCDF, and PCB Concentrations in Human Milk from Two Areas of Finland," *Chemosphere* 34(1997):2571–83.

264 Role of diet: K. Noren, "Levels of Organochlorine Contaminants in Human Milk in Relation to the Dietary Habits of the Mothers," *Acta Paediatrica Scandinavica* 72(1983):811–16; G. Schade and B. Heinzow, "Organochlorine Pesticides and Polychlorinated Biphenyls in Human Milk of Mothers Living in Northern Germany: Current Extent of Contamination, Time Trend from 1986 to 1997, and Factors that Influence the Levels of Contamination," *Science of the Total Environment* 23(1998):31–39.

264 Lake Ontario and New Bedford: P. J. Kostyniak et al., "Relation of Lake Ontario Fish Consumption, Lifetime Lactation, and Parity to Breast Milk Polychlorobiphenyl Concentration and Pesticide Concentrations," *Environmental Research* 80(1999, sec. A): S166-S174; S. A. Korrick and L. Altshul, "High Breast Milk Levels of Polychlorinated Biphenyls (PCBs) among Four Women Living Adjacent to a PCB-Contaminated Waste Site," *EHP* 106(1998):513–18.

264 Swedish study: R. Vaz, "Average Swedish Dietary Intakes of Organochlorine Contaminants via Foods of Animal Origin and their Relation to Levels in Human Milk, 1975–90," *Food Additives and Contaminants* 12(1995):543–58.

265 Breast-milk monitoring programs: K. Hooper and T. A. McDonald, "The PBDEs: An Emerging Environmental Challenge and Another Reason for Breast-Milk Monitoring Programs," *EHP* 108(2000):387–92.

265 U.S. program ended in 1978: Schettler et al., *Generations at Risk*, pp. 204–05. Some leading researchers had recently called for a breast-milk monitoring program to be relaunched in the United States, coordinated by the U.S. Department of Health and Human Services in collaboration with state and local groups (K. Florini and L. R. Goldman, "Mothers' Milk Should Not Be Such a Mystery," *San Francisco Chronicle*, 29 Nov. 2000), p. A27.

265 Canadian studies: Craan and Haines, "Twenty-five Years of Surveillance."

265 Mothers' Milk Centre in Sweden: K. Noren and D. Meironyte, "Certain Organochlorine and Organobromine Contaminants in Swedish Breast Milk in Perspective of Past 20–30 Years," *Chemosphere* 40(2000):1111–23.

265 Trends in Germany, Netherlands, Denmark, and Britain: Papke, "PCDD PCDF"; Schade and Heinzrow, "Organochlorine Pesticides and Polychlorinated Biphenyls."

265–266 Trends in Canada: Craan and Haines, "Twenty-five Years of Surveillance."

266 Dioxin trends: D. H. Buckley-Golder, *Compilation of EU Dioxin Exposure and Health Data. Task 5: Human Tissue and Milk Levels* (Oxford, U.K.: AEA Technology, 1999); J. S. LaKind et al., "Infant Exposure to Chemicals in Breast Milk in the United States: What We Need to Learn from a Breast Milk Monitoring Program," *EHP* 109(2001):75–88; A. K. Liem et al., "Exposure of Populations to Dioxins and Related Compounds," *Food Additives and Contaminants* 17(2000):241–59.

266 Signs of a plateau: S. S. Atuma et al., "Organochlorine Pesticides, Polychlorinated Biphenyls and Dioxins in Human Milk from Swedish Mothers," *Food Additives and Contaminants* 15(1998):142–50; P. Furst, "PCDDs/PCDFs in Human Milk—Still a Matter of Concern?" *Organohalogen Compounds* 48(2000):111–14.

266 Flame retardants: Hooper and McDonald, "The PBDEs"; Noren and Meironyte, "Certain Organochlorine and Organobromine Contaminants."

266–267 Aromatic amines: L. S. DeBruin et al., "Detection of Monocyclic Aromatic Amines, Possible Mammary Carcinogens, in Human Milk," *Chemical Research in Toxicology* 12(1999):78–82.

269 Animal studies: D. C. Rice, "Behavioral Impairment Produced by Low-level Postnatal PCB Exposure in Monkeys," *Environmental Research* 80 (1999, 2 Pt 2):S113-21; ibid., "Effects of Postnatal Exposure of Monkeys to a PCB Mixture on Spatial Discrimination Reversal and DRL Performance," *Neurotoxicology and Teratology* 20(1998):391–400; ibid., "Effect of Postnatal Exposure to a PCB Mixture in Monkeys on a Multiple Fixed Interval-Fixed Ratio Performance," *Neurotoxicology and Teratology* 19 (1997):429–34; D. C. Rice and S. Hayward, "Effects of Postnatal Exposure to a PCB Mixture in Monkeys on Nonspatial Discrimination Reversal and Delayed Alternation Performance," *Neurotoxicology* 18(1997):479–94. See also A. Brouwer et al., "Report of the WHO Working Group on the Assessment of Health Risks for Human Infants to PCDDs, PCDFs and PCBs," *Chemosphere* 37(1998):1627–43; R. D. Kimbrough, "Toxicological Implications of Human Milk Residues as Indicated by Toxicological and Epidemiological Studies," in Jensen and Slorach, *Chemical Contaminants in Human Milk*, pp. 271–83; D. B. Sager and D. M. Girard, "Long-term Effects on Reproductive Parameters in Female Rats after Translational Exposure to PCBs," *Environmental Research* 66(1994):52–76.

269 Quotes from popular handbooks: K. Pryor and G. Pryor, *Nursing Your Baby* (New York: Pocket Books, 1991), pp. 86; H. Lothrop, *Breastfeeding Naturally: An Approach for Today's Mother* (Tucson: Fisher Books, 1999), pp. 92; S. Kitzinger, *The Experience of Breastfeeding* (New York: Penguin, 1987), pp. 140–48.

269 1998 quote from researcher: van Birgelen, "Hexachlorobenzene as Possible Major Contributor."

269–270 U.S. studies: For an overview of these studies, see K. N. Dietrich, "Environmental Chemicals and Child Development," *J. of Pediatrics* 134(1999):7–9; National Research Council,

Hormonally Active Agents in the Environment (Washington, D.C.: National Academy Press, 1999), pp. 178–84. See also the references cited in the note for pages 144–46 under the key phrase "human studies showing adverse effects of PCBs on fetal brain development." Many studies that examine prenatal exposures also examine breast-milk exposures.

270 Inuit studies: J. D. Baxter, "Otitis Media in Inuit Children in the Eastern Canadian Arctic—An Overview, 1968 to Date," *Intl. J. of Pediatric Otorhinolaryngology* 49(1999, sup. 1):S165-76; E. Dewailly et al., "Susceptibility to Infections and Immune Status in Inuit Infants Exposed to Organochlorines," *EHP* 108(2000):205–11.

270–272 Dutch studies: Dietrich, "Environmental Chemicals and Child Development"; M. Huisman et al., "Neurological Condition in 18-month-old Children Perinatally Exposed to Polychlorinated Biphenyls and Dioxins," *Early Human Development* 43(1995):165–76; C. Koopman-Essebaum, "Overview of the Dutch PCB Study in Children: Effects on Neurodevelopment and Thyroid Hormone Levels in the First 3 1/2 Years of Life," in *Proceedings of the Atlantic Coast Contaminants Workshop 2000* (Bar Harbor, Me.: Jackson Laboratory, June 2000); C. I. Lanting et al., "Breastfeeding and Neurological Outcome at 42 Months," *Acta Paediatrica* 87(1998):1124–29; C. I. Lanting, "Effects of Perinatal PCB and Dioxin Exposure and Early Feeding Mode on Child Development," Ph.D. diss., Rijksuniversiteit Groningen, Netherlands; S. Patandin et al., "Effects of Environmental Exposure to Polychlorinated Biphenyls and Dioxins on Cognitive Abilities in Dutch Children at 42 Months of Age," *J. of Pediatrics* 134(1999):33–41; S. Patandin, "Effects of Environmental Exposure to Polychlorinated Biphenyls and Dioxins on Growth and Development in Young Children," Ph.D. diss., Erasmus Universiteit, Rotterdam, 1999; S. Patandin et al., "Plasma Polychlorinated Biphenyl Levels in Dutch Preschool Children Either Breast-fed or Formula-fed During Infancy," *Am. J. of Public Health* 87(1997):1711–14; N. Weisglas-Kuperus et al., "Immunologic Effects of Background Exposure to Polychlorinated Biphenyls and Dioxins in Dutch Preschool Children," *EHP* 108(2000):1203–7.

271–272 Quote by authors: Weisglas-Kuperus, "Immunologic Effects of Background Exposure."

272 Finnish studies: S. Alaluusua et al., "Developing Teeth as a Biomarker of Dioxin Exposure," *Lancet* 353(1999):206; A. M. Partanen, "Epidermal Growth Factor Receptor as a Mediator of Developmental Toxicity of Dioxin in Mouse Embryonic Teeth," *Laboratory Investigation* 78(1998):1473–81; J. Raloff, "Dioxin Can Harm Tooth Development," *Science News* 155(1999):119.

272 Dutch study: M. Forouhandeh-Gever, et al., "Does Perinatal Exposure to Background Levels of Dioxins Have a Lasting Effect on Human Dentition?" *Organohalogen compounds* 44(1999):279–82; Dr. Janna Koppe, University of Amsterdam, personal communication.

274 Formula kills 4,000 infants a year: Dr. Miriam Labbok, chief of nutrition and maternal health at the U.S. Agency of International Development, estimates that 4,000 more U.S. infants would survive each year if all U.S. mothers breastfed for at least twelve weeks. These represent additional lives saved from infectious diseases and S.I.D.S.

274–275 Early risk assessments: W. J. Rogan et al., "Should the Presence of Carcinogens in Breast Milk Discourage Breast Feeding?" *Regulatory Toxicology and Pharmacology* 13(1991):228–40. See also J. W. Frank and J. Newman, "Breast-feeding in a Polluted World: Uncertain Risks, Clear Benefits," *Canadian Medical Association Journal* 149(1993):33–37. See also the critique of early risk assessments in Schreiber, "Transport of Organic Chemicals."

275 Later risk assessments: Buckley-Golder, *Compilation*, pp. 2–3.

275 Quote from recent report: Ibid., pp. 2–3.

275 "Arguments for ignoring contaminated breast milk are no longer valid.": H. R. Pohl and B. F. Hibbs, "Breast-feeding Exposure of Infants to Environmental Contaminants—A Public Health Risk Assessment Viewpoint: Chlorinated Dibenzodioxins and Chlorinated Dibenzofurans," *Toxicology and Industrial Health* 12(1996):593–611.

275 "Officially, it is said that breast milk is safe. . . .": J. Yonemoto, "The Effects of Dioxin on Reproduction and Development," *Industrial Health* 38(2000):259–68.

275 2001 review: LaKind, "Infant Exposure."

275–276 Contaminants interfere with milk production: B. C. Gladen and W. J. Rogan, "DDE and Shortened Duration of Lactation in a Northern Mexican Town," *Am. J. of Public Health* 85(1995):504–08; C. I. Lanting, "Environmental Exposure to Polychlorinated Biphenyls

(PCBs) Is Negatively Related to Human Milk Output and Fat Content," in Lanting, *Effects of Perinatal PCB and Dioxin Exposure*, pp. 101–14; W. J. Rogan et al., "Polychlorinated Biphenyls (PCBs) and Dichlorodiphenyl Dichloroethene (DDE) in Human Milk: Effects on Growth, Morbidity, and Duration of Lactation," *Am. J. of Public Health* 77(1987):1294–97; W. J. Rogan, "Pollutants in Breast Milk," *Archives of Pediatrics and Adolescent Medicine* 150(1996):981–90; Schettler et al., *Generations at Risk*, p. 205.

276 Problems with vegetarian approach: Strict vegetarianism (veganism) means eating a diet with no milk, cheese, eggs, or any other animal product. In 1997, researchers tested two adult American vegans—one male, one female—for dioxins and PCBs. Their blood levels were one third to one half those of the average man and woman from the general population. However, both individuals had adhered to a vegan diet for nearly thirty years (A. Schecter and O. Papke, "Comparisons of Blood Dioxin, Dibenzofuran, and Coplanar PCB Levels in Strict Vegetarians [Vegans] and the General United States Population," *Organohalogen Compounds* 38[1998]:179–82). When dairy-eating vegetarians have been tested for dioxin, their blood levels are no different than those found in the general population (Linda Birnbaum, U.S. EPA, personal communication). See also Beck et al., "PCDD and PCDF Exposure"; P. C. Dagnelie et al., "Nutrients and Contaminants in Human Milk from Mothers on Macrobiotic and Omnivorous Diets," *European J. of Clinical Nutrition* 46(1992):355–66; F. Ejobi et al., "Some Factors Related to sum-DDT Levels in Ugandan Mothers' Breast Milk," *Public Health* 112(1998):425–27; J. Hergenrather et al., "Pollutants in the Breast Milk of Vegetarians," letter, *NEJM* 304(1981):792; Jensen, "Levels and Trends"; Papke, "PCDD/PCDF"; H. J. Pluim et al., "Influence of Short-Term Dietary Measures on Dioxin Concentrations in Human Milk," *EHP* 102(1994):968–71; A. Somogyi and H. Beck, "Nurturing and Breast-feeding: Exposure to Chemicals in Breast Milk," *EHP* 101(1993, sup. 2):45–52. Thanks to Jill Stein, M.D., Physicians for Social Responsibility, whose ideas helped inform my analysis of this topic.

277 Problems with avoiding weight loss: J. G. Dorea et al., "Pregnancy-Related Changes in Fat Mass and Total DDT in Breast Milk and Maternal Adipose Tissue," *Annals of Nutrition and Metabolism* 41(1997):250–54; C. A. Lovelady et al., "Weight Change During Lactation Does Not Alter the Concentrations of Chlorinated Organic Contaminants in Breast Milk of Women with Low Exposure," *J. of Human Lactation* 15(1999):307–15; Schlaud, "Organochlorine Residues in Human Breast Milk"; M. R. Sim and J. J. McNeil, "Monitoring Chemical Exposure Using Breast Milk: A Methodological Review," *Am. J. of Epidemiology* 136(1992):1–11; Schreiber, "Transport of Organic Chemicals."

277 Pumping and discarding: Center for Health and Environmental Justice, *American People's Dioxin Report*, p. 29.

277 Switching to formula: Beck et al,, "PCDD and PCDF Exposure"; Pohl and Hibbs, "Breast-feeding Exposure of Infants"; Sonawane, "Chemical Contaminants in Human Milk."

277 Formula more contaminated with lead: J. Newman, "Would Breastfeeding Decrease Risks of Lead Intoxication?" *Pediatrics* 90(1993):131–32. Furthermore, soy-based formula raises long-term health effects owing to high levels of plant estrogens, which has been shown in animal studies to alter thyroid functioning (National Research Council, *Hormonally Active Agents in the Environment*, p. 73; K. D. Setchell et al., "Exposure of Infants to Phyto-oestrogens from Soy-based Infant Formula," *Lancet* 350[1997]:23–27).

278 Nitrates and weed-killers: B. A. Cohen et al., *Pouring It On: Nitrate Contamination of Drinking Water* (Washington, D.C.: Environmental Working Group, 1996); J. Houlihan and R. Wiles, *Into the Mouths of Babes: Bottle-fed Infants at Risk from Atrazine in Tap Water* (Washington, D.C.: Environmental Working Group, 1999); L. Knobeloch et al., "Blue Babies and Nitrate-Contaminated Well Water," *EHP* 108(2000):675–78.

278 Leaching plastics: G. Hess, "Activists Push FDA to Remove Bisphenol-A from Baby Bottles," *Chemical Market Reporter* 255(17 May 1999):9; A. D'Antuono et al., "Determination of Bisphenal-A in Food-Simulating Liquids Using LC-ED with a Chemically Modified Electrode," *Journal of Agricultural and Food Chemistry* 49(2001):1098–101.

278 The method that works: Thanks to Dr. Jill Stein and to the members of the breast-milk working group at the Dioxin 2000 conference—Kim Hooper, Sharyle Patton, Allen Rosenfeld, Gina Solomon, Pilar Weiss, and Jane Williams—whose ideas contributed much to my analysis here.

278 Quote from U.S. researchers: Smith, "Worldwide Trends in DDT Levels in Human Milk."

278 Quote from German researchers: Papke, "PCDD/PCDF."

278–279 Quote from Swedish researchers: K. Noren et al., "Methysulfonyl Metabolites of PCBs and DDE in Human Milk in Sweden, 1972–1992," *EHP* 104(1996):766–72.

279 Quote from Dutch researchers: C. I. Lanting and S. Patandin, "Exposure to PCBs and Dioxins: Adverse Effects and Implications for Child Development," in S. Gabizon, ed., *Women and POPs: Women's View and Role Regarding the Elimination of POPs—Report on the Activities of the IPEN's Women's Group During the IPEN Conference and the INC3, Geneva, September 4–11, 1999* (Utrecht: Women in Europe for a Common Future, 1999), pp. 10–12.

279–280 Convention on Rights of the Child: Infant Feeding Action Coalition, "Breast-feeding: A Human Right," *INFACT Newsletter,* Winter 1997, p. 3.

280 States that consider breastfeeding a civil right: According to the American College of Nurse-Midwives, these states are California, Florida, Georgia, Idaho, Iowa, Minnesota, Missouri, New York, Oregon, Tennessee, and Texas (www. birth.org).

280 Case of Janet Dike: C. S. Shdaimah, "Why Breastfeeding Is (Also) a Legal Issue, *10 Hastings Women's Law Journal* 409(1999):5–34.

283 New Jersey fish consumption advisories: See www.state.nj.us/dep/dsr/njmainfish.htm. For fish advisories in any state, see www.epa.gov/OST/fish.

AFTERWORD

284 History of Precautionary Principle: C. Smith and C. Curtis, "The Precautionary Principle and Environmental Policy: Science, Uncertainty, and Sustainability," *Intl. J. of Occupational and Environmental Health* 6(2000):263–65.

285 Wingspread conference: C. Raffensperger and J. Tickner, *Protecting Public Health and the Environment: Implementing the Precautionary Principle* (Washington, D.C.: Island Press, 1999), pp. 349–55.

285 Rationale for Precautionary Principle: Smith, "Precautionary Principle and Environmental Policy."

285 "Kogai": Dr. Tomohiro Kawaguchi, School of Public Health, University of South Carolina, personal communication.

285 Precautionary Principle since 1998: C. Raffensperger et al., "Precaution: Belief, Regulatory System, and Overarching Principle," *Intl. J. of Occupational and Environmental Health* 6(2000):266–69.

286 Quote by Kjell Larsson: "Swedish Minister Talks Tough on Toxics Phase-Out," Reuters News Service, 25 Jan. 2001.

286 POPs treaty: J. Kaiser and M. Enserink, "Treaty Takes a POP at the Dirty Dozen," *Science* 290(2000):2053. For a detailed description of the treaty's contents, see http://irptc.unep.ch/pops.

286–287 Goal setting: Mary O'Brien, personal communication. See also M. O'Brien, *Making Better Environmental Decisions: An Alternative to Risk Assessment* (Cambridge: MIT Press, 2000).

287 Corridor of bellies: Thanks to Charlotte Brody of the Center for Health, Environment and Justice, which helped organize this event, for her vivid description.

Acknowledgments

No new mother writes a book without assistance of the most extraordinary kind. I thank first my husband, Jeff de Castro. Most of the words appearing on the preceding pages were written between 9 P.M. and 2 A.M., while Faith slept. This was possible only because Jeff arose at or before dawn every morning for nearly two years and cheerfully served as the primary parent during the first shift while I slept. During the months I was conducting library research, Jeff also carried on well into the second shift. It was Jeff who planned meals, washed dishes, laundered clothes, shoveled snow, hauled firewood, wrapped birthday presents, bought groceries, served baby food, scheduled pediatrician visits, sacrificed career opportunities, and accompanied Faith to play groups, music classes, and toddler reading hours. He also read every chapter of this book in draft form, prefacing his nightly reading sessions with the disclaimer, "Remember, if I fall asleep, it's not because I'm bored."

I gratefully acknowledge a crew of child-care helpers. Chief among them is Jan Jorrin, who is Mary Poppins by way of Twyla Tharpe. Thanks also to Caryl Silberman, Janet Collins, my sister-in-law Mary Ludwig, my mother-in-law, Bobbi Dennis, my sister Julie Jones, and my mother, Kathryn Steingraber, who also offered proofreading and fact-checking assistance and showed me how the book should end.

For the past two years, I have enjoyed a residency at Cornell University, which has provided me office space, computer services, access to a world-class library, and the encouragement of inspiring colleagues. I thank especially my coworkers in the Program for Breast Cancer and Environmental Risk Factors in New York State, on whom I tried out many ideas, and the program's past and present directors, Dr. June Fessenden-MacDonald and Dr. Rodney R. Dietert, each of whom offered me much support and good advice. I am grateful also to my two intrepid research assistants, Fan Lau and Tamar Melen, who spent countless hours ferreting out books and journal articles from various campus libraries, navigating electronic databases, fact-checking, photocopying, tracking down obscure sources, and generally cheering me up. Two brighter students I have never had occasion to work with. And for underwriting the cost of this research I thank the Jenifer Altman Foundation, which helped defray expenses ranging from conference fees to child care. Special thanks to Marni Rosen, its director, and Michael Lerner of Commonweal for putting us in touch.

I owe a considerable debt to many librarians, particularly those who process interlibrary loan requests at Cornell's Mann Library and those who staff the Somerville Public Library's reference desk.

Many colleagues contributed their expert knowledge to this project by commenting on all or part of the manuscript. For their invaluable feedback and advice I thank Michael Bender of the Mercury Policy Project; Dr. Linda Birnbaum, U.S. Environmental Protection Agency; Judy Brady, San Francisco; Margaret Lee Braun, Rochester,

New York; Dr. Pat Brown, Siena College; Dr. Bruce Carlson, University of Michigan; Drs. Bruce and Norma Criley, Illinois Wesleyan University; Dr. Lynn Goldman, Johns Hopkins University; Barbara Goldoftos, Wellesley College; Dr. Philip Grandjean, Boston University School of Public Health and University of Southern Denmark Institute of Public Health; Dr. R. Given Harper, Illinois Wesleyan University; Dr. Kim Hooper, California Environmental Protection Agency, Hazardous Materials Laboratory; Dr. Tomohiro Kawaguchi, University of South Carolina School of Public Health; Dr. Janna Koppe, University of Amsterdam; Dr. Caren Lanting, TNO Prevention and Health, The Netherlands; Dr. James and Anne McGowan, Bloomington, Illinois; Betty Mekdeci, Birth Defects Research for Children, Inc.; Pamela K. Miller, Alaska Community Action on Toxics; Dr. Peter Montague, Environmental Research Foundation; Dr. Peter Nathanielsz, Cornell University; Dr. Margaret Neville, University of Colorado Health Sciences Center; Dr. Mary O'Brien, Science and Environmental Health Network; Sharyle Patton, Commonweal; Dr. Fred Quimby, Cornell University; Dr. Barbara Katz Rothman, Baruch College, CUNY; Dr. Arnold Schecter, University of Texas School of Public Health, Dallas; Dr. Londa Schiebinger, Pennsylvania State University; Dr. Ted Schettler, Physicians for Social Responsibility; Dr. Suzanne Snedecker, Cornell University; Dr. Gina Solomon, National Resources Defense Council and University of California–San Francisco; Dr. Edward Swain, Minnesota Pollution Control Agency; Dr. Louis Verner, Texas Parks and Wildlife; Dr. Tom Webster, Boston University School of Public Health; Dr. Bernard Weiss, University of Rochester School of Medicine and Dentistry; and Jackie Wynne, California Birth Defects Monitoring Program. All responsibility for the accuracy of the text, of course, remains with me alone.

Three pregnant friends read chapters of this book in draft—one finishing forty-eight hours before giving birth. Their comments were essential to me, as were their words of encouragement and dinner invitations. I therefore express my abiding appreciation to Karol Bennett, mother of three; Monica Hargraves, mother of one; and Carmi Orenstein, mother of two.

Many scientists, researchers, and journalists too numerous to name here played an important role in this project by answering questions, sharing data, and alerting me to important new publications. I particularly thank members of the Children's Environmental Health Network, the International POPs Elimination Network, and the Mercury Working Group.

Two different editors helped shepherd this manuscript through to publication. For their steadfast support and keen editorial judgement, I thank Melanie Kroupa and Merloyd Lawrence. From Melanie I learned much about the carpentry of telling stories. Merloyd's broad knowledge of prenatal life and childbirth practices pointed me in many new directions; our shared wonder at the mystery of it all formed the basis of a close working relationship.

More than ever, I am grateful to my literary agent, Charlotte Sheedy, who believed in this project from its conception.

Finally, thank you, Faith, for patiently serving as both my muse and subject matter. Every day your name teaches me again its meaning. You are my heart's delight.

Further Resources

Here are some organizations I have found particularly useful in my own research and activism. (All World Wide Web addresses begin with http://.)

Birth Defect Research for Children, Inc.
930 Woodcock Road, Suite 225
Orlando, FL 32803
www.birthdefects.org
Provides parents with information about birth defects and support services for their children. BDRC also sponsors the National Birth Defects Registry, a research program that studies associations between birth defects and environmental contaminants.

California Birth Defects Monitoring Program
1830 Embarcadero, Suite 100
Oakland, CA 94606
www.cbdmp.org
A public health program devoted to finding the causes of birth defects, with a particular interest in understanding gene-and-environment interactions. CBDMP is funded through the California Department of Health Services and jointly administered with the March of Dimes Birth Defects Foundation. Its Web site makes available birth defect registry data and research findings on topics such as the relationship between birth defects and prenatal exposures to organic solvents, hazardous waste, and pesticides.

Center for Health, Environment and Justice
P.O. Box 6806 • 150 S. Washington, Suite 300
Falls Church, VA 22040
www.chej.org
Founded as the Citizen's Clearinghouse for Hazardous Waste by Lois Gibbs, a community leader at Love Canal, CHEJ helps citizens organize and fight against toxic contamination in local communities.

Children's Environmental Health Network
5900 Hollis Street, Suite E
Emeryville, CA 94608
www.cehn.org
A national project dedicated to pediatric environmental health, CEHN concentrates on the areas of education, research, and policy.

DES Action
601 Sixteenth Street, Suite 301
Oakland, CA 94612
www.desaction.org
Informs the public about DES and helps DES-exposed individuals.

Environmental Defense
257 Park Avenue South
New York, NY 10010
www.edf.org
www.scorecard.org (to access right-to-know data for your community)
Dedicated to protecting the environmental rights of all people. ED's "scorecard" Web site allows citizens to identify sources of pollution within their home zip code. It includes maps, chemical emissions data, and information about health effects of specific toxic chemicals.

Environmental Research Foundation
P.O. Box 5036
Annapolis, MD 21403
www.rachel.org
Publishes Rachel's *Environmental Health Biweekly* and provides research and technical assistance for those facing specific environmental problems within their communities. The ERF Web site is an excellent starting point for researching toxic chemicals and their effects.

Health Care Without Harm
c/o CCHW
P.O. Box 6806
Falls Church, VA 22040
www.noharm.org
Advocates environmentally responsible health care. HCWH works to transform the health-care industry so it is no longer a source of environmental pollutants—especially dioxin and mercury.

International POPs Elimination Network
c/o Canadian Environmental Law Association
517 College Street, Suite 401

Toronto, Ontario
Canada M6G 4A2
www.ipen.org
A global network of public interest organizations united in support of the global elimination of persistent organic pollutants. IPEN played a key role in the U.N. POPs treaty negotiations and is currently pushing for swift ratification and implementation of the Stockholm Convention.

Mercury Policy Project
1420 North Street • Montpelier, VT 05602
www.mercurypolicy.org
Raises awareness about the threat of mercury contamination. MPP works to promote policies that eliminate mercury uses and significantly reduce mercury exposure.

**National Coalition Against
the Misuse of Pesticides**
701 E Street, SE, Suite 200
Washington, D.C. 20003
www.beyondpesticides.org
Provides the public with information on pesticides and alternatives to their use, including on lawns, gardens, and golf courses, and in homes, day-care centers, and schools.

Natural Resources Defense Council
71 Stevenson Street
San Francisco, CA 94105
www.nrdc.org
www.nrdc.org/breastmilk/
An environmental organization with over 400,000 members. NRDC has recently launched "Healthy Milk, Healthy Baby," an on-line resource that offers well-researched information about chemicals in breast milk from a pro-breastfeeding perspective.

**Nightingale Institute for Health
and the Environment**
P.O. Box 412 • Burlington, VT 05402
www.nihe.org
Founded by a nurse, NIHE helps health-care professionals recognize the link between human and environmental health.

**Partnership for Children's Health
and the Environment**
P.O. Box 757 • Langley, WA 98260
www.partnersforchildren.org
PCHE is an international coalition of organizations committed to protecting current and future generations from harmful environmental exposures.

Pesticide Action Network
49 Powell Street, Suite 500
San Francisco, CA 94102
www.panna.org
Advances alternatives to pesticides worldwide. PAN is an international pesticide reform network. Its North American regional center, Pesticide Action Network North America (PANNA), coordinates public interest groups in Canada, Mexico, and the United States and provides an on-line guide to help with pests and pest problems.

Physicians for Social Responsibility
1875 Connecticut Avenue, NW, Suite 1012
Washington, DC 20009
www.psr.org
Works on issues of nuclear weapons, global environmental pollution, and gun violence. Recently, PSR has had a particular interest in raising awareness about fetal exposures to neurological toxins.

Science and Environmental Health Network
3704 W. Lincoln Way, Suite 282
Ames, IA 50014
www.sehn.org
A think tank for the environmental movement, SEHN focuses on the relationship between science and ethics and is the leading proponent in the United States and Canada of the Precautionary Principle. SEHN also operates a network for students interested in pursuing careers in public interest science.

Washington Toxics Coalition
4649 Sunnyside Avenue N, Suite 540 East
Seattle, WA 98103
www.watoxics.org
Dedicated to protecting public health by promoting alternatives to toxic chemicals. WTC provides practical information about preventing pollution in homes, schools, workplaces, agriculture, and industry.

World Alliance for Breastfeeding Action
P.O. Box 1200 10850
Penang, Malaysia
www.waba.org.br
Dedicated to protecting, promoting, and supporting breastfeeding around the world. WABA is a global network of organizations and individuals who believe breastfeeding is the right of all children and mothers. It works in liaison with UNICEF.

Index

About the Author

*S*andra Steingraber, Ph.D. is the author of *Living Downstream: An Ecologist Looks at Cancer and the Environment* and *Post Diagnosis*, a volume of poetry. She received her doctorate in biological science from the University of Michigan and taught biology for several years at Columbia College, Chicago. She has held fellowships at the University of Illinois, Radcliffe College, and Northeastern University, and has served as a writer in residence at DePauw and Illinois Wesleyan universities. As an ecologist, she has conducted fieldwork in northern Minnesota, East Africa, and Costa Rica. In 1999, as part of international treaty negotiations, she briefed United Nations delegates in Geneva on breast milk contamination. As a writer, she received both the Will Solimene Award for Excellence in Medical Communications by the New England Chapter of the American Medical Writers Association and the Jenifer Altman Foundation Award for "the inspiring and poetic use of science to elucidate the causes of cancer. She has been selected as the 2001 recipient of the Rachel Carson Leadership Award from Carson's alma mater, Chatham College. Currently on the faculty at Cornell University, she lives in Ithaca, New York, with her husband, the sculptor Jeff de Castro and their daughter, Faith. Please visit her web site: www.steingraber.com